Natural Progesterone
The World's Best Kept Secret

Dedication

*To God
and
the women*

Natural Progesterone
The World's Best Kept Secret

Jenny Birdsey

Published by Natural Progesterone Advisory Network.
8 Normanby Street,
East Geelong, Vic. Australia 3219.
Telephone: 61 (03) 5222 7145 Fax: 61 (03) 5222 7145
Registered Trademark NPAN World Owned Logo

Registered business name: Natural Progesterone Advisory Network (NPAN)
Founder and Director, Jenny Birdsey since April 20, 1998
This book is the sole property and copyright of Jenny Birdsey

Printed by: Sands Print Group, 2 Bayldon Court, Breakwater, Vic. Australia 3219

Cover design and layout by: Eric J. Stribley, email: esgraphics@bigpond.com

Web Host: Advanced Webcreations, emails: donna@domainhost.com.au
erez@domainhost.com.au   Phone: +61 3 9696 8800 Fax: +61 3 9696 8099

Edited by Andrea McVean

First published: October 2001
Second edition (Revised) July 2004

ISBN 0957955227

Disclaimer
The information and procedures contained in this book are based upon the research, observational
data, women's feedback and the personal and professional experiences of the author. Jenny
Birdsey.

The publisher and author although a registered nurse by profession is NOT a medical practitioner.
This book is for information purposes only and is not a prescription for your particular needs.
Consult with your medical or health care practitioner if in doubt or if you have questions. This book
Is the result of the reporting of hundreds of women and their data through Jenny Birdsey's
consultancy and the authentic NPAN information and its network founded and operated by Jenny
Birdsey.

Natural Progesterone Advisory Network/NPAN will not be held responsible in any way for the
fraudulent use of its name or fraudulent use of any information contained within this book.

All information can be obtained from my secure websites:

www.npan.com.au

www.natural-progesterone-advisory-network.us

Foreword

It is my great pleasure to introduce Jenny Birdsey to the readers of her exciting new book. I am sure that the information in this book will fill in many missing parts of the jig saw puzzle for women searching to find hormonal balance in their lives.

I have known Jenny personally for several years and have had the pleasure of working with her in Australia in our mutual quest to help women gain the knowledge they need to be healthy. Jenny is a nurse whose life was shaped by her own hormonal problems for which she could find no real help. This led her into a long journey of research to discover the real truth behind the hormonal chaos experienced by herself and millions of other women. The journey has not always been easy for Jenny, as is true with most pioneers into new territory however this has not daunted her indomitable spirit and passion to help others. Jenny Birdsey seeks the truth and will not settle for anything less. She has known rejection, frustration and isolation which has really helped her to become the woman she is today. Jenny is no longer the naive girl she was a decade ago - today she is a strong powerful force in the wilderness of hormonal disorders. She has a huge compassion to help women who battle with hormonal problems which has given her the drive to write this ground breaking book on hormonal problems. Jenny has also started a clinic in Geelong where she helps women with weight problems that are associated with the hormonal imbalance of Syndrome X. I have personally trained Jenny in techniques for weight control and she works closely with my Women's Health Advisory team in Sydney.

The hormone progesterone has been in the limelight for several years now and many women are now able to take advantage of its health promoting benefits. Jenny calls progesterone "the worlds best kept secret" and if anyone understands the tremendous benefits of progesterone, I would say it is Jenny Birdsey!

Jenny has worked tirelessly behind the scenes for years to bring progesterone to Australian women. She has worked with the WA government and TGA to make progesterone a legal and available prescription drug. She wanted the use of progesterone to be controlled from the top levels thus ensuring a high level of quality control and professional prescribing. Jenny Birdsey has taught several Australian doctors how to use progesterone to alleviate such problems as -

Premenstrual Syndrome

Postnatal Depression

Menstrual bleeding problems

Polycystic Ovarian Syndrome

Menopausal symptoms

and much more

In the year 1998, Jenny Birdsey founded The Natural Progesterone Advisory Network (NPAN) to enable women to have a comprehensive information base about progesterone and indeed all hormonal matters. NPAN is also working to see progesterone treatments made available on the NHS and to ensure that more doctors are aware of its tremendous advantages.

At last we have a comprehensive, down to earth, authoritative book on progesterone. This book is well researched and fills in the missing links that all women need to find the hormonal truth in their lives. This is now possible because of Jenny Birdsey, who would not rest until she had discovered the real truth about hormones. Thankfully for us she did!

Enjoy the book and "Don't Let Your Hormones Ruin Your Life"

Provided and Written by Dr Sandra Cabot

*The information in this book
is largely based on my work with my
organisation Natural Progesterone Advisory
Network (NPAN).*

*My work incorporates the use of particular
products and formulations.*

*I cannot guarantee that you will get the
same magnitude of results if you use
different products than the recommended
formulations of NPAN and what I have
used in my work, however the
principles remain the same.*

CONTENTS

Preface

Someone once said that the thing we teach best is the very thing we had to teach ourselves. In my case this is so true.

When a person is in harmony they function like a human being should. I have been a daughter, a mother, an auntie, sister and a wife. In all of these roles I played, I forgot about myself and so I paid the painful price. I began doing my own hormonal research when I couldn't find satisfaction from the supposed experts. I am not a doctor, chemist, university graduate or literary scholar who, no doubt, could find double definitives, incorrect grammar or spelling mistakes.

I do not write for the world of academia or the rocket scientist. I write for the woman in the street, who longs to be complete. The woman who remembers how it felt to be brimming with vitality and dearly misses that part of herself, to the woman who senses the absence of well being and sorely wants to reclaim that part of herself.

This book is about your hormonal balance and finding those elusive keys, the vital links.

I share with you my years of research and findings. I do not advocate that you become a hormone buff. I'm just asking you to come along with me for a while and see what I have to share.

I trust the contents of this publication will provide you with intelligent answers to your intelligent questions and present a new approach for a happier, healthier and fuller way of life.

With Blessings,
Jenny Birdsey
Author, Director and Founder of Natural Progesterone Advisory Network (NPAN)
Worldwide Trade Logo ®©

Introduction

The World's Best Kept Secret

"Twenty years ago a doctor asked me why I wasn't on progesterone and I responded, "nobody told me I should be". Within 3-4 days of commencing progesterone cream, I felt so much better about myself. More confident, more in control of my life. I've been using progesterone and feeling the benefits for twenty years without any side effects.

"During this time doctors tried to take me off the cream but I refused. I have suggested that maybe these doctors listen to the women who are taking progesterone and getting well.

"Many times I have shared my experience on progesterone cream with women but their doctors argue they don't need it. Such a pity! I personally wouldn't be without it." (supplied by a woman from the USA).

Natural progesterone has been around since the 1940s. In the past, the late Dr. John Lee had bravely championed its use along with Katharina Dalton despite the medical fraternities inability to embrace their theories. Millions of women around the world continue to be eternally grateful to them having discovered the benefits of its use because of their indefatigable stance. Thank you to these two incredible pioneers in progesterone. So, why are doctors reluctant to prescribe it? Why does mainstream medicine remain skeptical? Why is it so difficult for women to get their hands on reliable information? Or find a doctor who will honour their choice of natural progesterone? And why is it the world's best kept secret?

Perhaps resistance is largely due to the lack of published clinical trials and scientific evidence made available to doctors on natural-to-the-body hormones like progesterone. So what's hindering test trials that can change all this? Simply put, lack of funding. Pharmaceutical companies, in the interests of self-preservation, flatly refuse to inject millions and millions of dollars into research and development of a drug that cannot be 'owned' under a patent.

Meanwhile, the pharmaceutical industry is guilty of a massive campaign of misinformation in regards to the less 'natural' hormone replacement therapy drugs they manufacture and push doctors to prescribe.

There is growing evidence that synthetic HRT is perhaps not all it's cracked up to be. Clearly some medical claims are based on myth and not fact. The effect on Heart Disease is just one example. The dangers of synthetic HRT, especially on breast cancer, are only now being given any exposure as more and more women demand answers to their health questions.

Let's not fool ourselves here. What's best for women's health is not very high on the agenda. It's about patents and profits, and chemically-altered drugs that ineptly replace our natural hormones. It's about over-shadowing responsible information on hormone replacement therapy with test trials and data, in some cases funded by the multi-national pharmaceutical companies that manufacture these drugs.

Women globally are angered by this conspiracy. One has to ask why this information is buried so deep even the medical profession cannot find it? This is what inspired me to call my book 'The World's Best Kept Secret'.

As things now stand, women literally stumble upon natural progesterone by accident. And, in so doing, they struggle every step of the way to bring 'the world's best kept secret' to the light of day.

I seek to break the bonds of limited choices in HRT and replace them with the freedom to be treated individually and more safely. For is it not a woman's birthright to feel and celebrate a wholeness in mind, body and spirit?

Over my years of work and personal renewed health experiences I have discovered by talking, listening and working with hundreds of women, that natural progesterone is different from synthetic progestins currently used in conventional HRT. It has less dramatic side effects but has all the actions that nature intended for progesterone. It is the missing link back to optimal hormonal health and wellbeing.

This book will do much to ease your concerns and answer many of the questions you might have about natural progesterone. Drawing upon a compilation of several years consultation and observational data provided by women using progesterone, I will walk you through the various stages of progesterone replacement therapy and help you make sense of its action in the body.

This book will demonstrate, once and for all, why natural progesterone – our essence hormone, so vital to women's hormonal health is – the world's best kept secret which has now expanded to a second book to be used in conjunction with this book and gives greater detail to enhance your journey exposing more truths on progesterone usage and revealing more secrets

About the Author

Jenny Birdsey's Personal Story
Updated 2004.

To write my story was difficult as it challenged me to be honest about my beliefs, values and convictions. To share with the world who I am left me with a sense of vulnerability and exposure.

However, as I thought about it I realised that hundreds of women have done just that with me; opened their hearts and souls and entrusted me with their own feelings and experiences. For this reason I too feel compelled to reciprocate my truths to all those women that made this book possible, simply by telling them who I am.

My story is not much different from any other woman. My journey involves a lifetime of searching for answers for ill health, knowing there was something wrong but never being able to have a diagnosis to confirm what I felt in my body was in fact hormonal and not in my head.

I was approaching 35 when a naturopath gave me a diagnosis called Endometriosis. I felt such relief that day knowing that the pain and suffering I had experienced all those years actually had a name. That I was not psychotic and neurotic, and that this thing really did exist.

After that, gynecologists and doctors began to listen because I could tell them I had Endometriosis, and thus I started to get appropriate treatment such as Endometrial Ablation and all sorts of other pain management treatments, none of which were long lasting but certainly brought some form of relief.

Ever since my first period I can recall always having some form of pain and difficulty. My whole school life was spent walking around the schoolyard with a hot water bottle tucked in underneath my tunic. I can recall even throughout my pregnancy feeling fantastically well, and following the pregnancy the return of excruciating pain and problems with the return of Fibrocystic breasts, chronic pain, exhaustion and endless amounts of postoperative complications following my Caesarean – all very scary.

I tried to go back on the Pill without much success, so my husband at the time decided to have a Vasectomy. The doctors advised me that I would never be well enough or strong enough to have another baby but this was never a reality in my mind and the Vasectomy was only a temporary measure.

Ironically, within a year of that Vasectomy I still had to go back on the contraceptive pill, purely for pain management, which I stayed on for the next fifteen years uninterrupted until the diagnosis of Endometriosis.

By this point I was in a state of chronic fatigue, and suffered what I now believe was undiagnosed Fibromyalgia, and I was burnt out emotionally, physically and spiritually. My marriage had come to an end and I was incredibly unstable hormonally.

The implants that I had endured/undertaken along with synthetic hormone replacement tablets and other hormonal cocktails and medications (compounds which I cannot recall) taken in desperation sent me quite crazy.

I contribute a lot of that to my marriage breakdown, however, all I knew in my heart was that I had to find a way out, a way to get well other than the way I was going. My marriage ended sadly but in my heart I knew that somewhere out there, there were answers and perhaps there was another child waiting to be born, another man.

My husband had actually refused to reverse his Vasectomy years ago. Never did I think that I was not going to have another baby. I believed when I was leaving my marriage perhaps the opportunity would arise somewhere, somehow, some other time although I was not physically looking for another relationship.

To my blessing, three years later a wonderful man appeared in my life, a man who had never had children, who came with no excess baggage (ex-wives, children, maintenance), with a stable job and career as a clinical pharmacist. All he had was one mangy but beautiful, then 15 year old cat. My dreams had come true. We both wanted a child.

I stopped taking the pill prior to getting married, going back to a naturopath to prepare the way for fertility. Everything went haywire and drastically wrong. I started bleeding dreadfully, the pain was excruciating and it was unbearable. I knew my time was running out fast and I knew I had to seek medical attention so we chose to undergo the fertility program quickly.

Prior to that I was administered a 'Goserilen' implant by my GP (designed to block pituitary gland activity) which actually put me into a state of menopause. The side effects were horrific. My doctor claimed this would enhance fertility, and ignorantly I took it. I was so ill on that implant with severe side effects I thought I was going to die, and it took months and months to get it out of my system (it was supposed to be a three monthly course).

At that point I was getting scared about putting anything more into my system. I was frightened to take naturopathy because I had had a bad experience with the naturopath I was under. I didn't have answers - there was still a missing link I hadn't yet discovered.

I was married in June and by December that year (age 40 and weighing 5 stone) I was suffering chronic diarrhoea every time I ate. I was malnourished, sick and undergoing a lot of bowel tests amongst other things. The pain was so bad that I begged the doctor to do an emergency Hysterectomy. I couldn't cope any longer, wasn't thinking straight – desperate. I felt that I was running out of options.

In January I had a Hysterectomy and unbeknown to me at the time I released my ovaries without permission, as I was offered a Total Hysterectomy I assumed that I had no choice in keeping my ovaries. Had I known differently I would have retained my ovaries and cervix, knowing what I know now. In the hospital, unfortunately the pain didn't let up and I was devastated.

I actually stated that I took this Hysterectomy as pain management as I was advised it would actually sort out the pain and control the endometriosis. The doctor politely stood at the end of my bed (a young probably 25-26 year old) stating that "Sometimes these things don't work, its just the luck of the game". I said, "Do you mean to say I have gone through all this for nothing?". Her reply, "That's just the way it is". I said, "I don't think so, I don't think you have ever suffered period pain and that's just not the way it is".

I was furious, angry, crushed, mortified. My specialist visited and said he wanted to discuss HRT before I was released. I said "What for?". He said, "Now that you are in surgical menopause you will need to go on HRT to control the hot flushes". I replied, "I thought I couldn't go on estrogen because of the endometriosis", and he said, "No, you'll need to be on some form of estrogen". I said, "No, I didn't go through all this to go back on HRT, I went through this to get off HRT".

I honestly, even as a trained nurse, had not thought it through. No one had explained to me a Hysterectomy procedure, let alone what the consequences of a Hysterectomy were, and the extra health problems I was going to encounter following the hysterectomy.

With a medical background in nursing it was assumed that I understood the implications and I was too frightened to enlighten them, having never been exposed to hysterectomies or menopause in my training to any degree. I had always thought that once a woman had undergone Hysterectomy her periods stopped and it was the best treatment for Endometriosis. Because I was so desperate to get out of pain and not thinking straight, with pressures from the medical profession, family and peers, I went ahead oblivious of the consequences.

The type of pressure I was under included comments such as "You're being silly not to get rid of your uterus, it has no purpose for you any more, you won't be less of a woman because of it, you don't make love to a uterus" from my family GP, and "Who wants to put up with periods all their life". My family felt that I was being a martyr, and encouraged me to find a solution such as hysterectomy - get over it.

I had never even thought about the next step. I was just so desperate to eradicate pain out of my life. Clearly, I was not thinking straight. Submitting to peer and medical pressure, I agreed to the hysterectomy.

Four weeks after my Hysterectomy, the pain continued to increase. I went back to the specialist and she told me there was no possibility that the pain could be worse, it was all in my head. I lost it big time! I told her how dare she tell me it was in my head, it was in my body. I asked her to walk my shoes for a day. "It is my body, I know, I am not a hypochondriac, I am hurting" and I told her to "do something about it". She was a doctor, not to judge me and make innuendo and comments that I was psychotic (indicative because I was a nurse).

I was at that point getting angry and starting to fight back. I was taking HRT, getting hot flushes, experiencing estrogen dominance, palpitations, heartburn, agitation, weight gain, fluid retention, migraines, gastrointestinal upsets and other ghastly symptoms, which I'd never encountered to this degree. I felt I was getting back on the same treadmill again, but the problem was exacerbating.

All my instincts and alarm bells were going off and I felt the need to start defending and protecting myself. I started then to rebuke what was being offered to me medically.

As a last resort, I visited another gynecologist who was replacing my doctor at the time, who said "I don't know Jennifer, I just don't know what to do with you". She referred me to the Pain Clinic that had just started up at the hospital, because she really didn't know what to do for me, and because my husband worked at the hospital, I think she may have felt obligated to be seen to be doing more than what she had already done.

There I met a wonderful man called Steve Bolsin who ran the Pain Clinic at Geelong Hospital. I will be forever grateful to Steve who I had given such a hard time to. When he decided to give me an epidural I questioned if he knew how to do it, and if he was confident about the technique.

You see the last epidural I undertook caused me to haemorrhage from the site of the epidural after the surgeon accidentally hit a blood vessel. I was in labour, and these complications threatened both me and my unborn child.

Due to exhaustion and foetal distress, an emergency Caesarian was performed 24 hours later. Following the Caesarian, I experienced years of sciatica which I believe was related to the epidural experience, so I was a bit nervous again going under another epidural. I think by the time I finished lecturing Steve he was a bit nervous too. But being the type of guy he is, a man of principle, knowing his job and doing it so well, he proceeded with the utmost professionalism (guiding me beyond my paranoia). His technique was somewhat different from the first epidural I had had for child birth years earlier. (My son is will be 26 in October, 2004).

The epidural procedure covered 5 days, in which time the pain circuit was broken. I could not believe the difference. For the first time in my life since my periods started I was actually pain-free and I couldn't believe the difference – no more pelvic and back pain, or bearing down feeling and generalised discomfort. It gave me a glimpse of hope and light, and I was able to have a goal.

I then knew for the first time what health was all about and what I was meant to be aiming for. Up until then I didn't know what to grab hold of, I had nothing to aspire to, no measuring stick, no idea. All I knew was that I was trying to run away from my body, trying to escape, dull it out with analgesia, alcohol and cigarettes. Numb it, black it out.

I didn't know the difference between pain free and pain numbness. I had never experienced what it was like to feel at ease deep within my being.

Steve gave me an incredible gift that now I am able to impart to so many women, to give them a glimpse of hope and a light to work towards. I always say to women that there is light at the end of the tunnel and I endeavour to make sure I can guide them there. Once she gets that glimpse of health potential she can hang on to it and work towards it.

The epidural was so appropriate for me because I actually ran a chronic pain pathway. Steve explained that because I was Codeine dependant and addictive for many years it set off a pathway that actually enhanced my pain. Every time I took Codeine it was like an addiction that my body was withdrawing from. He also explained that this was probably one reason why I always fell very quickly into depression, being the same type of pathway.

I have been able to use this in my work. Understanding that these chronic pathways, depressive pathways, hormonal imbalances and addictive pathways are very similar and very inter reactive. (Being an addictive personality, giving up smoking did not come easily for me and I still to this day have to keep a check on my tendency to become depressed easily, as when I am out of balance hormonally).

As it turned out, the pain I was enduring was due to a massive Haematoma, post Hysterectomy, which sat in my pelvic cavity and took many months to dissolve. However while I was in bed with the Haemotoma I was able to begin working through issues of grief and remorse, clearing my head, dealing with the shock of not being able to have any more children, and dealing with my anger in my heart and soul, which I knew went back to sexual abuse, though I wasn't really ready to admit the degree of it.

Within one week, two of the Late Dr. John Lee tapes arrived on my bed from two different States. One from a person who loved me dearly, was a Christian and wanted to give me further hope, and another from an MLM company that had heard of my mishap with a hysterectomy and felt she could help me with a Wild Yam. I am forever grateful again for that person, who went on to sell me several jars of wild yam cream which I believed was progesterone!!!

This was not really helping me and intuitively I sensed that something was wrong and it was from there I started to pursue the truth about wild yams and progesterone and what it was all about.

I formed a Natural Progesterone Advisory Network (NPAN) initially with another associate who went her own way so I continued to build the then infant organisation to where it stands today. I pursued as a result of my anger, frustration and confusion, and the need for correct information and guidance of usage. I was like an island stranded without support, and the more I delved into the truth the more complex and complicated it became. Little wonder women remain confused and are open to exploitation.

When I heard The Late Dr. John Lee's tapes I cried for a day. I then got very angry and I haven't stopped being angry. I have channeled that anger into constructive rather than destructive forces. It was too late for me to have another baby and perhaps if I had had the progesterone cream five years earlier it would have been a solution or been beneficial easing my endometriosis problems. The horse had bolted and I was so mortified. I kept asking God, "Why did you give me this information now?" I had always asked for a miracle, prayed for one last opportunity to have another baby and I don't know why you should deny me this information and why you present it now - your timing is inappropriate.

I was angry at God, at the world, at myself for submitting to the hysterectomy, at the surgeons, at medicine, but more importantly I was angry with the drug companies. Angry that they could deny this truth from women and keep this, the best kept secret in the world, and as far as I am concerned the biggest crime of the century (having this knowledge of this molecule for over 50 years and modifying it for patentability).

I made a decision at that point that I was not going to let another woman suffer from lack of knowledge and information. That no one had the right to silence us any more. That maybe I couldn't have more babies but maybe other women could. Maybe if I could save one more hysterectomy it would be worthwhile. I had absolutely nothing left to lose.

I continued every day to deal with my emotions of grief, pain, and coming to terms with the God that I had known and felt betrayed me. I worked on the phone line answering women's questions, sending out information and keeping up a brave front. The women helped me survive and I helped them survive. It became like a co-dependency.

More importantly, there was this compulsion, an obsession that was beyond my own strength. I don't know where this driving force came from. I can't describe the force, but I can still feel the force and passion working through me every day. It was almost a God-driven strength. I get tired, drained, have often been kicked in the guts or challenged, and exploited for being too generous with my intellectual property.

And there have been many issues that have been battled along the way to keep the organisation going. I have experienced personal criticism, confrontation, opposition, and financial difficulties. Beyond all that, I feel there is a God-driven force that drives NPAN and directs women to seek & find NPAN.

Not least of all, the other driving force has been a magnificent man, my husband Garth, who not only nursed me back to health, unconditionally loved me and gave me safeness, strength and time to heal, but encouraged me to work endlessly with the women, having witnessed what progesterone was doing in my life and health and to other women. His mindset was being altered.

Initially he went searching for data in support of synthetic HRT usage, as he was concerned for my health in my refusal to use estrogen, particularly because of a family history of coronary Heart Disease (my father died at 39 following several heart attacks). Garth was apprehensive about me not having estrogen.

Like others, Garth felt that The Late Dr. Lee's work was biased, one man's opinion, no evidence or controlled studies or data to back it. Garth was trained to be conservative, objective and analytical being a clinical pharmacist and his specialisation and expertise was in working the cardiovascular arena consulting cardiologists on cardiac drugs. And suddenly he was confronted with an irrational wife refusing to take HRT and rubbing on cream that had no strong evidence of support for its usage.

As Garth searched the latest journals daily (and still does) he was astounded to find strong evidence although minute and scattered supporting progesterone. For example, his latest finding in 'Clinical Therapeutics', January 1999, Vol 21, No.1, pages 41-60, "widespread use of micronised progesterone in Europe since 1980, over 500,000 current users in France, no specific side effects have been reported."

His initial beliefs and training on estrogen and progestogens has changed, and he continues to do his research. So Garth joined my cause. In fact, at times when I wanted to walk away and felt the heartache and struggles, particularly financial sacrifices, he was the one that pushed me on. Contributed his wages and extra lecture income to keep me on the phones talking to women all day. Perhaps he believes that there is such an important place for this for women's health.

I ask women to visit the section on the spirituality of progesterone and perhaps they can understand a little bit more where I come from. Like hundreds of other women before me, I have travelled a journey that is inexplicable. It is a transitional and inner journey, a journey back to myself and a hormonal coming home to myself.

Perhaps destiny found me or I found destiny. Sometimes the bigger plan of our health is not always obvious, and we have to fight for it, be committed to seeking optimum health and answers. And only when I was prepared to peel back the many layers and deal with all the painful issues that had been poisoning my soul, could healing be manifested in my physical body.

All I know is that I now feel at ease with myself, my body and my spirit, and good health is not elusive any more. It has taken me 48 years to arrive here. So maybe there was a bigger plan in my search for health, other than having another child or children (a daughter in particular). To arrive at a state of wellness is a process; it was beyond my comprehension back then where this journey to good health would take me. I would have settled to be free of pain and, in so doing, would have short-changed myself.

Over and beyond the pain that I endured, the confusion, the search for missing links – all those years progesterone was the answer. When I heard The Late Dr. John Lee's tape it made sense, it resonated with me. It was the only thing that, for the first time, fell into place. Felt right intuitively. I have never ever stopped believing and knowing that truth. I walk over hot coals for women to deliver that truth. There is a sense of justice and truth that needs to be spoken out which takes courage and conviction. And this needs to be imparted to every woman as she undertakes her own personal journey. Be brave and honour your body and your truth and intuition. God only knows if I had done that maybe things would be different but then I wouldn't be here now.

Empower yourself by questioning, seeking and being informed.

I have witnessed many miracles in my organisation. I have seen women being blessed with beautiful babies (from cases of Polycystic Ovarian Syndrome, Endometriosis and other Infertility diagnoses). I have seen many women save their uterus by avoiding hysterectomies, restore their health and be pain free; Endometriosis and Fibroids successfully being managed and pain controlled. It has been a worthwhile journey but with untold sacrifices personally, physically, emotionally, financially and spiritually.

My story is about expressing, diverting and re-channeling my anger, compassion and sense of justice. Justice that perhaps was never given to me by drug companies. By doctors who didn't understand or know the difference. Justice from people I loved who never ever stood up for me with my sexual abuse, and then years later on recall. Justice about not being believed or heard. Justice in that progesterone - that's real progesterone and not synthetically modified progestogens - deserves to be instated in it's rightful place in hormone replacement therapy.

I have travelled a very incredible path and have exceptional health now. As each year goes by, I get healthier and healthier.

I have learnt how to find formulas that work for myself and for many women, know what it is like to be pain free, flexible and have mobility in my body, a beautiful figure back again (well I think so!!). I'm not Mrs Blimp, Mrs Wasted or Mrs Neurotic.

I have a joy for living, an abundance of energy, a clarity of thought (most of the time). I have a quality of life I have never had before, my sexuality and libido has returned (although I will never experience the depth of uterine orgasms like I used to, but I have learnt ways of restoring and replacing losses in many areas of my life).

I share my experiences indirectly with women around the world. I see so many women find their own miracles within. In a sense I have lost the opportunity of one baby but for thousands of foetus', embryos and seeds of hope have come to birth in thousands of women through my work and the NPAN organisation. Maybe not manifesting in the short term, but manifesting in quality of life and spiritual enlightenment.

I am humbled, honoured and eternally grateful to all those hundreds of women who shared their infinite knowledge and experiences with myself and my organisation, NPAN which I have been able to collaborate and pass on in a universal pool of knowledge.

When I was healing, particularly through my sexual abuse recall which actually came to surface eighteen months after my hysterectomy (I was just starting to get well again and I had to deal with this), I had an incredible need to return to the church and to worship. I sat there numb, week after week, and cried and cried. I used to ask God why, why all this emotional pain now, having gone through the physical. My soul was literally haemorrhaging and I never thought I'd stop crying. (This lasted a year).

Here I was helping hundreds of women and couldn't even help myself. There was a baby in the next aisle, probably a week old, and I had this overwhelming urge to go over and touch that baby. I crumbled into a thousand pieces. I have never shared this with any one, but that night I had the opportunity of having another baby in spirit.

Through that encounter with that other baby (and soul) it was like giving birth again myself, I could smell my own baby again, my first child which I had never bonded with. (I must have been suffering post natal depression on reflection).

I also never recognised that I could actually smell for the first time the birth of the baby and the feeling within myself as if I had just given birth. The experience was so overwhelming and awesome.

With a Caesarian Section and being anaesthetised, I could not bond with my baby. And, after 36 hours in labour, everything was dramatically disrupted. I'd haemorrhaged with the epidural, so lots of things went wrong. I realised all those years I was yearning just to experience natural childbirth.

It wasn't another child I wanted so much but to experience the totality of giving birth. The experience of completion and bonding. To have my baby passed through the vaginal canal, to smell him, and to feel the connectiveness post delivery as he is placed gently on my stomach. Not have my baby ripped away from me and brought back in a little supermarket-like shopping basket all bundled up. This was the introduction to my child. My only opportunity to bond with Scott was to have him nestled against my cheek. That was all I was allowed.

God gave me this incredible vision and experience of spiritual healing. The opportunity to relive the experience the way it should have been. My son is now 25. For the first time, I actually had a sense of connectedness with my son, my baby, and had this feeling of inner contentment and overpowering sense of oneness and peace. The feeling of having experienced motherhood and the birth of my baby. That night I came home and rang my son and shared the experience with him. I told him that I had never bonded with him and he said he was really glad that I told him because he felt there was always something missing in our relationship. I told him he was now free to get on with his life; now that we have connected we can disconnect so we can both move on and grow and love each other freely and unconditionally. (except on mother's day when he forgets to ring me).

My son and I are incredibly close and from that day we have been able to be honest and free to love each other on a different plane. I was able to move forward and project a sense of peace into my work and let go of the longing to have that other baby. I was able to find forgiveness in my heart to God for denying that miracle I always asked for, and find incredible gratitude for the one miracle I had, that is my son, Scott.

My healing consisted of many days of blackouts. The cause of these episodes were a part of coming to terms and dealing with childhood sexual abuse recall. Triggers and flashbacks were beyond my control, and I spent many hours in therapy over and above being at the helm of NPAN. After 18 months intense therapy, the wounds were less raw.

Each day I move further and further away from being the victim, and revalidating and rebuilding myself as a human being. It never ceases to amaze me how many women out there have been the victim of abuse which has been reflected in their self-worth, and manifested in their ill health.

My painful experience has helped me connect with women on a deeper level. I honestly believe in my heart that I could not have achieved the depth of self-actualisation without progesterone - the essence hormone - supporting my body and wellbeing throughout these horrific ordeals of dark days / nights of hell. Progesterone helped support my stress.

I realise that perhaps the formation and development of NPAN is a blessing for the women and a personal growth journey for me. I do the work because I feel passionate about these issues and the women's rights to make healthy informed choices on bio-identical hormones without being ostracised, patronised and intimidated due to misinformation, the medical mind-sets and inappropriate trials supporting the usage of progesterone. The rewards in my work and organisation have been manifested by seeing hundreds of women (and men) at different biological stages becoming well again and seeing the living evidence of how it has changed their life and the lives of their loved ones.

When I talk about NPAN, I often refer to "we". By this, I mean collectively the thousands of women who have been part of NPAN, not only me. Founder & Director of NPAN, I am here. I have self-funded and operated NPAN, now seven years, with some contribution and heaps of support from my husband. A registered business in my name, it is a one man band (myself), but collectively it is hundreds and thousands of women's experiences.

NPAN is about every woman who has rung and shared her story. In return I pass on this 'living entity and energy' that just goes on indefinitely. NPAN is not about me, its not about one individual, it is about every magnificent women.

Whenever NPAN is violated, whenever someone takes NPAN information (our collective knowledge or "my" intellectual property), or fraudulently pose as the Natural Progesterone Advisory network and tries to make money on it, I do get very angry. Not only does it impact on me personally, it violates the trust of hundreds of women who have brought their stories and information willingly and freely to this organisation.

It's about honouring their privacy, their fragility and vulnerability, and respecting their individuality and uniqueness. That's why I now feel compelled to write this book FOR YOU.

I have seen far too many people exploit what was handed out freely with love and pure motivation. I have seen my information and intellectual knowledge being revamped, misused, and unfortunately falling into the wrong hands, dangerously leading women to inferior products and information. In some cases, leading back to doctors to medicalise what shouldn't be medicalised, further disempowering women.

I have realised over the years the power of silence and its hold - to be silenced is to give up your freedom, identity and authenticity. Breaking my own personal silence has been an imposed process of character strengthening for me. I've stopped invalidating myself.

Speaking out about my sexual abuse has not been easy and has cost me the closeness of my family, personally in my relationship with my mother, sister, brother, their spouses and children. Breaking the silence is a very painful process to endure, and not without a high price to pay which, in my case, was losing my family. I had to do it to validate who I was and to find my freedom. In a sense, progesterone is a bit like this. And if I do not fight for it, speak out, it will fall back into silence, be overshadowed by patented HRT drugs. And what better spokesperson than someone who has already travelled this journey, taken the risk to speak out and seek the truth ... THE WOMEN. NO LONGER VICTIMS.

I will continue to fight government legislation, to question TGA, and to beg women to keep on voicing their opinions (and not just go along blindly). I will continue to lobby within Australia so that women can have access to a safe, reliable natural progesterone cream. One that is manufactured under drug conditions, batch controlled, ensuring physiological doses with the highest quality of micronised BP progesterone. One that women can use knowing they are going to be able to follow physiological doses and not take a calculated guess. A cream that has been trialled and is included in the doctor's drug manual.

Unfortunately though, in the process, I still need to continue to educate women and provide them with information and my knowledge, and I don't know what other way to do it. I thought by educating doctors it would be delivered correctly, but I have learnt differently.

I have learnt that this drug may again become so medicalised that women will be disempowered from the knowledge of how to use it. And how to gain the confidence to work out their own physiological doses according to their charts, journals, and to realise that the power is within their own hands.

I hope and pray that my motives always remain pure, that this information arrives with women as it should with NPAN's blessing. That NPAN's work always remains true to its origins, and the journey has not been in vain. That my ego will never let me lose sight of who I am - a lay woman on par with the women I reach out to.

It is my hope that all the observational data, painful knocks, hassles, harassment, exploitation, criticism, financial hardship and sacrifices come to fruition for every single woman. That this book helps every woman find her missing link, renewed hormonal health, and a quality of life so profound that she can rediscover, validate and reclaim herself.

I extend my blessings to you on your magnificent journey. Never, ever stop questioning or seeking the best for yourself. It is your birthright.

It is where my book began.

My story was written in 1997 it is now 2004. My first book started evolving in 1998 and my second book is on the way. Nearing 8 years work and consultancy and passion for my work. Due to my continuing passion in this field and my desire to help I have had to write a second book to cover the new knowledge that I have learned about and wish to share/impart. Their have been many more babies born to women who felt they would never achieve this miracle. I feel blessed that I have been able to help them in some small way or be part of it.

I am now busy with more consultations not just with Australian women but worldwide. It is a fascinating time for my own growth as a woman, I have stretched my own comfort zone to include public speaking at seminars on natural progesterone often incorporating Dr Sandra Cabot's weight control, body shapes and liver principles.

Last but not least our beloved cat BJ passed away at the grand old age of 17. He has been replaced by a flock of ducks, fantail doves and multitudes of dwarf lop eared rabbits, which provide me with a relaxing outlet, these are my babies. I have survived the onslaught of detractors with my last book and have revealed to myself and others the truth behind this chapter in my life by covering it in the revised update.

On reflection I have come to acknowledge that anger is a gift from God, an opportunity to utilise it and is not a negative, shameful emotion. It can bring transformation under grace. I have emerged stronger, wiser and more mature as a woman now 48 years old. I embrace my growth and future work with more excitement and enthusiasm than ever and realise the sky is the limit. I might be half deaf, now wear glasses but these are not handicaps just afflictions or annoyances. It is what is deep within desiring, expression, outlet and the need to impart to others that counts. It is about everyone giving what they can and not what they can't or haven't got. I believe everyone no matter who they are have a gift to give something of themselves. A wise friend once said "what the world needs best is what you can do best"."If you don't use it, you lose it". Be it a mother, a career woman or whatever it doesn't matter because you are special and unique and God holds a special place for all of us. I am just thankful that I have found a special place in my life a sense of value and contribution no matter how small. I'm grateful for the riches life has provided me and so many wonderful interactions with some many amazing men and women.

It is with great sadness that Gemma had to be put down on the 20th of May 2004 as she suddenly deteriorated with suspected acute onset arthritis or cancer to the spine and was suffering. Her essence is in all the pages of both books, as she insisted on sitting on top off all my drafts while I compiled the pages of these books. Her spirit keeps me going even though my heart is sad and I grieve her loss.

With love and blessings Jenny.

Acknowledgements

To True Friends

'Friends are angels who lift us to our feet when our wings have trouble remembering how to fly'.

You do not need to be named because you know who you are and you are very much loved.

A special note of thanks from Jenny .....

To the handful of precious women that are the nucleus, strength and inspiration beneath NPAN's wings.

To those ladies that arrived at my doorstep to give selflessly back to the organisation hours of voluntary help and loving friendship.

To those who propped NPAN up with a much needed donation in money, envelopes, stamps, books, photocopying, tapes, or a home cooked meal when I was sick or busy.

To those who took over my office and phones to give me time out or a quick vacation, all the while allowing me peace of mind and providing continuity and support to myself, NPAN and the women in need. To those that sent me flowers, gifts and words of encouragement. And not forgetting to mention here the 'unofficial committee gals' for your commitment and pioneering spirit attending monthly meetings in the early days, assisting, supporting and sharing answers to problems and extending fellowship with other women in similar situations. You are the foundation on which NPAN has been built and on which it has survived and grown.

Finally, there are a handful of special souls that have shown me how to realise my ideas by prompting and encouraging me to write this book and to put my work in words for other women. Without your input, belief and encouragement and your commitment to the bigger picture, this book could not have happened. I acknowledge and bless you with endless gratitude. This book is a reflection of your love, faith and encouragement of my efforts in NPAN's work and what it stands for.

To my very closest friends who believed in me, gave me strength to go on, endorsed my work, stood by me no matter what without judgement and endured my hormonal swings and insecurities and continue to remain loyal and true – thank you.

With all my love and blessings,
Jenny

To Every Woman belonging to and contributing to NPAN

There are just too many women to thank individually here, but each of you know who you are. Your unique contribution, including your active lobby work (formative years), is indelibly imprinted upon my heart. I am honoured and forever grateful to have shared part of your journey. Your contribution to NPAN is invaluable, and continues to touch other women in need. You are NPAN. Without you, this publication would not have been possible. Without you NPAN organisation would not have survived and flourished in true essence.

I thank you and it is my hope that as more and more women will continue to share and touch others that they too will discover their vital missing link, their essence hormone and unfold the World's Best Kept Secret.

A special note of thanks from Jenny to Garth

To my husband, thank you for sharing our home with hundreds of women in need. The countless hours spent on the phone, often late into the evenings and weekends. Your support to all the women, for the data and journal researching. And for personally funding NPAN, and now this publication at great sacrifice. Thank you for also assisting me to run NPAN.

From my heart there are not enough thanks or words to express my love for you. Your unconditional love and belief in me, my work and women's health allows me to heal, grow and reach my potential of expanding horizons and challenges.

Your spirit fuels my spirit enabling me to reach beyond boundaries I never knew existed.

God works in mysterious ways and you are just one example of his work.

I love, adore and cherish you. Thank you for being you. You are one of the kindest and giving person I have been blessed to know. Thank you for standing by me, the women, my work and NPAN when we stood to lose everything - even our home. You would not allow me to crumble nor NPAN to become dysfunctional through attempts of sabotage.

I feel proud of the man you are and feel lucky to be your wife and I'm more in love with you than ever.

You are my star that shines and guides me when I am lost, frightened, plagued with self doubt and exhausted. You are everything and more. You are 'my man!'

Your Jennifer Ann

To my son Scott

My miracle, my love, my life. Through your existence my life's purpose and totality have been fulfilled. Thank you.

Your devoted mum and friend,

always loving you, and always in awe of your uniqueness Scott.

'Jennie'

To my cherished friend Keith Hayes

Who believed in me, invested in my growth 25 years ago, encouraged me to be the best possible person I could be, impressing upon me that what the world needs is what you can do best. I can never thank him enough for believing in me and thus helping me to realise the greatness in myself and reach my fullest potential and to nurture my dreams and unfulfilled/unreached goals. From which the preface was written in the early morning upon sunrise at his and Jan's Queensland retreat/home on their verandah. This was the last time I saw Keith and he never saw my book materialise into hard copy. For those that know Keith he was one of those rare individuals who was able to touch mine as well as hundreds of other peoples lives in a positive and enriching way.

Keith Gregory Hayes, director of The Greatness In You Company established in 1972. (Which still thrives under the directorship of Jan Hayes, Gail and Lyle Gillett). This is where my self awareness journey began with these wonderful people. Website www.greatnessinyou.com

Died in 2001 at 64 years of age. Young in age but old in wisdom, missed by so many and loved by all for being who you were, an individual on you own destiny and a man who really knew yourself and beliefs, reflecting understanding, self awareness and clarity upon others. (Not always in a subtle way). You were a great teacher and taught me so much and showed me how to embrace my own self awareness, learn what commitment and taking responsibility for my own life was all about.

Thank you Keith and Jan and to the GIY company.

To Doctor Sandra Cabot - "The Flying Doctor"

Thank you for believing in me, my organisation and respecting my work and for providing the heartfelt forward. Years of mental support, encouragement, wise advise, medical guidance and imparting many invaluable hours of teaching and knowledge to me. Thank you is not enough, you are an inspiration to myself along with thousands of other women and men. Your work is appreciated, admired and respected by those who have followed your principles, advise and truth. I believe you are one of Australia's most unsung heroes in women's health.

With gratitude, "Birdie".

To my friend and dog Gemma

You will always be printed on my heart as much as in my books.

Thank you for being my ears in your younger days and my committed, loyal companion (shadow) all these years. You were always so tuned into every emotion I felt. You never let me down or deserted me.

I cannot believe or come to terms with how much I miss you, my darling dear old friend. Perhaps my closest friend of all. Your love was unconditional and unfailing you never betrayed me even when I scolded you. There was no room for hate, grudges or judgement in your heart - only room for love, food and you gave me so much joy and happiness.

Our animals miss you also and are lost without your leadership. It has been hard to finish these books without you in my life now. My heart is heavy and physically hurts, my chest feels crushed. My inspiration and energy has diminished in my indescribable deeply buried sorrow of enormity, which I dare not visit until these books are printed.

The hours feel so empty without you by my side and I miss your company when sometimes pushing into those early morning hours now without you.

Your loyal companionship, memories and your unconditional love, gave me such comfort and strength writing Book 2. I didn't realise how much I depended on your company which filled the long enduring hours and the consuming time. None of which you complained of but did insist on sitting over my drafts. When Book 2 is off the press I will lay you to rest, spread your ashes and say my final goodbyes to you and deal with this closure of this part of my life, allowing myself to express the well of suppressed tears, sorrow and great pain of your death that is so immense. For now I cannot bare to let you go and face this loss but want you to know how much I loved you and am eternally grateful for being there so much with me while writing Book 2 and revising Book 1. Go free in spirit Gemma and until we meet again goodbye with all my love, cherished memories of you and appreciation of your undying eternal devotion and companionship.

To Monica

My kindred soul friend on a journey, with my eternal gratitude.

Let me say - I hold you totally responsible for Book 2. I think you could see the prophecy well before I had started revising Book 1 and encouraged me to take my time and do it right starting another. Thank you for the shove and all your help.

To My Typist Andrea

Where would I have been without you - dissolved in tears, lost in all those drafts. After much desperate searching an angel on a prayer must have sought you out bringing you to my final hours of rescue.

Without your skills, dedication, hours of commitment (beyond what you expected) you have hung in and given more than 110% of your time, patience and endurance.

I very much doubt I could have kept going. Thank you so much for helping me finalise the books and inject so much of yourself, expertise and energy into this obsessional project. Thank you for your commitment and working ethics. Welcome to NPAN, Andrea and the women's network and natural progesterone, which you now type in your sleep! The women will be forever grateful because I suspect without you I may not have been able to get these back to print and would have had to abandon these books, giving up in despair. You've made this happen when so many others let me down you arrived at the door. The last part of the picture has been left in your capable hands and abilities. Thank you. Exhausted as I feel, it was an exercise in 'whatever you believe you can do!' The 'how to' comes second and life provides those real angels - you are one of them.

The humble beginnings of NPAN and the need for Information.

This book has come about as a result of the confusion between wild yam, progestogens and the lack of knowledge available on real progesterone.

In Australia, the Therapeutic Goods Administration (TGA) has classified Progesterone an S4 drug that is only available on prescription. This is NOT the case in countries like the USA where natural progesterone creams can be legally sourced through whatever channels are available.

Notwithstanding how women sourced their cream, and if in fact it actually contained micronised progesterone, there remained a million and one questions on how natural progesterone transdermal cream ought to be applied, what was the correct dosage, and how to interpret the signs and symptoms after commencement of progesterone replacement therapy.

The Natural Progesterone Advisory Network (NPAN) was conceived and registered by myself in 1998, in direct response to this cry for help! At the heart of its endeavours was always a fervent understanding of each and every woman's silent suffering.

In the early days when NPAN was first formed and the progesterone movement took off subsequent to The Late Dr. John Lee's visit to Australia October '96, I adopted The Late Dr. Lee's principles and relied solely on his books, tapes, newsletters, and occasional phone calls to discover how best to use progesterone. The women's isolation dictated the need to become resourceful and self-reliant. The Australian women willingly experimented with progesterone in pursuit of ways to improve their health.

My knowledge and observational data came about as a result of women being forced to network in my own home and depend on each other for assistance, feedback and validation. The women needed each other (still do) because we were out there on a limb without the blessing or endorsement of the medical fraternity.

For it had been made very clear to women here in Australia that if we were to be 'silly' enough to go down the progesterone pathway, we would be on our own, possibly compromising our health. Women in our country were breaking the law if they purchased progesterone without a valid doctor's prescription. And because progesterone was unknown, untrialled, and not drug company driven, only a handful of doctors agreed to issue a prescription, accompanied by scare-mongering. This just served to make women more courageous.

Over time, through my work, in my organisation NPAN, I began along with the women to identify the need to individualise dosage according to each woman's unique hormonal profile to treat her symptoms.

My information draws upon literally hundreds and hundreds of 'personal accounts' reported by women incorporating natural progesterone replacement therapy in their health regime. And there are many success stories out there that NPAN has been a part of, you may wish to read the women's testimonials of only a handful of women contained in my filing cabinets and records. These are not anecdotal or placebo, they are real case histories, many of which have been tracked and observed for nearly 8 years.

In Summary the compiling of the need for information evolved into hard copy books.

My first book condenses five years consultation into a handy, Q&A reference guide, now updated to include 3 more years of invaluable knowledge extending into Book 2, Natural Progesterone More Secrets Revealed. Positive feedback from the first print has indicated that little of my work requires alteration because most of the information is still relevant to the women who find this book a surprisingly refreshing resource for their particular needs. Book 1 is the starting point, providing the foundation of your knowledge and understanding of progesterone, its use and dosing.

Book 2 delves in depth on more subjects, accommodating and assisting at a greater level of understanding progesterone usage. It provides explanations on problems and confusion which some women have encountered on their own journeys. It adopts a holistic approach of putting together strategies and techniques, incorporating nutrition to enable a total package embracing a more successful journey. In this way it becomes a companion book to the first book.

Please note, I am NOT a medical practitioner (doctor), and strongly urge you to work in consultation with your own medical practitioner and healthcare professionals.

ABOUT MY SECOND EDITION REVISED

On 26th March 2004 I processed the last book orders for the first edition and placed the remaining few books aside to fill back orders. I felt a sense of relief (being an end of a phase) and panic. No more books left to meet the ever-demanding orders that now reach my website and desk daily.

The hard copy "Natural Progesterone, the world's best kept secret" was first published in October 2001. That was nearly three years ago and so much has happened since then. It was a risk I took at huge financial expenditure in printing, not knowing how the book would be received by the women, let alone whether I would ever move all those cartons of books, which I had to store elsewhere due to the lack of floor space at home.

The hard copy has been overwhelmingly received and as it is only being distributed by myself, it has gained enormous momentum through word of mouth. Being self published has its advantages as it gives me the freedom and flexibility to change information as it comes to hand (as it is not in the ownership of a printing/publishing company). The disadvantage is, however, that it takes longer to reach the marketplace and because of the expensive printing costs (not being mass/bulk printed), it does not give enough inbuilt margin to allow an appropriate required discount to the bookstores, whereby they are not interested in stocking it on their shelves despite public demand. Hopefully this will in the near future, change, as I can increase the number of books printed, thus reducing printing costs. However public demand is forcing libraries to keep increasing their stock of this book.

A lot has happened in the last three years in my work, my observational data and findings, in my organisation and my personal growth, all these factors warranting a revised update.

Because of the sudden surge of sales and demand for my book, running out of the books was not anticipated to be so soon. I am now on deadlines to get this book updated and back on to the print.

Sadly, to jeopardise the situation further, the printing company which I used (Rowick printers) has lost, through a sudden death, the proprietor Barbara, and of course are grieving their loss and attempting to restructure and continue on without her driving force and input. It is a very close family business and they have all helped and supported me tremendously as I was green at the beginning. To Barbara, I would like to publicly say thank you for helping me materialise my book, thus helping thousands of women. You will be missed and always appreciated for your input.

My book is being updated for several reasons and for those who have the original edition, do not feel short changed. Much of the progesterone information remains the same bar some variations of dosage on various problems such as Fibroids. These dose changes have been arrived at from observation, feedback, reports and results or non results.

I have extended more repetitive information or elaborated on topics in greater depth because some questions kept being raised around topics that indicated there was still a shortfall in understanding, or I was not making myself clear enough. Clarity was needed, which I hope I have successfully achieved.

I have also included a lot greater depth of information on topics that I steered clear of in the first book (such as libido and sexual abuse), but dare now to embrace simply because in my consultancy, it was plainly obvious there were problems that were of great concern with women, needing assistance, verbalisation and clarification.

I have also incorporated more nutritional and hormonal strategies and guidelines, assisting you in your ongoing understanding and success in progesterone usage. Many more questions have been addressed in answer format and common problems/obstacles tackled in greater depth.

As I continued to add to my knowledge the last 3 years of my work I found that it was virtually impossible to put all this in one book without information overload so I decided to create a second companion book.

I have attempted to close more gaps and open more doors, giving women more validation, information and opportunity for more choices.

More understanding to compliment and enhance women along their journey and fill in more of the missing pieces of the jigsaw puzzle.

Furthermore I decided that this would also define once and for all my intellectual property and remove any dangers of perceived ownership, although I am fully aware that this book will no doubt be condensed, reworded and core contents removed for plagerisation again.

I have allowed myself licence to be myself and the freedom to express, without intimidation, fear of criticism and/or disapproval. I have allowed myself to be real and totally honest, hopefully reaching out and touching others, sharing my experiences along with imparting many thousands of other women's experiences. To this end, connecting us all and providing a nucleus of belonging and being affirmed as magnificent, intelligent women/human beings, our fellow mankind.

I have endeavoured to reach everyone individually so you do not feel isolated, frightened, alone or floundering, silently suffering, anxious and confused.

As I cannot, through lack of hours, speak to everyone personally, I have incorporated my consultancy style and format as if you are personally in my lounge room or I am speaking to you directly. How I write is how I talk, teach, support and impart knowledge.

My writing style has been criticised by a few academics and literary conscious individuals. This I do not mind and yes, it can be annoying to some. I make no apologies for my writing style bearing in mind that this is a book on information not a literal work.

Having grown up in a world of 50% bilateral deafness, I have always found audio learning a struggle. I am fully aware my tenses and pronunciation can be incorrect, having not heard correctly in my formative years, relying heavily (subconsciously) on lip reading. I have been known to make up my own words and spell things my way in 'my language' I drive my typist crazy.

My hearing difficulty was never picked up until six weeks prior to my final exams in nursing, when I stumbled onto a ward in my training that had a sister in charge who was a mumbler. Because I was finding it difficult to cope with her instructions and consequently making an idiot out of myself, I confronted her, explaining I found her difficult to hear. She sent me off for an audiogram and the results landed me in the Matron's office, who told me to leave immediately because I was potentially a dangerous nurse! A petition throughout the hospital, unbeknown to me, overrode her decision and action, and I completed my final exams gaining a qualification as a State Registered Nurse WA. I was never allowed back at my hospital (Royal Perth Hospital) and the Matron stated that as long as she was alive, she would see to it that I would never enter a reputable hospital, so I worked in Nursing Homes following my graduation.

I always struggled through school and nursing, taking on extra tuition (at school, in English – joke!) and always copied lecture notes from my fellow students. Dictation was horrendous and still is. But I am determined, and always have been, to achieve and to be normal.

My hearing deficit is not a disability to me, just an inconvenience. The disability often lies with other people through their intolerance and impatience of my impaired hearing. I have been labelled ignorant, rude, snobby, arrogant and stupid. I am none of these. Mind you, it has put me in some awkward and embarrassing situations. It has also provided many numerous funny incidences. The latest being while at an Expo in Melbourne assisting for Dr Sandra Cabot a little boy of about 4 years old came up and said to me 'hey, lady you have something stuck in your ears'. (I was wearing my hearing aids that day). He could not fathom it. His mother was so embarrassed but I just laughed at his innocence, curiosity and cuteness.

My impairment has given me a greater gift, one of intuition which I believe has been a great asset in consultancy and working with people on a deeper level. In many cases I listen and hear from my heart.

In my preface, I do not claim or profess to be an academic or to write for the scholar. I am here for you, and invite you along to share the wealth of knowledge the women, my life's laboratory (my university) and the knowledge the universe has provided to me. God is gracious.

Lastly, but by far not least, I have taken back my power in this book, changing it to the present tense 'myself' and I would like to explain why to clear up some public confusion and misconceptions.

This work was always my intellectual property, based on my observation, my organisation, years of consultancy work and my own life's totality and quest for health.

When I wrote this book, it started with my story, well before a book was ever intended. The exercise in doing my story using a Dictaphone was for my therapy only. It was a healing exercise that I needed to conduct. After a year of crying and not coping internally (in spite of being there for the phones and women and being able to put some perspective back into their lives), I personally was floundering and lost in a void. My emotions had no words or a place of identity. It was time to verbalise what I was really feeling and to name these "things" that were so deeply hidden, crushing my soul and creating blocks which were not allowing me to move forward with my life and healing. My story was never intended to be published or exposed to the world, but it was the power and driving force behind my book, combined with my anger and frustration in my quest for answers.

Whilst conducting monthly home meetings in my lounge room of forty women, which was NPAN's original support nucleus (then voluntary), the women kept prompting me to put my knowledge into writing, stating I had a knack of explaining everything so easily, making sense out of progesterone and its usage. Being a person who has always learned from internalisation and once making logical common sense out of it, I found it second nature to easily re-siphon complex information back in simple, lay women's terms.

One of my then members, Cathy Van Loon, who was at the time recovering from a broken leg, offered her time and assistance to me to get the book started. She helped me get what was in my mind onto paper, using a dicta-machine. Van Loon also had a great handle on progesterone and was on my wave length, so we chose our living room problems and questions on progesterone as a base of approach. We realised women needed the gaps filled, devoid of medical jargon and mumbo jumbo confusion.

The KISS principle was adopted (Keep It Simple Stupid), and this is not to insult anyone's intelligence. It was obvious from the inundation of phone calls over the years to my advisory line that there was a common theme of the same repetitive questions and common problems being experienced by the women. I became aware that no one was really addressing these missing links and assisting women in interpreting and understanding progesterone usage.

All I seemed to be doing was working for authors of books written on natural progesterone or silently assisting the compounding pharmacist's customers, none of which were earning me an income.

So, the book evolved over 18 months, depending on the limited funds and availability of time. As I did not have an income, my home meeting door charges ($5) went towards typing and lobby work. It was a long haul.

The title of the original text was Natural Progesterone, A Woman's Guide to the Use of Natural Progesterone by Jenny Birdsey, 1998.©

When it came to the publishing, editing and formatting side, Van Loon and myself hit a brick wall. We had no inkling, so I approached a third previous associate to employ, to edit and to be the web master (being an IT computer whiz). She agreed to this but as a third partner and coerced us to take the electronic format, being the "way of the future", and justifying that it would not cost much to publish.

Thousand of dollars later (borrowed), the E book was launched and my work and my organisation Natural Progesterone Advisory Network, known as NPAN (in abbreviation) and my trade logo were lent for the purpose of launching. What I failed to realise at the time was the domain name was registered (which I gave permission for prior to this) in private ownership to this third party. Being internet ignorant, I did not understand these things then.

Van loon was pushed out by this associate, leaving me with a no win situation. Now my intellectual property and the domain name of my registered business and identity (of now eight years) was now seriously in jeopardy and a .com domain ownership/private to the third associate had not been handed over to the legal partnership as agreed (and never was!) Instead it was later taken by the third associate along with my intellectual property, registered business name and logo.

I pursued in good faith and trust, as I believed in a positive outcome. After all, the aim was to provide the women this information. It was never about wealth and fortune for Van Loon or myself. Our partnership intent was never in question so we did not have concern for a third associate until it was insisted that Van Loon was removed. I started to now question motives. I wanted to trust the partnership.

The electronic version proved to be user unfriendly, was erroneous and easily changed without my knowledge or consent. To a lot of women such as myself who knew nothing about computers, being totally computer illiterate, I insisted on a further risk investment, going hard copy, and after an intensive exercise in re-correcting errors which insidiously had crept in (upon my discovery) changing the total concept of the material contained within, I re-edited the errors. I also discovered editing had not been done as was supposed to be done by this third associate.

Urgent to get things back on track, I printed, only to find that legal action was taken against me and the .com domain name, owned by this third associate (never transferred to the common partnership), was taken away and removed, along with the website electronic version, my intellectual property and registered business name, as well as my world trade logo, NPAN. The Electronic version and the software was inaccessible to me and still is.

All funding of the entire enterprise was provided by myself and my husband.

It has been a huge learning curve and a lesson in boundaries, trust and betrayal, but NPAN, my organisation and my soul survived this gut wrenching ordeal.

The partnership was publicly dissolved and after twelve months I walked away from the solicitors and legal disputes (some thousands of dollars further out of pocket) as this was an endless bottomless pit with no opportunity for resolution (which my husband and I desired). Only the solicitors win. We felt shafted and manipulated in systems that I believe had no justice unless we were prepared to pay the high stakes in hefty court fees and battles which could have gone on for years. Money which we did not have, as it had been sunk into the book and electronic enterprise. It will take my husband and I years to financially recover from this, being a substantial cost against our mortgage.

To this day I am still bewildered and will never understand the reasons, motives or actions behind this whole ordeal and consequential destructive outcome and horrific sabotage, which I cannot deny, hurt deeply.

There are thousands of people who have experienced fraud and dishonesty and have been exploited, betrayed, hurt or used. It is an unfortunate part of life's expression of human traits, be it greed, power, jealousy, lack of self love, self worth, no consciousness or just plain predatorisation and exploitation (for whatever reason, our fellow humans see and believe fit). It is part of life's learning, challenging you to become a better person!! Humility is a strength. Not a weakness.

It is hard to forgive and let go but if you don't, anger and the need for justice eats at you, consumes your energy and makes you no better than the person violating and/or exploiting you. Non-forgiveness only creates illness. Forgiveness is a necessity for your own freedom, health and growth. A hard call! God knows my truth and I know my truth, and what is my God-given right, He knows my heart, my work and my motives. So do the women who know me and have been involved with my organisation, Natural Progesterone Advisory Network, or myself.

I emerge today, back on track, wiser and more resilient, ignoring those who use my intellectual property, claiming it is their own, or those "passing off" my organisation Natural Progesterone Advisory Network, NPAN. Women's discretion always wins out and karma is real and truth conquers (even if it is within).

I believe in progesterone more than ever. I believe in myself, and my work more than ever and I believe in truth, justice and the giving universe, and the need to keep on giving, no matter what to enable the flow to keep on going.

I am passionately committed to women's hormonal health and in every woman who wants her freedom, vitality, empowerment and her truth.

God bless you and thank you for being a part of my life's journey, enriching me as we connect as fellow human beings.

The information packed in this updated book and the companion book has astounded me. I am so excited how it has evolved and cannot wait to give it all back to you.

With love, Jenny

How to understand and obtain the most out of this book and companion publications

Use this book like a manual, index sections applicable and work at your own pace, eventually tackling the whole book. It is not a novel. The second Book 2 Natural Progesterone More Secrets Revealed is the companion book to this one and will assist you to journey further along the way in the near future. This Book 1 Natural Progesterone the Worlds Best Kept Secret is the foundation book.

Disclaimer

This book is not a medical book, nor should it be treated as a medical guide. It is a book based on my observational data, case histories and women's experiences using progesterone.

It is not censored, controlled or owned by drug companies or progesterone manufacturers. It is unbiased and derives no remunerations from sales of progesterone creams. My husband is a clinical pharmacist (specialising in cardiovascular) and lecturer and he does not make progesterone cream. I am self funded and independent from any other organisations, companies or operators. All information can be obtained from my secure websites: www.npan.com.au and www.natural-progesterone-advisory-network.us There are no branches or umbrellas operating under my organisation Natural Progesterone Advisory Network (NPAN), registered since 1998.

What compels, inspires and influences me as a woman, as a progesterone advocate, consultant and author.

What compels me as an author and the reason for the style I have adopted.

When I started to revise Edition 1 "Natural Progesterone The World's Best Kept Secret" (Book 1) and update (in December 2003), I had no idea what I would be in for, or the extra hours involved.

Reflecting over the last three years of numerous consultancies, case studies, emails and conversations with women, I could not contain myself or resist the temptation of going deeper, with more inclusions for the revised updated book. Due to enormous information another book obviously was being compiled - Panic! However I decided not to compromise information nor did I wish to delete old information or take shortcuts to meet unrealistic deadlines. The solution to my problem was to retain Book

1, update/revise and follow on with Book 2. Natural Progesterone More Secrets Revealed. The workload, brain power and limited typing resources and mounting costs (due to me constantly adding more material to their pile) has been a marathon.

My Consultancy work and income earning has had to be put on hold during this time to avoid distractions and energy expenditure. I hope I have met your needs. I apologise to the frustrated women who have been neglected these past 6 months, I too am guilty of self neglect, consumed in this project.

The aim of my books and work has always been to reach thousands of women, impart my knowledge, findings and observations that come to hand – shared and disclosed by thousands of women who have made progesterone usage and this book and book 2 possible – **Thank You.**

The Aim of Book 1 "Natural Progesterone The World's Best Kept Secret and Book 2 "Natural Progesterone More Secrets Revealed:

This first book is designed to teach women how to use progesterone to assist them on their self journey successfully, answering every possible scenario, providing possible solutions to individual problems, which may be encountered along the way with their progesterone usage and related health problems. *It is the foundation book which focuses on how, when, where and why guide to natural progesterone.*

The aim of Book 2 Natural Progesterone More Secrets Revealed is to assist you further along the way, delving in greater depth and answering many of the most commonly raised questions and problems from various angles. It also offers total packages to hormonal health incorporating strategies and demonstrating where nutrition and other related issues fit into the bigger picture. No stones should be left unturned hopefully. I have approached book 2 on the same methods of work I use in my consultancy and the suggested management plans I put together, bringing together the total picture, fine tuning diet, weight, body types, nutrition and hormonal balancing. I assist in helping women become empowered with common sense knowledge, confident in applying skills, technique, strategies, dosage adjustments and supplementation to achieve their own optimum health. I do not retain any secrets instead I reveal them.

Through my eight years of work and involvement with amazing women of all walks of life, I have discovered there is no easy way to explain or answer one question or problem. The same question may need to be answered in many ways, or from different angles tailored to suit different situations and circumstances. Each question and answer is complex as are every individual's circumstances, medical history and hormonal constitution.

For this reason, the same question may warrant the same answer from a slightly different perspective, thus the need for extensive repetition, which may drive some of you crazy ("Yes, she has already said that"!). Due to the extensive information required by various women I have split the books for easier access to information to enable you to gain a complete comprehension and understanding of progesterone usage.

Things that I have had to take into account along the way

Many women do not read the book from cover to cover, believing some areas do not apply to them, whether it be Infertility or menopause. Thus, they may miss vital points along the way. A classic comment "I lent my book to my girlfriend who is going through menopause problems and I didn't think I needed it now but next week I am having a complete hysterectomy and have been told my menopause will be induced. Now I wish I had that book as I do not know much about hysterectomies or menopause". Alternatively women do not have the ability to focus and concentrate when in hormonal disruption (understandably so!). Answers need to be simple, short and effective appropriate at that given time.

For these reasons I have taken these points on board (and relate to them) and the need to delve more in many specific areas, so information is not missed (often cross sectioned in other subjects), therefore requiring more repetitiveness and your patience.

Also, it is impossible to segregate progesterone to one thing/organ or problem exclusively, as the body is a magnificently fine-tuned machine of sophisticated interrelated message systems. These message systems are relayed throughout every cell of the body required for constant adjustments to maintain bodily function and balance. Hormones are part of the regulating message system, constantly being adjusted for bodily requirements and as progesterone receptors are found throughout the whole body, it is impossible to segregate progesterone, being so multi factorial in its behaviour.

So many people have suggested that I write a handbook on progesterone – WOW! – that's challenging (and will be done soon), as the more I work with progesterone, the more intriguing and complex it becomes. How do you summarise such a magnificent clever hormone and do it justice?!

However, to assist women in getting the most out of both books they are designed to be indexed in sections that are applicable to them. I go back to my earlier days when I started my progesterone journey and recall how I felt and have also sensed the same resistance from women when I suggest they read my book first. This is why I chose to write in this style because I myself could not focus or concentrate.

I can recall post hysterectomy and instantly induced menopause, my state of being – exhausted from hot flushes, disinterested in life, depressed, grief-stricken (with the prospect of no more children), loss of identity of who I was any more, unable to function, focus or concentrate. My mental faculties and ability to multi task job skills had disappeared totally.

The last thing I wanted was an academic medical book. I just wanted the quick fix and an easy, logical road map out of this dreadful place of barely existing. I wanted to find a dentist to remove my aching tooth, so to speak, and was not the least bit interested in how he did it, as long as he removed the pain. This was where I stood.

It took me a year to read, let alone decipher the material contained in the late John Lee's book "What your Doctor may not tell you about menopause" – a must to read. I could only read two or three pages and even then couldn't remember what I had read (scary!). I wondered if I'd ever become normal again whilst I watched my size 8 figure disappear in a dispersed body shape and weight gain (what I call the 'Spayed Look' – I even felt like a dog after sterilization). Yes, life was the pits.

Somewhere within my flickering spirit (a candle that I feared was going out), was a ray of hope. Faith and fate played a tremendous part in my life and helped me find a way out of my maze. God hung on to me, which was my daily payer, for I could barely hang onto myself. Suicidal thoughts were frequent. I surrendered to my struggles and threw my heart over that unknown line, trusting somehow the rest of me would follow.

I reached out to my fellow women and gave more than I had. My mission, talent and destiny found me. I certainly wasn't looking. All I wanted was a lifeline.

It was my anger, frustration and inquisitive, belligerent and diligent nature that compelled me forward in my quest for answers and solutions and the desired need for more information on progesterone. Intuitively it resonated with me.

This is where my work was born, from the seed of fertilisation, which embedded in by being. NPAN evolved.

Where my desire came from as a Progesterone advocate in seeking out the truth and justice about Natural Progesterone

I can still recall my initial reactions when I discovered this so-called hormone which I knew nothing about other than being a pregnancy hormone. My nursing career certainly didn't cover this topic – or menopause for that matter – perhaps I wagged or slept through those lectures?! Now suddenly I found myself confronted with menopause, with the need for more knowledge on this hormone, progesterone, that was now in my awareness.

My feelings were mixed and my alarm bells were ringing. It had my full attention and fascination and even focus – nothing else did! "Curiosity got the cat" so to speak. Underneath the curiosity was a sense of panic and fear – of finding hidden truths, perhaps challenging my belief system and my medical background and current medical status.

I recall my first thought was scepticism. If this was so good and the miracle worker it claimed to be, with so many multi-factorial benefits, why was it such a secret and why was all this information hidden from women for over 50 years? If it was perhaps the vital missing link and answer to so many of our health problems (mine in particular), why was it not used and available in mainstream medicine? Why hadn't I heard?

My second reaction was anger (rage) at the prospect that the answers were there right in front of me, yet took 40 years of my life to find them (a trained nurse who knew nothing about progesterone and had just undergone a now questionable Hysterectomy). I remember looking at the possibility that if this was true and a baby could have been conceived, a Hysterectomy avoided and an answer in treating years of suffering with Endometriosis and related gynaecological and emotional problems (including a resultant collapsed marriage) what would I do with the reality that someone or somebody was responsible for denying thousand of women including myself, accessibility to this hormone and its related knowledge on its uses and benefits!

Women like myself needed a place to turn to, to decipher this confusion! A 1800 line was installed. 'Natural Progesterone Advisory Network' (NPAN) and 'Natural Progesterone Support Information Group' was set up from my lounge room. Membership was created to cover running costs. The phone line proved costly. Many women assumed being an advisory network that it was government funded, not so! It was set up by myself out of compassion to help women.

The motive behind NPAN and my advisory line was to provide truthful answers:

My brain was full of questions such as:

- Why all this confusion and mystery?
- What or who was behind this conspiracy and who was protecting whom! – certainly not the women.
- Why so much difficulty in getting to the bottom of the bull-ant's nest?
- Why so much difficulty in getting progesterone?
- Why was it classified an S4 drug, being natural and bio identical to our own progesterone hormone?
- Why was it so difficult to find out information on where to get it and how to use it?
- How did we know it was real natural progesterone?

All these thoughts and questions and more possessed and plagued me.

Now outraged and stifled with sickened grief, I went on a mission - to get to the bottom of this (that was eight years ago, and I'm still on the mission). "Surely it was wrong" I said, trying to reassure myself, sensing in the pit of my gut and soul that it was true. What if that Hysterectomy was unnecessary? I moved between anger, denial, bargaining, aggression, grief and despair. I sensed that progesterone was perhaps the answer I had been looking for all these years and I was determined to prove it right or wrong, whatever it took.

I could not settle, rest, or leave it alone. I became obsessed and compelled, turning over every stone, often attacking people who fed me mistruths or lies on products. I was no longer compliant, gullible or pacifiable. I wanted straight, honest answers. I wanted accountability from so many people – doctors, MLM distributors (who were at the time selling progesterone in Australia), wild yam manufacturers claiming their products were progesterone, progesterone distributors selling creams in Australia with reluctance to come out and state the progesterone contents, passing them off as wild yam creams. There was so much secrecy around it, almost black marketed not to mention the confusion that reigned here in Australia.

The reasons behind my lobby work:

More importantly, I wanted answers and accountability from drug companies pushing HRT on us as opposed to natural progesterone. I wanted answers from our Health Ministers and TGA and the political status and regulations involving this so-called natural product.

Thus the commencement and involvement in my active lobby work to politicians, health ministers and "the politics" surrounding this hormone. I wanted to know why it was an S4 drug, which required a script, was classified as such if natural and more importantly, being an S4 drug, why were doctors were so reluctant to prescribe and why so difficult to legally access. Why the big deal no one had died yet cigarettes could be bought over the counter.

It all seemed contradictory, confusing and unjust. It didn't make sense. So many riddles to sort out. So much confusion to decipher. I didn't know where to start. The more I delved, the more confused I became. It was like opening a can of worms.

Here I was, from a medical background with access to doctors, nurses and pharmacists within my own family, yet unable to get answers. It concerned me deeply that what hope did a lay person have, because I certainly felt shipwrecked, even with the resources I had at hand.

NPAN found expression and flourished:

This is were my ignition started. Anger and frustration eventually grew to passion, commitment to women's health and dedication to truth and information. This was the foundation, from which NPAN (Natural Progesterone Advisory Network) was born, in answer to my own and thousands of other women's pleas and cries for help, taking all the riddles out and making sense of the kafuffle.

My first book has been a natural progression:

My first book evolved from years of searching for the truth, lobby work and knowledge gathered from home meetings and running a '1800' advisory line the incorporation of my consultancy work, phone work and now seminar work. It was also a totality of my own experiences and quest for health.

These books are designed to be as user friendly as possible, accessing where applicable at your pace. They are also designed to take out the guesswork. As you journey in progesterone therapy, you will find yourself visiting more sections and grasping more information. Learning how to apply it to your own particular needs. You will also learn new thing that are not in the book and discover certain truths about yourself and your body.

Do not worry if you don't understand it all at the beginning. Remember it is a journey and it will make sense as you use this amazing hormone and keep referring back to both the books, as so many women have reported from Book 1. But as there were still gaps, which I was made aware of by the women calling, book 2 has been written to fill these hopefully so women can continue to progress on their journey and usage.

I commend every woman who takes it upon herself to get well and embrace this journey. Book 2 has been dedicated to the Courage and the Women who have been courageous.

Walking with you through my book and your journey:

I trust that I can walk with you at each stage, assisting you in your journey and filling in the gaps (which in my own manhours, I cannot possibly do personally). I endeavour to reach you through my heart and books.

I want you to become the captain of your own ship and travel vast oceans capturing the beauty along the way. Our hormones are like the sea, everchanging, evolving and unpredictable. Storms and rough seas may erupt, but do pass, so please hang in there.

The progesterone journey is worth it, as thousand of women before you have taken the adventure, discovering remarkable benefits and inner power (empowerment) and deriving continual health benefits over the years!

Progesterone is as fascinating as it is amazing, being so multi factorial, it is your essence hormone. Please read the Spiritual Side to progesterone.

Catching up on the last three years:

Updating this edition has been so exciting for me and has given me tremendous joy. This hormone never ceases to astound and intrigue me and yes, I do have a lot of mileage on my mouth, after eight years of rewarding, fulfilling and enriched work.

Many women ask me don't I get sick of it, and the answer is no. Tired perhaps, frustrated with limited funds but not sick of this fascinating hormone and how it has helped thousands of women get well.

It is a giving universe and give you must, and I am so privileged that I have been able to share and give much of my life, myself and my work to assist many women find their essence and way home to themselves.

I trust you will enjoy this book and Book 2 *'Natural Progesterone More Secrets Revealed'* as much as I have enjoyed writing it for you.

CHAPTER 1

Testimonials from Women...

supplied to Jenny for book publications
and her use only©

Brigitte Muir, Australia - 1st Woman to climb Mount Everest.

Main Symptoms: PMS and Lack of energy.

"What do you do after you climb Everest? How many times did I hear that one after I came back from becoming the first Australian woman to reach its top? And how would I deal with the aftermath? I wrote a book about it, "The Wind in My Hair", published by Penguin in 1998. Well, that's what you do after you climb Everest I thought, and I should have been happy with it. So why was I feeling so much anxiety and such mood swings, and why was I bursting into tears for no reason whatsoever?

I spent the best part of a year alternating between Mrs Muir and Doctor Bitch, and generally 'making' my husband and my life a misery. It was at a women's forum in Western Victoria that I first heard about natural progesterone. One thing led to another and I eventually ended up giving Jenny Birdsey a call and asking her about that famous progesterone cream.

I had just found salvation. Jenny assessed me, she talked to me for hours about the benefits of the cream, and the reasons why a lot of 21st century women cannot do without it. I have been using natural progesterone cream for more than two years now, and it has given me a new lease on life. Gone the PMT, gone the debilitating moods, welcome peace and balance.

As long as I exercise enough, and stick to my cream regime, adapting it to my needs (gosh, you sure know when it is time for another dollop!), I stay out of trouble. I can live life to the fullest. I am definitely taking my cream to the South Pole when I pioneer my new route there!

Natural Progesterone cream is not something you can keep to yourself. Like all the other members of NPAN before me, I have been raving about it to all my female friends. Try it, and you will as well! But please, read Jenny's words first. She is the one expert I trust and recommend in a world too often directed by greed."

Anne, Australia

Main Symptoms: PMS and perimenopausal symptoms.

It is with great pleasure that I tell my story.

"I was sharing with a very dear friend about my problems with PMT and becoming menopausal. My friend is Brigitte Muir the adventurer. I have been filming her pursuits over the last 11 years and also helping her with Sponsorship.

She was passionate about Natural Progesterone cream and encouraged me to make a trip to Geelong to see Jenny Birdsey. My quality of life and not to mention my husband's has been so drastically improved, thanks to the advice I received from Jenny. Her knowledge of Women's Health Issues is immense and I have put literally dozens of my friends and colleagues in touch with her.

Thank you Jenny for your ongoing support and advice. I trust that your book will help many others."

Nina, Australia

Main Symptoms: Estrogen dominance, xenoestrogen sensitivity, heavy bleeding and the importance of a quality cream.

"I discovered NPAN about a year ago when I first used a locally compounded progesterone cream for a very severe hormonal imbalance.

The locally compounded cream did not alleviate any of these symptoms. Instead it made them worse. That's when I turned to NPAN for help. NPAN came to my aid immediately with practical suggestions to alleviate my symptoms, phone support whenever I needed it, and provided me with informative up-to-date information on natural progesterone, its use and availability. I am now using an excellent natural progesterone cream made in Australia under strict drug regulations and stringent quality control. Since using it all my symptoms have gone.

I am now more in tune with my body and have learnt to recognise what triggers a hormonal imbalance - for me its estrogen vaginal cream, paint chemicals (even "no-fumes" or "no-odour" house paints), and carpets and underlays.

Thanks to NPAN I feel more in control of my health."

Debbie, Geelong

Main Symptoms: Mouth ulcers and nail problems.

Since using Pro-Feme Cream I have noticed a dramatic improvement in my fingernails. No longer are they constantly splitting and breaking.

Another significant improvement has been in the mouth ulcer area. It has been a common problem starting a day or two before my period and lasting up to 5 or 6 days.

Thank you Jenny &Pro-Feme.

Julie, South Australia

Main Symptoms: Endometriosis and Hysterectomy.

"For years I have been dealing with Endometriosis which has involved several operations, different drug treatments (and all their wonderful side effects) and finally a Hysterectomy. All of which only worked for a limited time and then the disease would come back.

Then at 37 years I started going through menopause, which I thought was going to be the answer to all my prayers, but some of the menopause symptoms were becoming almost as bad as the pain of the Endo. My doctor put me on HRT and it did help with the hot flushes but not with much else. And I started getting bad headaches almost every day which I had never experienced before. I was wondering if I was ever going to feel well again.

Just before Christmas last year I had reached rock bottom and heard about a naturopath, Denise, who had worked in the Endometriosis Clinic in Perth. I had been to many naturopaths before but because of Denise's Endo experience I thought I'd give this one last go.

Denise told me about Natural Progesterone and suggested a book by Dr. The Late Dr. John Lee called, " What doctors don't tell you about menopause". It helped explain a lot of things that had happened to me over the years, and at last I felt that there was some long term help available.

Denise told me about the Natural Progesterone Advisory Network and suggested that I ring Jenny Birdsey. I filled in a profile of my medical history and sent it off to Jenny.

With her help and advice I started on the Natural Progesterone cream. Not everything ran smoothly in the beginning and I had some severe estrogen dominance symptoms and crippling joint pains, but with Jenny's help and her understanding of my symptoms, we have worked our way through the tough times.

If it hadn't been for Jenny's thorough knowledge of Endometriosis and Natural Progesterone cream, and her reassurance in what we were doing, I wouldn't have continued past the first week of using the cream. Once we sorted out the dose that my body could cope with, I just had to ring her to tell her that after nearly 18 months of a continual headache/foggy head and numerous visits to the doctor with no answers, I finally woke up one morning feeling wonderful and without a headache!! At last I feel that there is a light at the end of the tunnel and I know that with continued support from the Natural Progesterone Advisory Network, I will finally get my life back (and my ever patient husband hopes so too!!)."

Julie, Australia

Main Symptoms: Osteoporosis at 37 years of age and bone building.

"I first found out about natural progesterone at the end of 1999, through a friend who was finding it helpful for her menopausal symptoms. My ears pricked up when she mentioned that natural progesterone could help improve bone density.

Although I was only 37, I had already discovered that my bone density was dangerously low, and my doctor had told me that I would need to go on HRT when I got to menopause to help prevent my condition from becoming worse.

I was fortunate to have been picked out at random and asked to take part in the Geelong Osteoporosis Study, which was subsidised by the government. Had it not been for this study I most probably would not have even considered the need to have my bone density checked until I reached menopause.

I made an appointment to see Jenny Birdsey at the Natural Progesterone Advisory Network, who I found to be extremely helpful and very thorough.

She asked me lots of questions about my health history, and gave me a detailed questionnaire to fill in so that she could get a total picture of my health status. She suggested several dietary supplements, as well as the natural progesterone cream which I started using in January 2000.

I might add that Jenny has been particularly helpful along the way since then, answering numerous questions for me either over the phone or in person. I'm really impressed by her level of commitment!

My previous bone density scan results were as follows:

September 1996: 1.029g@cm2 (Just below the acceptable range for my age)

December 1998: 0.965 g/cm2 (Well below the acceptable range for my age; a decrease of 6.2%.)

I had given birth to my first child 10 weeks before the second scan. I figured that it was probably normal to lose bone density during pregnancy, but at the same time I was quite worried as I thought perhaps I shouldn't try for more children, if this was going to happen with each pregnancy. I had supplemented my diet with extra calcium since the first scan and especially throughout my pregnancy, so the second bone scan result was particularly deflating for me.

For many months after giving birth I suffered with back pain, with having to carry the baby around, and especially when having to lean forward to do things like bath him or change the linen on the cot. I felt like I had no strength in my back. Many times this pain almost drove me to tears. Nineteen months later I was asked to have another scan. At this point I had been using the natural progesterone cream for 6 months. The results were as follows:

July 2000: 1.097 g/cm2 (Within the acceptable range for my age - an increase of 13.7% since my previous scan and an overall increase of 6.6% since my first scan.)

I was thrilled with these results! I realise that since having my baby I've had the extra "exercise" of weight-lifting every time I have to pick him up and carry him around, and that this in itself may have had a small positive impact on my bone density, but I am convinced that the biggest single positive influence on my bone density has been my use of natural progesterone cream.

I am sure that the natural progesterone cream has helped me in other ways too such as reducing my symptoms of PMS, helping me to sleep better and generally have more energy, and an improved ability to cope with day-to-day living.

Two months ago we decided to try for another baby. I decided to go off the natural progesterone cream altogether, which wasn't necessary but I was curious to see if I would notice any changes. This month I've been particularly aware of general aches and pains, (including back pain with associated loss of strength) and increased symptoms of PMS. This month I'll definitely be back on my natural progesterone cream!"

Klara, Australia

Main Symptoms: Infertility and diagnostic premature menopause.

"Hi! My name is Klara and I have had problems with my hormones all of my adult life.

After we were married I couldn't get pregnant and after many tests, tablets and injections I finally got pregnant two and a half years after starting treatment. After our daughter was born we started trying again. Then after six years and one miscarriage I stopped all treatment and two years after that at the age of 35 I had my tubes tied. I'd had enough.

I was put on HRT (Premarin.625 mg) and for about 9 years I was doing all right. When

I turned 45 I started having major symptoms: panic attacks, anxiety attacks, mood swings, I was teary and unsociable. I wouldn't go out anywhere, I tried to cope by myself.

I was talking to a girlfriend of mine, telling her what was happening to me. She told me she was seeing a lady called Jenny Birdsey. Her daughter was having trouble with Endometriosis and with Jenny's help with natural Progesterone and vitamin supplements was starting to feel better. I saw Jenny and talked with her for two to three hours about everything that was happening to me. She gave me a video tape to watch from America and I was very impressed with it.

I was sent to have blood tests by a doctor to assess my hormone levels. After that I went off my HRT and was put on natural progesterone cream and some vitamin supplements. The vitamin supplements helped to tone down my estrogen dominance. Approximately two to three weeks later I started to feel my old self.

I went back to Jenny once a month to make sure I had my dosage right. I made up a chart with all the symptoms I was having and Jenny could tell me to either increase or decrease my dosage. If I had any problems I was able to ring Jenny any time to talk to her.

Eventually I learnt to read my own body signals. I talked to my family doctor about the progesterone cream and he was happy for me to use it, as he could see an improvement. I gave my doctor all the information Jenny gave me about progesterone cream which reassured him about me using it.

I have been on progesterone cream since April 2000 and I'm feeling great. I still have my off days but they aren't as severe and as often as they were in the beginning.

I don't know what I would be doing today without the progesterone cream and Jenny Birdsey."

Margaret, Australia

Main Symptoms: 10 years on continual HRT (incorrect premature menopause diagnosis) and Fibroids.

"It was four years ago when I first met Jenny. We were both desperately needing to find an alternative to mainstream medicine which was not working for us. We felt angry and deprived of our choices and no longer believed that we had to continue to follow the paths that our doctors had led us along.

After ten years of continual use of HRT I had decided that enough was enough. I had realised that if I stayed on it for much longer, my already failing health would deteriorate to the point of no return. I was attempting to 'wean' myself from it, going alone, without help or support but determined not to give in.

I met Jenny at a social function and we immediately connected. Jenny was one step ahead of me and she gave me Dr The Late Dr. John Lee's book to read along with one of his tapes. I was amazed, intrigued and so inspired with the information that I found myself dialing The Late Dr. Lee's telephone number in the States and lo and behold he answered!

He was extremely kind and considerate, he listened to my 'plight' and gave me very valuable advice. Without going into detail the words which rang clear and have stayed with me were 'just keep slapping on that cream'.

All sounds easy - but I struggled. NPAN came into force, and because of Jenny's persistent hard work, her fight for knowledge and her desire to help other women like myself, I started on the road to recovery. NPAN supported and guided me through a very difficult and emotional roller coaster. I had been using inferior creams which had created problems and after being diagnosed with Fibroids Jenny introduced me to Pro-Feme. I have not looked back and would not be where I am today without it.

I cannot speak highly enough or thank Jenny enough for her wonderful service, not to mention her husband Garth for his understanding, patience and advice, which he has undertaken to give me on numerous occasions regarding the use of medications which may or may not be harmful and their effects. All a very integral part of the 'healing' process.

Well done Jenny and Garth in helping me to get my health back again. There should be more people like you in the world!"

Fiona, Australia

Main Symptoms: About her mother's breast cancer.

"I found NPAN through Jenny Birdsey when she came to me as a massage client. The timing was spot on, as not long after my mum discovered she had breast cancer for the third time.

From many chats with Jenny willingly sharing her profound knowledge on progesterone, and the availability of books, video's and audio tapes from the network library, I began to understand the bigger picture.

My mum used the progesterone cream daily throughout her radiotherapy, while at the same time being guided by a naturopath who saturated her body with antioxidants, vitamins and minerals. She survived the radiotherapy beautifully only really suffering from burns. Nine months later she was all clear, the tumours had gone.

I have an 11 year old daughter going through puberty. I am at the other end of the cycle in my 40's and its a comfort to know that the network and progesterone is there if and when we need them. As a massage therapist I see a lot of women who share in confidence with me their health problems, and as I recognise imbalance related problems I offer them the network's pamphlet and encourage them to call.

For those that do I often check in with them and find that the progesterone, dietary changes and natural supplements from the network have made a huge difference and they are eternally grateful that they found the network before accepting other options of surgery, HRT etc."

Monica, Australia

Main Symptoms: Chronic Fatigue Syndrome, adrenal exhaustion and hormonal disruption.

"I came across the Natural Progesterone Advisory Network (NPAN) through the medical network in Geelong. My gynecologist referred me to a clinic in Geelong."

NPAN is an excellent women's health resource. It embraces a total health approach to women's health. NPAN's holistic approach to life and healing, values nature's products and the natural phases of a woman's life, and teaches women to honour, understand, and take control of her health and biological wellbeing.

A reproductive life cycle interrupted by several traumatic gynecological episodes and a continuing unpredictable biological clock, culminated in, and led me down the path to, preimenopausal hormonal disarray and a personality transformation bordering on the "dragon" syndrome! Natural Progesterone (as distinct from its chemical imitators) and NPAN's holistic approach to women's health, helped me feel in control and enjoy a wellbeing I had not enjoyed for as long as I can remember.

I know now that feeling constantly tired, emotional, and out of control, was not my imagination or me being emotional, but a signal from my body to listen to the changes of the life process.

Total health is a combination of feeling well in body, mind, emotion, and in spirit - a woman's spirit. It is easy to lose touch with our women's psyche and natural intuition in a world where logic and fact prevail. But the truth is, on a daily basis, women nurture others in our homes, our work, our schools, and our communities.

To give nurturing, we must know it is okay to also nurture ourselves. To do this we must find balance by listening to the needs of our body, or we shall lose sensitivity to what our bodies need and the totality of who we are. There is no substance to a skeleton.

My heartfelt thanks and congratulations to Jenny Birdsey, Founder and National Co-ordinator of NPAN, for a wonderful service. There IS life after Hormones!"

Pamela, Australia

Main Symptoms: Menopausal symptoms (hot flushes).

"At the age of 40 I started menopause - hot flushes, irregular periods, etc. I didn't want to go on HRT and was looking for alternatives. A girlfriend was telling me about the Natural Progesterone she was using and how it'd helped her, so I was very eager to look into it and phoned Jenny Birdsey the next day.

Jenny spent a couple of hours informing me about Natural Progesterone and its benefits as well as giving me plenty of information on women's health issues and the importance of nutrition and how much that plays a role in our wellbeing.

It's now 3 months since I started the Natural Progesterone cream as well as the herbal powders which Jenny tailored to my particular needs, and I'm feeling so much better. The hot flushes have reduced greatly and my general health has improved - my energy levels have increased so much so that my family have commented on the change! I'm also thrilled to know Jenny is only a phone call away if I need an answer to any query I may have."

Tracey, Australia

Main Symptoms: Skeptic of progesterone usage and benefits.

'I was feeling quite ill and went to the doctor who believed I was showing signs of estrogen dominance and sent me to NPAN. The information was great, although it was a lot to take in. It was very interesting reading. Learning to look after and read your own body, it takes a bit of getting used to. Once you've got the power its great.

I started on progesterone cream and felt great. I went off the cream, still felt good for a couple of months then it started all of a sudden. I went downhill fast, my symptoms came back - headaches, mood swings, fatigue, breast tenderness, sweet cravings. Back to NPAN for a talk. I went back on the cream and nutrition and I am back on track again. I was a skeptic but am now a true believer."

Kelly, Australia

Main Symptoms: A young sufferer of polycystic ovarian syndrome and endometriosis.

"Since I started my period at the age of 13 I have had severe pain before and during my period. Heavy bleeding due to complex cysts on my right ovary, extreme fatigue and mood swings. After three years of blood tests, ultra sounds, doctors and gyno visits I found no solution.

At this time I was also under extreme stress due to bullying at school and found this made my problem even worse. I heard about NPAN through a friend of mum's. She had great results I had nothing to lose by trying one more avenue.

After spending two hours talking to Jenny Birdsey she pin-pointed my problem. She gave me heaps of information on Endometriosis & PCOS giving me a better understanding. I can call Jenny any time I need advice.

I have been using the progesterone cream for three months and have found the results fantastic! No longer am I getting period pain or heavy bleeding and now my periods are only lasting 3-5 days instead of 2-3 weeks as before. Along with the herbal medicine to boost my immune system the progesterone cream has been a God send for me."

Madelen, Australia

Main Symptoms: Mastering awareness of symptoms and the value of charting.

"Jenny's NPAN has provided me with fantastic knowledge both physical and psychological. Lots of research information she provides - personal one-to-one dealings at initial interview and on the telephone regularly. The calendar for monitoring my 'balance' plus her knowledge of oral vitamins to take as well, has been fantastic.

The organisation NPAN is professional, a wealth of information - more than what general doctors know! I've been using the progesterone cream from WA for 18 months now. It has helped me with my PMS. I feel better taking something that's natural and has no side effects now or later. It has regulated my periods and eased my periodic depressed days. Jenny's help and knowledge has saved me from a lot of work (research) and she genuinely cares about this subject and her clients."

Maggie, Australia

Main Symptoms: Perspective from a Professional Electrologist.

"As an Electrologist, my clients come to me to remove their unwanted hair. Menopausal clients do present with unwanted hair, however, symptoms present which are most distressing and answers they have received have not eased their distress.

Hormonal imbalance is not restricted to the Menopausal woman. In these times of stress and uncertainty, I find many young clients are not considered if they ask questions which challenge the status quo.

They want to know about their bodies, why they have superfluous hair, why they cannot maintain a stable body weight, and vague feelings of being unwell that lead them to feelings of frustration and depression because answers are not forthcoming.

When I met Jenny Birdsey, I was so thrilled to meet a dedicated researcher and fanatical collector of data. This was the safety line my clients were looking for; a safety line that could talk their language.

I am constantly amazed at Jenny's knowledge and her information, her sources she shares generously. Her dedication to women makes them feel valued. Jenny empowers people to help themselves, and I must admit scattered amongst the clientele are some very happy men.

I can only speak highly of Jenny. It is great to be part of her Progesterone Network."

Fiona, Australia

Main Symptoms: Facial hair and self esteem.

"I found out about natural progesterone and NPAN through a friend who owns a healthfood store in Narrabri, but at the time was an employee working in the sandwich bar. It was such a relief to finally find an organisation and a contact person - Jenny Birdsey - who understood how I was feeling, and what I was going through.

My main reason for searching for an answer was in my early thirties I had excessive facial hair and dark facial pigmentation, excessive tiredness and PMS every day of every month. I found all of this to be really embarrassing (you cannot hide your face!). And because of PMS, I was not the person I wanted to be, and I couldn't hold down a full-time job.

Through NPAN I found the information and emotional support to be excellent. Previously I had read many books and I had been unable to fix myself. This support is ongoing which is really helpful if you do have a relapse. I feel so much better now and much more aware of my hormones and my need for supplementations, herbs, diet and exercise to compliment Natural Progesterone.

I am now studying at TAFE and applying for full-time jobs. And I am feeling much more positive and happier within myself. NPAN proves that there is light at the end of the tunnel through natural means. Thank you NPAN, and thank you Jenny."

Lurien, Australia

Main Symptoms: Chronic depression and hormonal problems.

"I have suffered with depression, heavy periods, pain and irregular bleeding. Surgery revealed adenomyosis, Fibroids and cervical erosion. These problems have all been alleviated with the regular use of natural progesterone, along with many other vague symptoms.

I first heard about natural progesterone through my counsellor, and received wonderful support from Jenny Birdsey in evaluating what nutritional and hormonal help I needed."

Marie, Australia

Main Symptoms: Breast cancer and ex Tamoxifen user and experienced side effects of estrogen administration.

I've just finished reading a book on natural progesterone loaned to me by a friend in New Zealand who, after meeting you, is now using the cream and has had a remarkable improvement in her menopause symptoms. I must say, the book made interesting reading and if I had had access to the information years ago, I would never have taken synthetic hormone replacement therapy. Why didn't my doctor assess me for hormone and progesterone levels or at least tell me about the cream!!! She put me on Ogen and just over 3 years later (1999) at the age of 57, I was diagnosed with grade III estrogen receptive breast cancer requiring 6 doses of chemo and 30 doses of radio. My life was turned upside down as you can well imagine. I don't see that doctor now !!!

My GP has reluctantly given me a prescription for progesterone cream which is hard to obtain and has suggested I speak to my breast surgeon before using it as I am taking Tamoxifen for 5 years, and although there seems to be no information as to whether the cream will affect the benefits of Tamoxifen, I need to be very, very sure. Having had cancer, I am reluctant to take even a headache tablet!

And so I write to you seeking information on the progesterone cream, its benefits and its side effects. At the moment I am struggling with hot flushes, night sweats, memory loss, sore joints, bloating, disturbed sleep, complete loss of libido, and weight gain. Sound familiar?

I am quite happy to pay for any information and look forward to your reply.

Klara, Australia

Main Symptoms: Appreciative client and NPAN's "Kiss Principle" (Keep It Simple Stupid).

I've had hormonal problems most of my life, and the hardest thing that I have found is to understand all the 'technical jargon', which goes right over my head. When your hormones are all over the place (over 20 years) your brain is not always in gear, and you find it hard to comprehend anything too complicated.

When I started seeing Jenny Birdsey I felt like I've been 'walking in fog' most of my life, and after talking to her (for 3 hrs) the fog started lifting and everything started to fall into place. Her simplified version of everything that was going on with me started making sense. I'm not a stupid person, and I think the average woman likes to be able to read information without it being like a big puzzle. If it's too hard to understand she will just put it in the "too hard" basket, and won't bother finishing it. Scientific words put people off reading anything.

Jenny has helped me understand the things going on with my body by explaining it in "plain English". Complicated and scientific words are hard to understand at the best of times. Jenny put me on the right track by explaining everything, step by step.

Monica's Update

Main Symptoms: Breast cyst of ten years disappears.

I am happy to say that my last mammogram in April 2004 showed that a 2 cm breast lump in my right breast which I have been carrying for more than 10 years, has completely disappeared after 4 years on "Pro-Feme" Natural Progesterone Cream.

Although being mammogrammed for many years because of a previous breast lump found in my early 20's together with excessive breast tenderness and no family history to indicate breast cancer risk, a review diagnostic mammogram was done because of suspected new fibrous and lumpy breast tissue strands.

I couldn't believe the lump had completely gone after all this time plus the all clear of any new concerns!

My next challenge is to completely resolve my uterine fibroids. They have been hanging around longer. They are not gone but I am happy to say they have not increased in size while on Natural Progesterone Cream.

Thank you Jenny for your continuous support and counselling.

CHAPTER 2

Attitudes towards progesterone

Why are so many people unwilling to address or come to terms with the hormonal problems afflicting women and men today?

As women are discovering across the globe, progesterone is proving to be their missing link to hormonal health and well-being in general. And this excitement and newfound knowledge is contagious. More and more, women want to share this revelation with their fellow sisterhood.

There is, however, a resistance out there, despite the fact symptoms appear to be associated with 'estrogen dominance' - a term coined by The Late Dr. Lee where progesterone levels are inadequate and estrogen dominates the hormonal environment. This can be caused by synthetic HRT, obesity, eating habits, fatty liver, lifestyle, or exposure to toxins in their environment.

Our society has given rise to the 'quick-fix' approach, where we reach for a tablet to rid ourselves of pain or to lose weight, get rid of, regulate or halt menstruation, protect against fertility or remove any likelihood of pregnancy the morning after. We are a society that has learnt there are quick, easy solutions which ultimately remove us from the responsibility of dealing with, and perhaps preventing these health problems.

With the advent of HRT, we have become conditioned by drug companies and the billion dollar industry that finds its target audience in the baby boomer generation, that menopause is something we do not have to worry about because when we arrive at it, we just visit our GP, get a script of HRT and that's the end of the story. And in many cases, we may be given HRT as the standard form of treatment. Incidentally with the published HRT scare and evidence to prove to some of its dangers the standard HRT approach in prescribing and treatment is insidiously changing. Still medicalised I am now seeing via the women new trends appearing such as the adoption of prescribing anti hypertensives (in the absence of high blood pressure) to attempt treating hot flushes. See Medical References.

What women fail to realise, in this 'one size fits all' treatment of menopause and menopausal symptoms, is that at the end of the day huge health problems continue to plague women. HRT hasn't provided a solution but rather generated 'repeat sales' for the drug companies and GPs who's business thrives as a result of the follow-up consultations and medication prescribed to treat secondary conditions that exist because women have been encouraged to take HRT in the first place.

If a woman is serious about embracing natural hormonal balancing techniques that include progesterone therapy then she is going to have to do the work. Hormonal health and well-being takes hard work, commitment, time and responsibility for the part you play in keeping yourself well. There is no quick fix or magic bullet on the immediate horizon.

It's not different for our teenage children. Mothers bring their daughters to my organisation with problems such as acne, irregular and/or painful periods, the absence of periods, sudden weight gain, daughters who are presenting with symptoms that indicate Polycystic Ovarian Syndrome and Endometriosis, girls who are exhibiting huge androgen effects in their body as a result of their eating habits and hormonal disruption.

By the time they come to me, some mothers have already tried putting their daughter on The Pill only to experience further problems, or they just don't like the idea of giving their child synthetic drugs, especially at such a tender age when their reproductive organs are still maturing. When it's suggested these symptoms may indicate hormone imbalance, it comes as an absolute shock to the mother and her daughter, and the following comments are not unusual, "but I've had her tested out","the endocrinologist says she is fine","there is no reason for her to be going through all this".

When a woman comes to me with a history of migraines and PMS, I suggest it may be a peri-menopausal symptom, an estrogen dominance symptom, or the result of hormone imbalance subsequent to a tubal ligation, etc. Invariably, the response goes something like this, "No way, my doctor says I'm too young for menopause". Again, a shock to the system. Or, if a menopausal woman comes to me after HRT failed to provide relief, or she is actually suffering debilitating side effects because of HRT, she'll turn around and say, "This isn't right, my doctor said that I wouldn't have to go through menopause", or "I thought I was through menopause".

There seems to be a lack of awareness and knowledge. A tremendous gap in education that makes it rather difficult to help a woman through the various transitional stages of hormonal changes within her body and throughout her life. We seem to know a great deal about puberty. It's now taught in sex education classes at school. And it's now common practice, mothers teaching their daughters that when they reach a certain stage of their young life they'll get their period, their figures will change, they'll get breasts and rounded little figures. Boys will notice their voices will change and maybe they'll be the victim of acute acne, and so it goes on. Just as a woman may have been moody in adolescence, she may be also that way again. Changes in hormone levels (estrogen) seem to be responsible at both stages of life.

But no one out there teaches a woman that the ebb and flow of her hormones will continue throughout her lifetime. And can be markedly influenced by the chemicals and toxins in her environment, her eating habits and poor nutrition, her state of mind, her sedentary and somewhat stressful lifestyle, all of which can create endocrine disruption to the body.

It is little wonder then that when we mention the word 'menopause' or 'hormonal imbalance', people automatically make the association, "Oh my God, that doesn't happen until you're in your fifties and sixties", locking it into their mind as some form of unwanted disease or unwanted stage of life that no one wants to hit. In some people's mind, it's a barometer that they are over the hill and heading down the pathway of osteoporosis and redundancy. (2 million Australian women are approaching menopause).

Consequently, the comments that come back to me through my organisation are quite phenomenal, and are more the norm than the exception. Here are a few examples, "I don't have that problem, I just have irregular periods"; "My boobs are just sore, it's got nothing to do with my hormones"; "I want a breast reduction because my boobs are too big, but it has nothing to do with the fact that I'm on HRT or that I'm estrogen dominant"; "I'll jump that hurdle when I come to it"; "Oh no, it's not a hot flush, my body is just hot and overheated"; "It must be the clothes I'm wearing", "I mustn't be very well"; "It must be the environment I'm working in"; "It's stuffy at work", "My husband gives off too much body heat and I get hot at night time".

Other more close minded comments include; "I don't want to know about that stuff"; "We don't talk about those things"; "I'm too young for that"; "It doesn't relate to me"; "Progesterone isn't what I need"; "How could progesterone possibly help my problem?"; "How can it possibly help my mood swings?"; "How can it possibly help my osteoporosis?"; "I've been through menopause, I don't need hormone replacement therapy"; "I tried that once before and it didn't work"; or "I'm already on hormone replacement therapy". "My Doctor tells me progesterone won't help my problems".

There seems to be pervading sense of embarrassment and social myth surrounding women's hormonal health that we suspect is driven by drug companies to keep women in the dark and fear stricken for monetary gain. Sadly, we wait until we are met with a health crisis in our life before doing something about it. It usually takes some life threatening situation or confrontational issue before we will actually change our life or change our style of living and eating patterns. And for this to occur, it usually takes a tragedy rather than being generally informed. What smoker doesn't know about the risk of lung cancer, and yet may wait until she has emphysema or a life threatening disease before she actually considers giving up the cigarettes. I find hormones are very much similar to that. NPAN generally sees women at the point when they have exhausted all options and have got nowhere left to go. I am often the last resort. Fortunately as more and more women share their revelations in new found health and wellbeing, they are spreading the word, more women are seeking me out or my book. By taking this step they are addressing symptoms earlier or taking preventative measures, witnessing their friends or associates extreme problems and not wishing to go down the same pathway.

Over a period of time I have witnessed some fantastic, remarkable things occurring throughout the network that connects women with friends and relatives. Women are helping women. They are educating others purely by spreading the word gently. Often women ask me, "How can I get my mother or how can I get my sister to use progesterone"? The fact is, you can't. All you can do is give her the information and leave it with her. Because when the time is right, when she needs it, she will come back to it. The seed is sown. The only thing a woman needs to do is offer her mother, sister or friend an option (in this case natural progesterone) beyond what they are currently aware of.

Whatever path she ultimately takes is her own decision, and it's not unusual to see women who have stubbornly ignored all information eventually embracing progesterone 12-18 months later, perhaps commenting, "Look, I heard about this some time ago and didn't believe it"; "I had to try HRT"; "I thought it was too simple, too good to be true, just couldn't be the real thing"; "My doctor told me I was being silly and that I shouldn't be considering products that haven't been tested on the marketplace".

One of my greatest joys and challenges at NPAN has been the advocation of natural progesterone to every woman I meet such that each has an opportunity to embrace a more natural, safer form of hormone replacement therapy. Furthermore, I jump at the chance to help educate young teenagers because it is not so much this generation, but the younger generation I along with many others are most concerned about. Polycystic Ovarian Syndrome is evidently in plague proportions along with Endometriosis.

More and more, we are seeing problems emerge where girls and boys are entering puberty earlier, where they are battling uncontrollable weight gain and in some cases severe hormone problems. Cases of Infertility are doubling, there seems to be a growing risk of Breast Cancer, Endometriosis, Ovarian Dysfunction. Menstrual problems that require synthetic HRT (The Pill) are on the rise. Basically, adolescents are suffering hormonal imbalance like never before in history.

I have seen hormone disruption across all age groups, not just the aged. I have seen it from as early as 9-10 years of age, right through to 80, but unfortunately the problem seems to be accelerating perhaps correlating with our fast-paced lifestyle and reliance on fast foods, refined sugars and carbohydrates. We have been trained to accept that there's a drug out there to fix all our problems, the advent of antibiotics being a prime example. But there is often a high price to pay for quick fixes.

So, if someone is resistant to your suggestion of progesterone, don't be offended by it or put off. Pat yourself on the back and say, "I've at least passed on a little bit of awareness". When they are ready, the right information will present itself, or they will come back and ask for more. I say to a women, you are the walking evidence. It will be your results that shine through. It will be your renewed hormonal health that will be the proof of the pudding, not your words.

In effect, "Walk the talk". Don't make the mistake of lecturing in the blind hope, you will reform the world. ("Monkey see what Monkey do" as the saying goes). Instead, just take responsibility and reform yourself. Take some action in protecting your environment, your immediate health and family, and news will spread. And when there are enough women out there doing this, a paradigm shift will occur. But change cannot be instigated until we make the change within ourselves.

Every day, I see more and more women making this internal change, which gives me faith and hope that the future might yet promise optimal health for our grandchildren. That we might yet educate young women to protect their ovaries (and testes in men) from further damage, and that of their unborn child during embryonic development, which has already lead to hormonal disruption in so many of our teenagers today. Classic example of drug therapy consequences used in the past now surfacing on the future generations has been the use of DES. Which was prescribed to our grandmothers and mothers to prevent miscarriages. Evidence is now coming out that this is one of the suspected causes of vaginal cancer, Breast Cancer, Infertility and premature miscarriages in women today (three generations later!) With such knowledge it is time to head the warning signs particularly with the usage of HRT and the oral contraceptive pill and perhaps we should be seeking safer options and considering the future ramifications.

CHAPTER 3

The Spiritual Side of Progesterone

The essence hormone of being a woman
A message from Jenny ....

I would like to share my observations over several years of work with women involving what I call the 'spiritual essence' of progesterone. It is purely my own viewpoint.

I would be doing the women and this book a disservice if I didn't disclose the inner soul and inner spirituality of what I believe is the progesterone journey from a holistic point of view, covering not only the physical benefits and usage of progesterone, but the spiritual side of progesterone and the emotional side of progesterone. I believe that they are all interactive and there is no clear defined line between what is hormonal, what is emotional and what is spiritual. They all interplay, and they all have a place of importance and need to be acknowledged and recognised.

I believe that to give a woman back her progesterone - her mother hormone, her essence hormone - you give her back an opportunity to reconnect with herself. Many women have become so hormonally imbalanced that they have no clue as to what their true essence feels like. Often stress, a very busy lifestyle, or family can and do distract her.

However, the one thing in common with every woman who has come through my lounge room for counselling, or picked up the phone to call me directly is that once a woman gets her hands on this vital hormone, she begins an incredible journey. Often she doesn't even understand what's going on herself but it's so powerfully obvious to the person witnessing the transformation.

I know that as soon as a woman puts progesterone into her body there's an incredible physiological reaction to that hormone. It's as if it resonates immediately, and she can 'tell' progesterone is central to her renewed health, not necessarily because of what she's read but how it intrinsically feels in her body. It's as if she's coming home to herself.

Even for those women who may experience incredible discomfort for the first 10 days to 2 weeks, when estrogen actually wakes up and estrogen dominance symptoms are exacerbated, she is determined to keep applying progesterone cream because she wants the end result. There is an intuitive 'knowing' that something good has been introduced into her body and she wants it to stay.

Unfortunately, some women abandon progesterone at the point of discomfort, not knowing how to get through the debilitating stages of estrogen dominance, which can occur at any stage. It is my hope this book helps you work through the setbacks so that you can stay with progesterone long enough to enjoy the true essence and benefits from both a physical and metaphysical viewpoint.

It is likewise understood that women who started HRT and felt dreadful in the initial period gave it up because they knew intuitively it was 'bad' for them. Often women don't even get to the point of opening that packet of HRT, or it sits in their handbag, often the script doesn't even get filled. Clearly, there is something that just doesn't feel right for these women. I say to women, "Honour your intuition. Honour this innate intelligence. Use your discernment".

During initial group meetings spanning 18 months, I had observed transformations that I now draw on during individual counselling sessions. I had seen women enter my lounge room (for group meetings) behaving like doormats – shrivelled, dripping with sweat, like a little dog shivering in the corner, insignificant, helpless, lost and frightened. Women in their 40s and 50s with families, careers, a wealth of experience and knowledge, and tremendous gifts to offer the world appear to lose all semblance of their true self because of incorrect or untreated hormonal imbalance.

Within months of progesterone use and balancing various aspects of their life, which I talk about in this book, and encouraging a woman to acknowledge herself and honour her body, I had seen these very same women start to plump up spiritually, become vocal, find their voice, express an opinion, exude confidence, and take back their self respect and a degree of assertion.

I have also witnessed husbands dragging their spouse in to my lounge room (office), distraught and desperate, looking for solutions to their wife's behaviour; her inability to cope, remember, focus, communicate, socialise. Interestingly, these same men have been the controllers in their relationship, having taken over their wife's capacity to think for herself and she has, in turn, become co-dependent.

These fuzzy-headed, tentative women, once they get 12-18 months into progesterone supplementation, often ended up being in a position of defining new boundaries and standing up to their husbands. They become assertive and very independent, and finally learn how to say "no". In fact, one such husband rang me and asked what the side effects of progesterone were, to which I enquired, "Why is that?" He stated that his wife hardly ever stays home now and that she never irons his clothes any more. Mind you, both of them were retired.

The wife suddenly found that she had interests outside of the home and returned confidence and had made a life independent of her husband. The husband, on the other hand, was quite angry that in getting back his wife's hormonal balance and capacity to function again, he had lost the control of his wife. I stated to this man that there are side effects but they certainly weren't ironing, or the lack thereof.

I see women come to me in a very vulnerable state. They are obviously out of tune with their bodies and their needs. They come distraught, exposed, fragile. They come exhausted physically, emotionally and spiritually. Women often sit for the first hour in my presence and cry. This alone is a relief and validation for them because they have finally found an outlet. They don't know why they are crying but they are crying and I always state that they have every right to express themselves. Something they may not have given themselves license to do for years. Tears don't come from nowhere. Tears have a purpose. Tears serve as a barometer, as guidance, as an expression of what's really happening in our body. Tears are also the cleansing of our soul!

Hormonal imbalances seem to weaken the emotional profile of a woman, meaning that what once was dealt with or excluded or in control, or put away, handled or not handled, is suddenly exposed and rears its ugly head. It's almost as if when a woman is going through a hormonal imbalance, whether she is in her early teens, or whether she is in her early twenties, or whether she is in peri-menopausal years of thirties to forties, or whether she is in post menopausal years of fifties onwards, she still has issues there that need addressing and hormones seem to have a way of bringing to surface grief, sadness, depression, lot of tears, emotional roller-coasters, sessions of hate, anger, frustration, belittlement, resentment, guilt and shame, and the list goes on and on.

We all too often tend to fob off or claim that it's hormonal, and that it's our hormones that are creating these things and that we're not normally like that. I would debate that and often I ask women to challenge that within themselves. I say the way to do that is first address your hormonal imbalances, get your progesterone back in, your mother hormone, your essence hormone, ground yourself. Get your nutrition and exhaustion in order so that you're feeling stronger in yourself and physically more able to cope with stress, infections and all the traumas and the impact that your body is exposed to on a daily basis. Then, deal with the emotional issues that arise, or are there and need re-addressing. Often women find that they now have to revisit events that they thought were in the past and resolved. Often they find that these conflicts are there and get worse and are uglier and more out of control and more irrational because the hormones are out of control.

Hormone imbalance creates emotional instability, but I also say emotional issues often create hormonal imbalances. There's always a connection with the adrenals when stress is involved (adrenal exhaustion can cause hormonal imbalance, hormonal imbalance can create adrenal exhaustion). I witness women who have had a shock, a death in the family, a loss of a child, a sudden divorce, a husband running off with a younger woman, suddenly going into menopause or her menses stops, and yet having no previous symptoms or signs. This goes to show how powerful the messages and chemicals of our brain and body are and how they impact so deeply and so cruelly on our delicate organs, and can throw the whole endocrine system upside down. And how stress can cause our body to lose balance, rhythm and connectivity.

One woman sat in my office sobbing bitterly because her mother wasn't going to be around for her menopause. And I thought to myself sadly, this poor women needs her mother now just as she needed her when she was going through puberty. It brought home to me how important support is for women at this, and various stages of their life. How important it is to have our mothers and our loved ones around us. And also how important it is that we go through life addressing and dealing with each phase. If we fail to progress through our natural phases like puberty and menopause in a healthy way, they can become for us a dis-ease (ill at ease with our body).

This applies to so many of us. Hormone imbalance appears to be a catalyst for visiting painful and hurtful conflicts and memories, thus isolating and alienating us into further despair and depth of depression, or for others triggering anxiety and panic attacks. There is this overwhelming helplessness and distortion of reality that is compounded by hormone imbalance, but seems to be easily addressed once progesterone is introduced. Mind you, progesterone doesn't mysteriously make the problems disappear. It just seems to give most women the ability to tackle her problems with a different perception and a more methodical approach.

For myself, mine was sexual abuse recall. Why it came up at menopause I don't know.

Again, it related to the filing cabinets being thrown open, my defence mechanisms being down, the fact that I went through so much stress with the Hysterectomy and surgically induced menopause that my body just broke down and so did my emotional filing cabinet. I personally sat in my lounge room for 12 months feeling I wanted out. I was looking for suicide every day. And I was frightened that I was thinking that way, and none of it made sense to me, I was in a void (abyss) and feeling totally helpless.

I was only able to start getting a handle on my life and my spirituality once I started to get the progesterone back into my system. For the first 6 months I was on Wild Yam cream. But once I soaked in the progesterone, I started to feel a bit calmer and more connected, and I felt I was coming home to myself. It didn't get rid of my grief, my emotional issues, traumas, and turmoil. In fact, upon reflection, it gave me the strength and clarify of thought to deal with them. It also gave me opportunity to deal with my internal grief that was so deeply buried in my subconscious and stored in my body. I cried through my emotional pain which lasted a year, it was my essence healing.

I always say to women, if there are issues there – grief, unresolved conflicts, burdens, sadness, relationship issues - then allow them to surface and use your menopause, use your hormonal imbalance as an excuse to have a damn good cry. Tears are for healing. Tears are the way of cleansing the soul. And then get on and deal with it.

This is a time of shedding. It is a time of re-building your body, and a time when women can actually re-build their persona. These are women perhaps suffering from the empty nest syndrome, or where the husbands are busy on their careers or have retired, abandoned or passed away. And suddenly they ask themselves, "Who am I? What am I?" and they feel this emptiness. An ambivalence as to who they are over and above their labels/identity as a mother, a lover, a wife, cook, friend, work colleague, confidante, and all those other magnificent skills which they too often take for granted. But they cannot comprehend who they really are, so they have great difficulty serving themselves after a lifetime serving others. It's almost like they are silently screaming out, "Give me attention. Serve me!" But too often no one's listening or they're not understanding. Often she cannot even ask precisely for what she needs. Instead, her needs are manifested as symptoms. These get the focus, not her. Surely this is an obvious cry for help. She knows she's floundering, and she's desperate to get to the other side.

Truly, it is sad to witness the many women who ask, "How do I love myself? How do I nurture myself? I've known how to be a wife, a daughter, a sister and a mother, I've known how to procreate, how to be a healer, a lover, a cook, a taxi driver, career woman, a super woman, a survivor, an organiser and all those wonderful multi-skilled roles that we women fill so readily, but when it comes to how do I look after me or how do I help me meet my needs, the score card comes up blank". Little wonder that women are crying in silence and suffering such bleak emptiness. That they feel such pronounced loneliness, confusion, grief, anger, sadness, and perhaps frustration because they've never taken enough time to listen to their own inner child. And we, as women, have not been taught that it's ok to be self-nurturing without feeling 'guilty'.

I explain that when a woman becomes pregnant, her progesterone is the most predominant hormone. When she is pregnant, she just automatically knows how to protect herself, to nurture herself and to keep herself stress-free. All these things ensure the baby's survival. Is it the hormone itself that gives her that sense of calmness so the world could be falling around her and she would be in a state of "Oh well"? Pregnant women absolutely flourish and they have that inner glow, their beauty radiates and their happiness is subliminal.

I liken this type of metaphoric process that occurs during pregnancy to what often I feel could be happening to a woman when she starts re-introducing progesterone back into her own body. It's almost like the body is so starved of that hormone that it needs to be reacquainted and, once this happens, then the body settles down. But, in the meanwhile, just introducing progesterone alone can do absolute wonders for a woman's spirituality and her sense of completeness.

When women start this journey they enter an 'awakening' period (some are more aware than others). She can use the same principles when she starts her journey with progesterone (that promotes life) to nurture and develop her own inner child perhaps neglected until now.

I say give a woman back her hormones - her progesterone - and you give her back her spirit. She will then inevitably start dipping into the 'too hard basket' and sort all these things out as they appear because she's rediscovered herself, her oneness, her self esteem and her ability to feel that she belongs in this world. That she has a purpose again. She also learns to become assertive and say "no". Invariably, she reassesses her values, her beliefs, and her position in life. She also learns to redefine her boundaries again, and to abandon things that no longer serve her. This may even be marriage or relationships; I have observed women actually come to a point of realising that their marriage is no longer appropriate, or may require reconstruction. They arrive at this decision with confidence.

I have seen women become more "selfing" (not selfish), to respect their needs rather than put themselves last, to realise that they need to recover and get well, that they need to spiritually nurture their souls, to heal their tired, stressed-out bodies. They need to take some responsibility for their own health. They acknowledge the need to devise plans that are going to target health, eating and nutrition, and lifestyle adjustment that will serve them and carry them through to old age. These are the same women that learn to take up new hobbies and interests. Basically, a whole new way of thinking and approaching their remaining years.

Often I see women, after they start the hormonal balancing journey, going back to school, undertaking new careers, taking on huge challenges, or returning to society to give of themselves in some serving form, and adopting new strategies in expanding their inner growth. I see these women starting to look for the greater meaning of life. I call these their 'croning years' and, in tribal times, these women crones were most respected and looked upon for their wisdom, knowledge and guidance. Within these tribal times, women anticipated this milestone as both an honour and measure of their worth within their community. Sadly, Western society does not venerate this epoch.

In our Western society, women enter their menopausal years fearful that they will be looked upon as redundant, no longer useful, and without value. And we bought the package! Again, women lose their own sense of value by buying into this unfounded social myth surrounding hormonal imbalance and menopause.

However, in my observation, I have seen that this may not be the case once a woman finds help, and a hormonal balancing infrastructure put in place. Anything and everything seems possible! And I've seen so much that nothing surprises me anymore when it comes to women's personal growth. Amazing, wonderful and miraculous things are happening to many, many women worldwide as they discover, and use this wonderful multi-factorial hormone called progesterone. As each woman reunites with herself, there's an internal shift of power and renewed energy which vibrates within her soul and is reflected in her energy field.

Often you'll hear me tell women, "don't underestimate the power of progesterone on a different level other than physiological symptoms". There is a wonderful, magnificent side of progesterone that I don't think we really understand. And, as I said earlier, it is purely an observation that never ceases to amaze and bemuse me. For every woman has her own special journey with progesterone. In time, you will probably take it for granted and it won't be so significant. But guaranteed, over the years, as you go through the years of croning and wisdom, you will find that perhaps progesterone has had some impact. That it was, in a way, responsible for both your growth and your journey, or at least it supported you.

You may look back, reflect, and realise that progesterone marked a significant milestone in your life such as pregnancy, your hormones for puberty, and your hormones for menopause. We sometimes fail to respect the importance of our hormonal persona and how it plays out in our life. How important it is for use in our life. And how important it is for us to connect to ourselves.

The fluctuations of our hormones throughout our life have been responsible for our growth and our physiological being. I encourage women to embrace imbalances so that they can understand who they are and what they are all about. And to find some points of balance and correction so that they can actually empower themselves with each milestone; as it occurs within their lives, as it was when they were pregnant, and when they were going through their first menses, etc.

I believe that women need to respect the progesterone hormone. It is a very, very powerful hormone. It is your nurturing hormone. It is your hormone of essence. It is the mother hormone to all the other hormones. But more importantly, it is the hormone that makes the difference between a woman and a man. A man has more testosterone, a female has more progesterone and estrogen.

Progesterone is often referred to as the happy hormone, and that is quite right (it's actually a mood enhancer and modulator). Because it's a happy hormone, I encourage women to find their own happiness and inner contentment, and to recapture the joy and bliss in their own lives as they journey with this hormone and discover its remarkable powers. Embrace these changes and utilise them for your own magnificence.

Often I hear that menopause covers the best years of a woman's life. Of newfound freedom and awareness. I really believe that this can happen, but sadly, with so much exposure to hormonal disruption like xenoestrogens in our foods and the environment, and the stress that we are subjected to - chemically, internally, and through the demands the world puts on us, or the speed at which the world is going, and the fast foods that are part of our lifestyle now - that we won't get past all these dreadful obstacles and symptoms.

Symptoms that keep us locked in our diseases, rather than realising the greatness that awaits us.

Without dealing with all the issues, a woman's treatment in hormonal balancing and health will not be as effective or as advantageous as one would like that woman to experience. It helps if women become very aware of their bodies through charting and through education, and open to its usage and how to get the most mileage out of progesterone, combined with attitude adjustment, dietary, nutritional, and lifestyle modifications. One thing that is necessary to include here is the importance of her spiritual and emotional journey and awareness.

I forever remind women that hormonal imbalance is not a disease but rather a transitional stage of life. If menopause arrives prematurely, then it's a signal either your lifestyle is not right or your eating habits are inadequate, perhaps your ovaries have been damaged through some unfortunate incident, or what you're doing to your body here and now in impacting your health. Whatever the reason, you still need to journey through the metaphysical and psychological aspects that go hand in hand with the physical changes of hormone imbalance.

From this viewpoint and experiences of woman associated with NPAN, I believe progesterone can perhaps support this transition, over and above what has been written and acknowledged to date on progesterone and its multi-factorial benefits.

On a closing note, I and my organisation NPAN, would like to extend my blessing, limited wisdom and love to all readers on your personal journey towards empowerment and awakening.

God bless you on your spiritual journey, Jenny

CHAPTER 4

Natural Progesterone and its relationship with other hormones

- *What is progesterone?*
- *The Steroid Hormone Pathway*
- *Women who are most likely to suffer with progesterone deficiency are*
- *Diagram - Monthly Hormone Cycle in a preimenopausal woman*
- *What is a progesterone receptor?*
- *Why do women need progesterone?*
- *If I am estrogen dominant, what are the benefits of using natural (to the body) progesterone?*
- *What is estrogen dominance?*
- *Symptoms of estrogen dominance*
- *How come I have estrogen dominant symptoms and yet I still ovulate?*

What is progesterone

Progesterone is a steroid hormone, often referred to as a sex hormone. Steroid is a generic name for dozens of body regulators (hormones) made from cholesterol.

Cholesterol, the basic building block for the steroid hormone, gives them all a similar structure. Switch a few atoms around and the role of the hormone can change dramatically.

Without sufficient cholesterol, we can't make sufficient steroid hormones. Some of the more familiar steroids are estrogen, progesterone, testosterone, the corticosteroids, and DHEA.

Progesterone is one of two main reproductive hormone groups, the other being the estrogens, made by the ovaries of menstruating women. It is primarily a hormone of fertility and pregnancy.

The three major functions of progesterone in our body are:

·   to promote the survival and development of the embryo and foetus

·   to provide a broad range of core biologic effects

·   to act as a precursor (building block) of other steroid hormones

Progesterone is produced upon ovulation. It is also made in smaller amounts by the adrenal glands in both sexes and by the testes in males. Progesterone is a precursor of other hormones such as estrone, estriol, estradiol, testosterone, and all the important adrenal cortical hormones. The hormone diagram demonstrates this and explains how cholesterol is converted into steroid hormones.

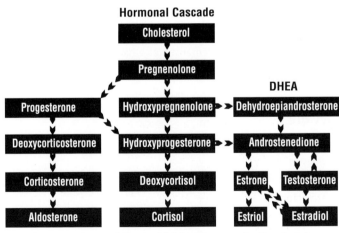

Production of Steroid Hormones in the body

THE STEROID HORMONE PATHWAY

Supplied & printed with permission specifically for Jenny Birdsey's use from- 'Ask Dr Sandra Cabot Newsletter', Edition 6

79

Progesterone is also made in mammals. In fact, progesterone was obtained from the ovaries of pigs and later from human placentas. Both these methods were expensive and only yielded small quantities of progesterone - therefore uneconomical to market.

In the 1940s, however, Dr Russell E. Marker discovered a chemical process by which he could economically manufacture progesterone from saponins (oils and fats from plants) harvested from the Mexican Wild Yam and Soy plants.

The levels of progesterone in a woman's body rise and fall dramatically with her monthly cycles. At ovulation, the production of progesterone rapidly rises from 2-3mg per day to an average of 22mg per day, peaking as high as 30mg per day a week or so after ovulation. After ten or twelve days, if fertilisation does not occur, ovarian production of progesterone falls significantly. It is this sudden decline in progesterone levels (as well as estrogen levels) that triggers a period/menstruation, and another menstrual cycle will begin.

If pregnancy occurs, progesterone production increases and the shedding of the lining of the uterus is prevented, preserving the developing embryo. As pregnancy progresses, progesterone production is taken over by the placenta and its secretion increases gradually to levels of 300-400mg per day during the third trimester.

If, however, a woman fails to ovulate during her cycle the result would be too little progesterone in her body, and estrogen dominates the hormonal environment. For your understanding, progesterone is manufactured by the empty sack left behind by the released egg. This sack is known as the corpus luteum. **Unless ovulation takes place and the egg is released, progesterone will not be manufactured.**

A fundamental key to hormone balance is the knowledge that when estrogen becomes the dominant hormone and progesterone is deficient, the estrogen can potentially become toxic to the body; thus progesterone has a balancing or mitigating effect on estrogen.

The diagram (page opposite) demonstrates what actually happens to a woman's body and the hormones estrogen and progesterone during her 28 cycle.

Women who are most likely to suffer with progesterone deficiency are

Those not ovulating monthly or anovulatory

Unexplained Infertility

Premenstrual syndrome (PMS or PMT)

Post Hysterectomy

Diseases such as Polycystic Ovarian Syndrome (PCOS), Endometriosis

Menstrual irregularities and bleeding concerns

Menopause natural or induced (chemotherapy or premature menopause and other causes)

Amenorrhea/ primary or secondary causes (discussed in the second book)

Estrogen dominance and associated symptoms

Post Tubal Ligation

Women with painful, lumpy breasts (Fibrocystic Breast Disease) and those

Other reasons for example hair loss, painful menstrual periods, Fibroids or Osteoporosis.

Monthly Hormone Cycle in a Preimenopausal Woman

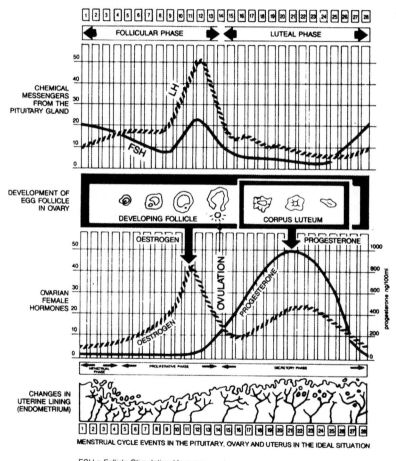

FSH = Follicle Stimulating Hormone

LH = Luteinising Hormone

Supplied & printed with permission specifically for Jenny Birdsey's use from- 'Ask Dr Sandra Cabot Newsletter', Edition 6

What is a progesterone receptor?

It is a physical structure on the cell membrane that attracts the progesterone molecule / hormone, and responds to its effect at that receptor site.

Because there are literally hundreds of progesterone receptors (sites) throughout the body, progesterone will have a major impact on your body as each receptor relays a specific message.

Why do women need progesterone?

Progesterone has a comprehensive role in a woman's body. And when levels drop, your body is going to react in a big way. This can be evident as seen in PMS, Post Delivery - childbirth, or insidious from years of progesterone deficiency resulting in a multitude of diseases and symptoms.

We now know that if we allow estrogen to dominate the hormonal environment, there is significant risk of Breast Cancer and reproductive cancer. So one of progesterone's most important roles is to balance or negate the effects of estrogen.

At menopause, a women's estrogen level will drop by 40-60% (or can be lower in cases involving thin women). Just low enough to stop the menstrual cycle. Progesterone levels, however, may drop close to zero in some women.

This wouldn't have bothered a woman at the turn of the 20th century who rarely lived beyond her reproductive years. But these days a woman can expect to live to 85 years and beyond. Coupled with living in an estrogen laden environment of this century (xenoestrogens).

She needs to give some thought to how she's going to rejuvenate her 'ageing' endocrine system. Natural hormone replacement will become a vital anti-ageing tool for both men and women, and progesterone supplementation is a good place to start.

At menopause, the adrenals and other organs take over the manufacturing of hormones, particularly testosterone and estrogen, and some progesterone. However, in cases of adrenal exhaustion and other health problems, the body often cannot compensate adequately, thus causing further hormonal havoc to the body.

Progesterone is a precursor (or building block) to many other steroid hormones such as cortisol, testosterone and estrogen (estriol, estradiol, estrone). Because it is a modulator, its use can greatly enhance overall hormonal balance.

Progesterone supplementation will stimulate bone building and help protect against Osteoporosis, not overlooking the numerous positive roles it plays in the body. For women who suffer hormonal imbalance but are not necessarily menopausal, progesterone is equally important. Even young women in their 20s and, on occasions, teenagers may need progesterone if they are not ovulating regularly and present with an array of estrogen dominant symptoms.

During pregnancy, rising progesterone levels prevent the premature shedding of the uterine lining (pro-gestation). If progesterone levels drop due to inadequate progesterone production, then a premature delivery could result, or bring about a miscarriage in the early trimesters.

In fact, feedback from women suggests *progesterone is very effective in opposing estrogen dominance symptoms of all ages.*

If I am estrogen dominant, what are the benefits of using natural (to the body) progesterone?

The progesterone benefits are as follows:

- Maintains the secretory endometrium
- Protects against fibrocystic breasts
- Helps use fat for energy
- It is a natural diuretic
- Natural anti-depressant / mood enhancer
- Facilitates thyroid hormone action
- Normalises blood clotting
- Restores sex drive (improves libido)
- Normalises blood sugar levels
- Normalises zinc and copper levels
- Restores proper cell oxygen levels
- Possibly prevents endometrial (uterine) cancer
- Helps prevent Breast Cancer
- Simulates osteoblast for bone building
- Restores normal vascular tone
- Necessary for the survival of the embryo
- Precursor of corticosteroids and other hormones
- Modulates other hormones helping to restore balance
- Promotes sleep
- Contributes to reducing anxiety and panic attacks
- Reduces estrogen dominance symptoms (refer to list on page)
- Other benefits: hair thickens, skin texture improves. Reduces breast pain, endometriosis (and pain), premenstrual headaches, painful heavy bleeding.
- Helps assist controlling mitigating estrogen driven diseases such as Fibroids, Endometriosis and hormonally related cysts
- Promotes and maintains full term pregnancy if there is a progesterone deficiency and no other underlying causes
- Softens breast tissue

- Can promote ovulation and restore ovarian function and menstrual regularity
- Balances the estrogen/progesterone ratio
- Helps manage aches and pains associated with hormonal imbalance
- These are just a few of many of the benefits reported by the women using progesterone.

What is estrogen dominance?

Estrogen dominance is a term coined by The Late Dr. John Lee in his first book on natural progesterone. *It describes a condition where a woman can have deficient, normal, or excessive estrogen but has little or no progesterone to balance its effects in the body.* Even a woman with low estrogen levels can have estrogen-dominance symptoms if she doesn't have any progesterone.

Estrogen is a name for a class of hormones that take part in regulating a woman's reproductive system. Estrogen is the dominant hormone for the first week or so after menstruation, stimulating the build-up of tissue and blood in the uterus as the ovarian follicles simultaneously begin their development of the egg. Levels peak and then taper off just as the follicle matures and just before ovulation.

Progesterone is a single hormone that is produced by the follicle after ovulation. It is a major reproductive hormone during the latter two weeks of the menstrual cycle. It keeps the inner lining of the uterus ready to receive a fertilised ovum, and later provides the nurturing for the development of the embryo. If the egg is not fertilised, progesterone levels drop dramatically causing the uterus to shed its lining and a menstruation flow results.

Even low estrogen levels can result in estrogen dominance if a woman's body fails to produce progesterone month to month. Conversely, during menopause when a woman's hormone levels drop as a natural protective mechanism, estrogen dominance might yet be a concern if she is exposed to foreign estrogens (xenoestrogens) via her diet, environment or HRT.

Symptoms of estrogen dominance

The symptoms and conditions associated with estrogen dominance categorised by The Late Dr. Lee are listed below. Later on, I'll go into detail how to chart/ journalise your cycle to better ascertain whether you are, in fact, estrogen dominant. If that is the case, outlining why progesterone therapy ought to be introduced to safely bring your hormone levels back into balance.

- Acceleration of the ageing process
- Allergy symptoms, including asthma, hives, rashes, sinus congestion
- Autoimmune disorders such as lupus erytherometosis and thyroiditis, and possibly Sjögren's disease
- Breast Cancer

- Breast tenderness
- Fibrocystic Breasts
- Cervical Dysplasia (abnormal cervix cells)
- Cold hands and feet as a symptom of thyroid dysfunction
- Cold buttocks (NPAN"s observation)
- Copper excess
- Zinc deficiency
- Decreased sex drive
- Depression with anxiety or agitation
- Dry eyes, gritty or watery, puffy eyes
- Early onset of menstruation
- Endometrial (uterine) cancer
- Fat gain, especially around the abdomen, hips, and thighs
- Fatigue
- Foggy thinking
- Gallbladder Disease
- Hair loss or thinning
- Headaches or Migraines
- Hypoglycaemia (low blood sugar)
- Increased blood clotting (increasing risk of strokes)
- Infertility
- Irregular menstrual periods
- Irritability
- Insomnia (difficulty in sleeping)
- Magnesium deficiency
- Memory loss, inability to focus or recall (not Alzheimer's)
- Mood swings
- Osteoporosis
- PMS/PMT
- Polycystic ovaries
- Premenopausal bone loss
- Prostate cancer (men)
- Sluggish metabolism
- Thyroid dysfunction mimicking hypothyroidism
- Uterine Hyperplasia (excessive formation of tissue)

- Uterine Fibroids
- Water retention, bloating

The Natural Progesterone Advisory Network has collated, through documented observation, a cluster of hormone imbalance symptoms including estrogen dominance not easily found in mainstream publications. And the list continues to grow, as more observational data comes to hand. They include the following:

- Twitching eyelid, puffy swollen eyes/eyelids, skin tags on eyelids etc
- Blurred vision, inability to focus and/or watery eyes, difficulty focusing
- Tender heels and/or feet, from sensitive to burning
- Restless legs - particularly at night-time (in bed) or Restless Leg Syndrome
- Itchy, burning, sore ears
- Sensation of foreign object in ear such as bees or insects, Tinnitus
- Vertigo, particularly around ovulation time onwards (more profound lying down in bed)
- Heartburn, indigestion, abdominal pressure, bloating
- Low resistance to infection
- Sinusitis, head congestion, flu-like headaches
- Premenstrual asthma and/or Sinusitus
- Painful, throbbing face, one side more than the other often reported
- Aching teeth - dental check-up inconclusive, cyclic mouth ulcers
- Cyclic throat problems - too many sore throats around ovulation time, throats that don't clear, consistent sore throats every month, tonsillitis, Asthma, upper respiratory problems
- Acne or pimples, particularly just prior to menses, also in older women
- Premature wrinkling or loss of skin elasticity, skin problems
- Chronic recurrence of Thrush, Cystitis, Vaginitis
- Reports of acne on the vulva that flares at menses and or cyclic vaginal boils
- Chronic Candida (systemic/vaginal)
- Bouts of diarrhoea prior to the menses, some alternating constipation, especially with women who have cysts and Endometriosis
- Leaky Gut Syndrome
- Inflamed bowel problems - Colitis, Irritable Bowel Syndrome, Leaky Gut Syndrome
- Inability to lose weight and shift fluid
- Loss of control over bladder (Stress Incontinence), inability to empty, tender & sensitive (absence of bladder infection), fluctuation/variation of bladder paralysis

- Palpitations (not cardiac dysfunction related)
- Mild - Extreme agitation and anxiety
- Panic attacks with or without other symptoms
- Inability to focus, foggy thinking
- Inability to concentrate
- Loss of short term memory, recall, word or name select
- Alienation and loss of confidence, self esteem
- Androgen side effects: facial hair, increased body hair, thinning scalp hair/hair loss
- Increased thickening and blacking of limb hair
- Atypical periods alternating from shorter or extending to longer, cycles become erratic, can alternate from heavier to lighter, or can be a combination of both - heavy clotting (no Fibroids)
- Fibroids (estrogen promotes fibroid growth - many women with estrogen dominance have Fibroids unknowingly)
- Aching joints present in the form of rheumatism or arthritis, joint and muscle stiffness, nerve endings feeling very fragmented and fragile and tender to touch, imitative of fibromyalgia syndrome, neuralgia problems
- Pins and needles, sciatica, deep hip pain down one side predominantly quite common although bone mineral densities and hip x-ray tests are normal
- Painful ovaries upon ovulation or groin pain
- Painful ovaries in the absence of ovulation, confusing women that they have ovulated
- Obsessive, irrational thought and behaviour patterns: finding a lost item, trying to think of someone's name, being aware on one level but unable to stop yourself on another. Some suicidal thoughts
- Lack of lateral thinking and ability to multi-task
- Fragmented physically, emotionally and spiritually
- Cyclic headaches and Migraines, sharp pains through top of head
- Overwhelming panic attacks and unfounded fear or phobias
- Social phobia, sense of loss of social skills, withdrawal, alienation
- Unrelated grief & sadness. Uncontrollable episodes of tears/depression
- Sluggish liver (aggravated by hormonal overload, overuse of synthetic HRT medications, xenoestrogens)
- Vocabulary / speech difficulty - 'tongue tied', verbal stammer or difficulty in word finding
- Constant lingering headache that wont shift likened to a tight elastic band around the head which will not be alleviated with analgesia

How come I have estrogen dominant symptoms and yet I still ovulate?

Many women know they are ovulating, on average, day 12-14. Some women ovulate earlier and it is obvious with the mucous discharge, however, they still show signs of progesterone deficiency because their estrogen is much higher than their progesterone, thus producing symptoms. In such cases it is because (on examination or observation and history delving) these women have had, in some cases, a tubal ligation 5 or 6 years prior, or have damaged ovaries as a result of other factors, and the amount of ovulation is fading out as they age. They are still ovulating but not producing high amounts of progesterone.

This is why it is important to do a saliva assay 5 to 10 days after ovulation (day 21 is usually the best time), if you are in doubt. Because if you did your salivas around ovulation (day 12-14) chances are it would indicate you have sufficient progesterone and your doctor wouldn't consider giving you progesterone.

If, however, that same saliva was done a few days later, there's a good chance, based on your symptoms, that your progesterone levels have, in fact, faded out. That is why it is wise to keep this in mind when you are looking at all the reasons, and to question if you need progesterone, particularly if you are ovulating. It is also suggested you address circumstances that exacerbate estrogen dominance. (Food, weight, liver state, environmental toxins and stress)

In the event you have followed all these suggestions and on-going symptoms indicate you are still estrogen dominant, then this is usually very strong evidence the ovaries just aren't functioning in the way they should and your adrenals, in particular, may be exhausted. These are some of the aspects that need to be looked at.

Exposure to estrogens via diet and the environment (xenoestrogens), and the body's production of excessive estrogen due to weight gain must also be considered. This is where understanding your body type and hormonal constitution associated with your body shape, has great significance as it determines where and how you utilise and store your hormones. Which is covered in greater depth in Natural Progesterone More Secrets Revealed.

CHAPTER 5

Natural Progesterone and what to be aware of

- What is a compounding pharmacist?

- What is the difference between a compounding pharmacist and a herbalist?

- How can I tell the difference between a Wild Yam cream and a Natural Progesterone cream?

- My naturopath tells me Wild Yam creams are safer than Natural Progesterone because the chemical process required to make Natural Progesterone could possibly be toxic to my body.

- Can my cream go off?

- How do I know if the cream I am using is a reliable, high quality cream?

What is a compounding pharmacist?

In Australia and New Zealand we depend on compounding pharmacists to formulate our bio identical hormones unlike in the USA where numerous progesterone creams are manufactured and available to buy over the counter or from various suppliers, without requiring a Doctors prescription.

A compounding pharmacist is a term used to describe the art of preparing medication to a specific formula. They are, by demand, returning.

A compounding pharmacist has the freedom to work with therapeutic drugs, scripts, scheduled poisons and also the freedom to work with natural herbs. He is licensed to tailor make drugs to the needs of the individual. When a doctor orders a script, the pharmacist can make up that formula according to that requirement. This is the original art of the pharmacist. Compounding is an art and science.

Over the years this art has all but disappeared from the dispensary, replaced by mass produced products from huge multinational companies.

Many pharmacists are not equipped with the modern technology to compound. In the days before the giant pharmaceutical companies began to patent their products en masse, each and every pharmacist was a custom compounding pharmacist.

The doctor instructed the pharmacist to formulate/tailor make the medication required in the treatment of a patient's illness. Modern pharmacists can still do this, however, only custom compounding pharmacists have the day to day experience with the method of treatment, equipment and training.

When it comes to compounding a natural hormone into a cream, only a handful of pharmacists in our country have cultivated the skills and training. Some may claim they are qualified. There are many pharmacists who ring me over this dilemma. I have lost count of how many pharmacists have rung me and asked me how it is made? or what is in it? I am bemused each time.

A few years ago, when NPAN would go out in search of reliable compounding pharmacists who knew how to prepare progesterone cream, i.e., use the correct bases, use only the highest quality ingredients and correct micronised progesterone imported from overseas, the pharmacists we discovered willingly submitted to our organisation's request for analytical reports and records of authenticity. This was of great benefit, relief and reassurance to the women.

More recently, we've seen an increase in compounding pharmacists who claim they can make cream. In the absence of analytical data supporting cream preparation, I recommend women err on the side of caution. They must be reputable and experienced as there are so many pharmacists jumping on this lucrative band wagon with no experience behind them in compounding bio identical hormones.

In a nut shell I explain it like this to women who get confused with their compounding pharmacist if they are new at compounding bio identical hormones. Everyone can qualify to become a Baker, Cook or Chef. But not all Bakers can make sponge cakes even though they all know the principles and the ingredients! Making good progesterone creams in my opinion is an art. Few have mastered making high performing quality progesterone transdermal creams, based on the results and feed back reports I have received from women over the years using various creams from different sources. Seminars on compounding are now beginning to appear in the doctors medical journals.

What is the difference between a compounding pharmacist and a herbalist?

In a sense, the herbalist has basically taken over the role of the pharmacist, prescription drugs excluded. There is a difference in the two methods of treatment and the purpose. A pharmacist will meet the script of a doctor while a herbalist can tailor make for the individual but does not necessarily have to meet the requirements of a doctor. *A herbalist is licensed to make herbs and use natural remedies, not S4 drugs or S4 scheduled herbs and he cannot make therapeutic claims.*

There are many talented herbalists out there who can balance a woman's hormones specifically through herbs. And herbs are something that cannot be underestimated. The power of herbs is unique and incredible, and dates back many centuries. In the right combination, they can do some miraculous things in our body.

Many women realise remarkable results with hormone balancing without the need of progesterone replacement therapy. Often I suggest a woman try a well recommended herbalist, particularly if she is ovulating and is not showing severe degrees of estrogen dominance. We know from experience that herbs such as Vitex and Macca can often bring a woman's hormones back into balance, in some cases increasing her fertility, without the need for natural progesterone treatment.

This approach treats hormonal imbalance by stimulating the pituitary, in turn getting the body to regulate, stabilise and normalise its messages rather than putting the progesterone molecule back into the body.

A woman who believes she is using 'real' progesterone cream compounded by her herbalist, be warned. Your herbalist is either not telling you the whole truth or breaking the law. Herbalists are NOT permitted to incorporate micronised progesterone into their preparations. To imply otherwise is bending the truth.

If, however, he is adding micronised progesterone to your cream, it would be illegal. Further, it is highly unlikely the insignificant levels of progesterone (often referred to as homeopathic) would be of benefit to a woman suffering severe progesterone deficiency.

It should be understood that if your adrenals are functioning optimally, they will produce progesterone but maybe not at the levels required to offset the fact you are no longer producing progesterone month to month through ovulation.

Once you enter menopause your adrenal glands will provide minute amounts of progesterone, however, not nearly enough to counter-balance the effects of too much estrogen in your body and the bombardment xenoestrogens from the food chain and environment.

How can I tell the difference between a Wild Yam cream and a Natural Progesterone cream?

Every woman, at one time or another, including members of NPAN myself included, have incorrectly thought wild yam extract creams and progesterone creams to be one and the same. The fact is they are not. They represent the same compound at two very different stages of conversion.

To make a Wild Yam Extract cream, plant sterols (oils & fats) are extracted from the Mexican Wild Yam and Soy plants. We know that Wild Yam creams have a 'phytoestrogen' effect on the body, but there is no scientific proof that when cream is applied to the skin (or ingested in tablet or powder form) the active ingredient (diosgenin) derived from Wild Yam creams can be converted by the body into progesterone. Because the active ingredient - diosgenin - is not identical to the progesterone molecule found in the body, it cannot do the work of progesterone.

Wild Yam Extract creams can exert estrogenic benefits on the body (phytoestrogenic) but it is not the same estrogen that our body makes. Basically, Wild Yam Extract creams cannot do the work of progesterone.

The active ingredient can latch onto estrogen receptor sites, hence the estrogen benefits, but cannot latch onto progesterone sites. When women understand the differences between these two molecules, and that there are two individual hormones - estrogen and progesterone - performing separate roles in the body, they then appreciate that one active ingredient cannot be touted as performing two different hormonal roles.

The argument goes that using Wild Yam Extract creams are more 'natural' because the molecule is unaltered and, therefore, safer to use as progesterone therapy, being a precursor (which I've just explained above is incorrect). A chemical process is still required to extract these saponins from the Wild Yam and Soy plants and *Wild Yam is **not** a progesterone precursor in the body.*

Chemicals ARE involved in the extraction process of Wild Yam Extract. By definition, an EXTRACT means that a chemical process is involved. I clarify this point now because many women have been encouraged to stop using natural progesterone by their natural therapists stating the natural progesterone creams have involved chemical processes that could be harmful. But they omit to mention that a chemical extraction process is involved even with the 'purist' of natural Wild Yam Extract creams. Discern for yourself, and check the motivation behind these statements.

Progesterone DOES come from Wild Yam or Soy Extract, but let me explain the process involved so you are not confused. The very fact that progesterone is derived from Mexican Wild Yam is coincidental. Since the 1940's scientists have been using soya beans, wild yams and other plants from the tuber family to make progesterone.

To make natural progesterone, Wild Yam Extract must be taken into the laboratory and synthesised with the aid of an enzyme, rendering it a hormone. This laboratory conversion is necessary because, as I stated above, the body has no means by which to convert the raw plant sterols into progesterone.

You can, at this stage, safely introduce synthesised progesterone into the body because your body sees this 'real' progesterone as having the same molecular configuration. No further conversion is necessary by the body. It's a perfect match. The key fits the lock. Because it's such a perfect match, the body recognises it as natural, and you don't experience any nasty side-effects that occur with some synthetic hormones. Further still, because it IS real progesterone, the body can use it to make other hormones.

Women get very confused, largely because The Late Dr. John Lee's work on progesterone has been promoted alongside Wild Yam creams. If you do see Wild Yam creams being marketed as a precursor of progesterone, steer clear (if you are after a genuine progesterone cream) because it does not contain real progesterone. It's just another way of confusing women into buying a product they didn't ask for in the first place.

Feel free to use a wild yam cream if you wish to, however, be aware you are not going to get any progesterone benefits. It's more likely Wild Yam cream will have a phytoestrogen effect on your body. Of some benefit, certainly, but not in the same league as natural progesterone.

The body cannot uptake the substance 'diosgenin' and convert it into progesterone because there is no enzyme in the body for this process to happen that scientists (and laboratory tests) are aware of. Many a marketing sales pitch will tell you that diosgenin is a precursor to progesterone and the body is capable of converting.

You'll remember in a previous chapter I outlined how diosgenin, derived from Wild Yam and/or Soy, is synthesised in the laboratory with the aid of an enzyme to render it a molecule your body can interpret. How then can the body convert this raw substance into a human hormone once it enters the body? The fact is it cannot. There is no enzyme in the body to do this.

One popular brand of Wild Yam Extract cream making these claims here in Australia was put to the test by a reputed research institute and found that there was no evidence that the body could convert diosgenin into natural progesterone.

Yet a significant number of herbalists or naturopaths believe in the body's ability to do the conversion, resulting in a flood of questions from women claiming that their homeopathic and herbalist remedies will increase or supplement the body's progesterone levels 'naturally'. Again, a play on words. Yes, Wild Yam Extract is a building block in the manufacture of progesterone. But NOT in the body - in the laboratory. Wild Yam constituents cannot be converted into progesterone by the human body. It does not happen.

"...Claims have arisen in the popular literature that the female body can manufacture progesterone from diosgenin, particularly if a wild yam cream is applied to the skin... no evidence exist for mammalian enzymes which are capable of effecting what is a difficult chemical conversion. The evidence that does exist strongly disputes the possibility of this conversion. In fact, diosgenin appears to have estrogenic properties in mice and lacks progesteronic effects." (Herbal Medicine, Principles and Practice of Phytotherapy, Modern Herbal Medicine, Simon Mills, Kerry Bone, Published Churchill Livingstone)

This confusion arises out of the fact that all **our steroid hormones are made in our body from cholesterol.** And the oils and fats extracted from the Wild Yam and Soy plants are very similar to our body's cholesterol molecule. That's where the similarity ends and the arguments stop. The reason they use Wild Yam, Soy, extracted oils (Saponins) is because it is economical to harvest these plants commercially.

On this hypothesis Wild Yam creams would be a precursor to ALL the steroid hormones, not just progesterone. Rubbing cholesterol onto our skin would have the same effect? Clearly, it's more complex than that. However, if you introduce natural progesterone into the body, you WILL manufacture other steroid hormones, because it's a bio-identical hormone (please refer to the Steroid Pathway insert in Chapter 4, What is Natural Progesterone, page 79).

How you can recognise if it is a Wild Yam quickly is it will have the various names on its contents Dioscolera Villarosa or Diosgenin or Wild Yam.

My naturopath tells me Wild Yam creams are safer than Natural Progesterone because the chemical process required to make Natural Progesterone could possibly be toxic to my body.

Even though Naturopaths will state that Wild Yam (diosgenin) is in its 'natural' state, a process is still required to extract these saponins from the Wild Yam and Soy plants.

Chemicals ARE involved in the extraction process of both Wild Yam Extract and Natural Progesterone. By definition, an EXTRACT means that a chemical process is involved !! Also many Wild Yam creams **do have preservatives** in them! If any creams do not have preservatives in them they will go off very quickly, usually before the contents of the jar is finished.

Can my cream go off?

Yes, it can. Ingredients in any product can go off, and you wouldn't know until perhaps a month or two when your bodies stores (reserves) drop and you begin noticing the effects of progesterone deficiency with perhaps the return of estrogen dominance symptoms. Oxygenation, for example, will break down the progesterone, as will extreme temperatures i.e. Heat.

Progesterone creams dispensed in tubes do not, by design, expose the entire batch to oxygen, sunlight or bacteria, where jars of cream can be easily contaminated when you dip your fingers, and the entire content is exposed to oxygen each time you unscrew the lid.

This is not to imply jars are inferior to tubes of cream. It's a matter of ensuring your applicator is free of bacteria, you tightly replace the lid, you leave your progesterone cream in a dark, temperature-controlled environment, and during extreme temperatures you store your cream in the fridge.

A pure progesterone cream formulated well does not have an odour. Therefore, if your cream has a rancid smell, then you can be pretty sure it's off or formulated with the wrong base. Cream separating or feeling gritty may be another sign.

Suggested hints: It's sometimes advisable to split your cream into two jars and work on half a jar at a time. Store the other half to prolong its shelf life, limiting exposure to oxygen.

Check expiry date. Cream can last unopened for up to twelve months if stored correctly. This can be confirmed by your cream manufacturer. A cream with no preservatives will go off very quickly within weeks, you will recognise this by the rancid smell or separation of contents. They can also go off with preservatives in them!

It always wise to store your cream in a controlled environment not exposed to light, heat and oxygen.

How do I know if the cream I am using is a reliable, high quality cream?

Quality progesterone cream, whether mass-produced and quality controlled batch to batch, or compounded by your local pharmacist, needs to meet certain criteria if it's going to work. I mentioned in a previous chapter that not all compounding pharmacists understand, or are sufficiently skilled at compounding progesterone.

Your cream must contain micronised BP progesterone/US Pharmacopoeia grade progesterone, in a stable fat soluble base, not a mineral oil base (Paraffin oil i.e. Aqueous cream or Sorbolene cream).

Otherwise it won't absorb and be assimilated correctly in the body. Too many women are rubbing on progesterone yet fail to derive the full benefits, largely because it's not compounded correctly, or, possibly it does not contain micronised progesterone.

There are different grades (i.e. quality) of micronised BP progesterone. If it's gritty, oily or greasy it often indicates that cream quality is sub-standard.

Batch control is especially important. There are recorded cases where women accidentally overdosed on locally compounded creams simply because they increased their dosage when cream failed to provide relief of symptoms week in, week out. It's why I recommend women purchase creams that are quality controlled and batch manufactured.

Even when you are bringing cream in from overseas, a good quality cream would have all the ingredients and the batch number, expiry date etc recorded on it. Ensure that you buy a pure progesterone cream with no other additives. You also should be aware of the physiological dosage your progesterone cream is delivering.

Be careful of creams that have been enhanced with essential oils and fragrances, and other unknown additives, as it is not understood the interactive behaviour these substances can have on the effectiveness of progesterone or skin sensitivity. For genuine progesterone benefits, don't play around with inferior creams. Your cream manufacturer should support the benefits of all ingredients and ensure progesterone quality is not compromised.

It has been found from experience and women's feedback that a high quality cream displays the characteristics of being readily absorbed, non-greasy, odourless, and doesn't stain or leave a greasy residue on the skin. It's important these features exist so that the micronised progesterone molecule can be readily absorbed through the pores of the skin and not be stuck on the surface trapped in a greasy base. Also a residual build up on the skin may prevent absorption of cream if it is applied over that area again.

I am under the belief that quick and easy absorption of the cream over a small area is indicative of a superior cream.

Simple test: Put a dab of cream on your skin. Do not rub, and see how quickly it soaks into the skin naturally. One minute is a good sign. Try different application areas to test also your own body's absorption rates. Some areas are better than others and can vary with individuals.

CHAPTER 6

Sourcing Natural Progesterone and The Law

- *Drug laws in various countries*
- *USA drug law does not apply to progesterone usage*
- *Why is Progesterone labelled an S4 drug even though it is natural?*
- *Can I buy my cream overseas without a script?*
- *Can I get a rebate on cream if it's bought on prescription?*
- *Listing of various natural progesterone creams that are mass-produced*
- *If you are importing creams from overseas*

Drug laws in various countries

The Australian Therapeutic Goods Administration (TGA) has classified Progesterone an S4 drug that is only available on prescription. Anyone using progesterone, whether in the form of a cream, troches, drops, pessaries or orally without a doctor's prescription are using it illegally.

The TGA's ruling on progesterone was in some respects necessary. Not too many years ago 'Down Under', women could buy genuine local and imported progesterone creams, while the law of the day slapped a muzzle on cream manufacturers such that little ingredient information was available to the general public.

In other words, women could get all the progesterone cream they needed (without a prescription), they just weren't allowed to know how much real progesterone was in a jar or tube. Some Wild Yam creams contained little more than diosgenin - a phytoestrogen - but how could a woman tell?

Progesterone creams and Wild Yam extract creams were all lumped under the 'Wild Yam' umbrella. Confusion and exploitation reigned.

Irrespective of progesterone's considerable safety margin, deliberately keeping women in the dark yet permitting self-medication, was totally unacceptable. The Natural Progesterone Advisory Network called into question the TGA's duplicity and change soon followed.

Some would argue we shot ourselves in the foot. Perhaps so. Certainly we all lost access to our preferred progesterone cream. Nonetheless, some attempt by the TGA to regulate was well overdue.

NPAN did its utmost to walk women and healthcare professionals through all the confusion, providing a resource centre of known progesterone cream outlets (compounding pharmacists) and doctors prepared to write scripts. I helped women, in my organisation NPAN, interpret their symptoms through charts and journals, distributing this collated information along with medical reports and articles, and I opened up a toll free number so women Australia-wide could tap into my network. This is still in operation however I ask women to respect this line as it is very costly to run and women use this mainly for ordering books, nutrition information or to make appointments.

Now that's not to say ALL creams disappeared from the Australian market. Locally compounding pharmacists, or at least the handful were already preparing progesterone creams.

Pro-Feme, a quality controlled progesterone cream produced in Australia by an Australian-owned pharmaceutical company was already manufactured but under existing State law, unavailable to women living outside the state of Western Australia. While Pro-Feme is registered under Western Australian drug law, it is not federally legislated. Until this occurs and the manufacturers of Pro-Feme go through TGA, sale of this cream will be restricted to Western Australia or overseas. There are ways legally to obtain it outside WA.

NPAN has lobbied vigorously these past years to bring about legislative change using a provision in our drug laws that was hoped would speed up this process. This was recently overturned in parliament.

Paradoxically, if your GP resides in a state other than WA and is prepared to pay the annual registration for inclusion in the Western Australian listing of General Practitioners, then all subsequent scripts for Pro-Feme issued by your GP can be legally processed in WA. Be warned though.

If the past few years are any indication, only a handful of doctors are prepared to write a prescription for progesterone, much less go to the trouble and expense of registering in WA.

American based companies marketing premium progesterone creams in the United States have not yet applied to Australian authorities for TGA approval. That's unfortunate really because thousands upon thousands of Australian women trialled these creams some years back and realised outstanding results. Some women, in fact, continue to import their cream from the US despite its hefty price tag. A note of reminder you still *must legally hold a script in Australia or New Zealand if you import for personal use*. You will not be able to obtain a rebate if you import creams from overseas even with a receipt. So most women have elected now to use local compounding pharmacists to source their cream so they are able to get a rebate back from their Private Health Insurance. A Doctor's script is necessary to obtain progesterone so if you can buy it over the counter or from another person it is not progesterone or it is illegal. (In Australia and New Zealand).

USA drug law does not apply to progesterone usage

While regulatory laws on progesterone exist in the UK, Canada, New Zealand and Australia, a doctor's prescription is NOT required in countries such as the USA. Natural progesterone creams can be legally sourced through whatever channels available - over the counter, via marketing distributors, or on-line over the internet.

Progesterone has been used safely in women's cosmetics and moisturisers in the United States for years. So, for the time being anyway, a US drug law does not apply to progesterone usage.

There have been rumblings, however, that America's Food & Drug Administration (FDA) is soon to impose changes to current drug law, restricting ad-hoc marketing of creams. The consequence of this decision will possibly push distribution underground and compromise the manufacture of quality controlled progesterone creams. Pretty much the scenario forced upon Australian women some years back.

Here in Sydney, Australia, randomised, double blind, placebo-controlled test trials have been underway for years in preparation for the registration of Pro-Feme through the TGA. Emphasis is now on trialing testosterone.

While our current situation is indeed deflating, we could yet be the first country to install progesterone in it's rightful place as an effective, well documented component of Hormone Replacement Therapy (HRT). Its listing in doctors' reference manuals such as the Australian Medicines Handbook, P.P. Guide, and MIMS Manual announces progesterone's therapeutic properties to the medical fraternity, making it readily available to all women. It's my hope this Australian breakthrough ripples out to women world-wide.

Why is Progesterone labelled an S4 drug even though it is natural?

As stated, S4 drugs are classified a poisonous substance. All therapeutic drugs and products in Australia must first pass through the TGA. The TGA, a Government body established to screen and approve drugs and to regulate standard criteria control on products intended for the market place, exists to protect the general public.

Even natural products such as vitamins found in your local supermarket must apply for registration through the TGA. Further, any therapeutic claim associated with products sold over the counter must first be approved by the TGA.

Please note, products said to contain an S4 drug (progesterone creams being a good example) should never be readily available 'off the shelf', at least not here in Australia. Certainly, my research and observation has borne out the fact that progesterone has a great safety margin. It still doesn't change the fact that progesterone falls under the S4 Schedule.

There exist at least two mainstream references to the word 'natural'. 'Natural' in that a substance is found in the body, and 'natural' in that it is found in nature. Cream is labelled Natural progesterone because the hormone it contains - progesterone - is found in the body. And the body sees as 'natural' that which has the same molecular configuration. In other words a perfect match so the body *interprets it as a real progesterone* hormone thus delivering the right messages to do the work it intended to do.

The progesterone that goes into a tube or jar of cream has undergone a process in a laboratory whereby it is synthesised or converted from one substance - diosgenin (oils & fats derived from Mexican Wild Yam & Soy plants) - into United States Pharmacopoeia (USP) grade progesterone.

It is referred to as 'natural' because the end result represents the same molecule naturally occurring in the body. It can, therefore, be introduced into the body with a relative margin of safety as progesterone replacement therapy with minimal side effects because the body recognises it. You can now appreciate the difference.

It is pointed out that *any substance that occurs naturally in nature cannot be patented*. In this case, we're referring to a hormone that can be produced in the laboratory by stages of chemical conversion, thus rendering it identical to the progesterone molecule in the body. No one can own a natural occurring molecule that our body makes. Drug companies, as with natural estrogen patches own the technology/deliverance "the patch".

This is why drug companies must alter, through further chemical processes, the molecular structure of natural progesterone such that it is no longer natural to the body (bio-identical) but can be patented known as progestogens., i.e. Provera or develop a technology in deliverance e.g. Gel, patch containing natural estrogen but the progesterone is progestogens, claiming progesterone like benefits. It is not natural progesterone and does not deliver real natural progesterone benefits.

A final word before moving on. To claim that a substance is derived directly from nature is no guarantee of its safety. What we ought to be more concerned with at all times is how our body interprets the substances we introduce, whether through diet, hormone replacement therapy, or over the counter products in healthfood outlets. Even Vitamin E can be natural or synthetic!

Can I buy my cream overseas without a script?

No, you cannot 'legally' import progesterone cream into Australia without a doctor's prescription. Again, Customs may intercept your package, check to ensure you hold a current prescription, and if you do not, instigate legal action. Many women have reported that their packaging was opened and inspected by Customs.

So be warned. If you intend to source your cream from overseas, it is recommended you obtain a prescription. And please be aware, the law only permits importation for personal use. You are not allowed to distribute to others.

Again the above specification DOES NOT apply to use in USA and other countries where no such drug laws imposed on progesterone exist.

Assuming then that you are importing your creams legally, that cream ought to come with a comprehensive list of ingredients. I strongly suggest women make sure they know what they are buying.

If not listed on the side of the container, ensure you receive product specific information outlining exact percentage of progesterone per jar or tube. If not, how can you be absolutely sure you are buying a genuine progesterone micronised BP or USP grade progesterone cream? How can you possibly know what dosage you are introducing into your body? You can't!

In some cases, companies and individual distributors have imported cream, changed the labelling content and packaging to disguise its S4 content to get it through the TGA, and then sell to you. If the salesperson can't be up front with a cream's specific ingredients, don't buy it!

If you are ordering through the internet or via mail order overseas, you are NOT required to submit your prescription to that country. Simply keep it current and in a safe place just in case Customs want to come and check that you are genuinely permitted to import an S4 substance for personal use.

Can I get a rebate on cream if it's bought on prescription?

In countries such as Australia where progesterone is classified an S4 Drug and only available with a doctor's prescription, there are *private health insurance schemes* that offer a rebate. Women with insurance can expect a rebate of around AUST$20 or more with proof of purchase (receipt) & duly marked prescription verifying your physician's Provider Number. Receipts from overseas will not provide a rebate in Australia. Rebate only applies to those covered fully (Top Cover) by their health insurance company. Medicare and those holding a pensioner card do not qualify.

Rebatable amounts vary with different health insurance companies, so it pays to shop around if you are thinking of joining one. It may be far more beneficial to ask for one receipt instead of individual receipts per container or tube however check with your Insurance Company as it may be more profitable to buy two items on the one receipt for a higher rebate claim.

It has yet to be substantiated that receipts for progesterone creams ordered through overseas distributors are 'official' enough for private health insurance companies to attract a rebate.

Listing of various natural progesterone creams that are mass-produced and are being distributed internationally

Because NPAN operates from a neutral stance, women feel comfortable asking me about various creams and their contents or which creams to buy. It is difficult to comment on many overseas creams. I have though, provided a comprehensive list located on page 407, where website visits will keep you updated.

I suggest that you may wish to refer to The Late Dr John Lee's list of cream guidelines also and the categories in which they fall regarding their dosage levels (too much progesterone, not enough, etc). These lists can be obtained by subscribing to The Late John Lee Medical Letter via Dr Lee's website or through his series of books also available on-line - http://www.johleemd.com. (Virginia Hopkins may also be able to assist).

About the Late Dr John Lee and the misconception of his endorsement of progesterone creams.

Please be aware although THE LATE Dr. Lee's talks WERE often sponsored by companies that sell progesterone cream, The Late Dr. John Lee did not endorse any one progesterone cream, nor did he make money from the sale of any progesterone cream. So if any company or person states otherwise it is factually incorrect!

Many Australians get confused with the product **Endau** cream, produced by Neways International. *In USA it is progesterone* and is listed in The Late John Lee's book but this is **not** the same product as the Australian version Endau, even though they are both made from the same company worldwide, keeping in mind that the laws that govern each country are different. To obtain Endau, it must be purchased through an independent distributor.

If you are Importing creams from overseas - Just a reminder, if you import your cream from overseas into a country where progesterone is listed as a scheduled drug, you will need to hold a current doctor's prescription. With so much sports drug controversy these days, it's not worth the risk of being without a prescription.

PRO-FEME AUSTRALIA AND EXPORTING LICENCE

Pro-Feme holds an export license and can export this product overseas. Import tax may apply in some countries for persons purchasing. If you wish to import (countries other than Australia), you can do this via their website.

LISTING COMPOUNDING PHARMACISTS IN AUSTRALIA AND NEW ZEALAND

As there is no product federally legislated at this point progesterone creams must be **obtained from compounding pharmacists with a Doctor's prescription. This also applies if you import your cream from overseas.**

Australian women who previously had difficulty getting their doctors to write a script for natural progesterone can breathe a little easier. ***Pro-Feme is now listed on their doctor's computer as a recognised prescription drug*** with dosage clearly defined. What cream you end up purchasing is entirely up to you! It simply means you have fulfilled your legal obligation to obtain a doctor's prescription.

Lawley pharmaceuticals is a Western Australian compounding pharmacist. Their product complies to the Western Australian Law which allows them to manufacture Pro-Feme. Whilst at this point of time they cannot trade interstate they can export legally.

Please find at the back of this book a list of various Australian compounding pharmacists and contacts that may assist you in sourcing your cream. *See pages 405, 406*

Current lists will be placed on my website and updated when necessary.

AUSTRALIAN AND "ENDAU" LAWS

Endau in Australia and New Zealand is **not** progesterone. It is a phytoestrogen of wild yam with many other valuable ingredients assisting in restoring balance and harmony. Ingredients complies to TGA regulations in Australia and New Zealand, modified to that of USA to comply with our strigent regulatory bodies and laws.

If you purchase Endau in Australia from an independent distributor you do not require a script, as it is not progesterone. If you purchase in USA, cream obtained from an independent distributor without a script and it is Endau USA progesterone, you are breaking the law and so is the person who sold it to you.

The Australian and New Zealand company Neways view this seriously and does not condone any misconduct and product misrepresentation.

If you wish to purchase wild yam Endau Australia contact Donna Chisholm for more details:

donna@premiumaromas.com.au
Phone: 61 3 9696 8800   Fax:61 3 9696 8099
Mobile: 0413 003 717

CHAPTER 7

Approaching your Doctor

- *The Patterns I have observed in the prescribing habits of Doctors*

- *How do I approach my doctor?*

- *What happens if I am having trouble getting a script?*

- *Possible reasons why Doctors have become resistant and cautious about writing scripts*

- *Why are Doctors so reluctant to write scripts for natural progesterone?*

- *This letter received from a lady recently is just one of the reasons demonstrating the existing problems women are facing with their Doctors*

- *Suggested guidelines on how you may wish to approach your Doctor*

- *Winning over a working relationship with your Doctor*

- *How will the special tests and my doctor's examination benefit me if I want to use progesterone?*

- *I feel guilty using progesterone behind my doctor's back because I know he does not approve of natural progesterone. Is it harmful to withhold this information, being a natural product?*

- *My doctor will not prescribe progesterone on the grounds that I am testing positive to estrogen receptors and progesterone receptors.*

- *How does the doctor know what progesterone dosage to put me on, and when to adjust?*

- *Adjustment Guide*

- *How do I know whether to buy a 1.6% or 3.2% or 10% cream? Which is the one usually recommended?*

- *Now that I have my prescription how do I process it?*

The Patterns I have observed in the prescribing habits of Doctors

What I have observed in the past several years in Doctors attitudes and their reluctance to write natural progesterone scripts, is founded in their training, I will explain why I think this merry-go-round has happened, and why this rift is widening.

In the beginning when I started NPAN and I amongst hundreds of women began circulating Doctor Information Packs provided by my organisation, Doctors began to start adjusting and relaxing over writing prescriptions for progesterone. It was then a case of finding reliable sources of progesterone from reputable compounding pharmacists.

So I then requested analytical proof of progesterone from these pharmacists who were compounding these creams. A handful of reputable pharmacists supplied my organisation their proof of authenticity and analytical data. To this end I amongst other women were happy to hand out this list of compounding pharmacists to assist women in obtaining their natural progesterone cream. With this list, prescribing doctors were also circulated. As natural progesterone could not be,(and still cannot) be advertised NPAN was an invaluable free advertising resource for these pharmacists. Because I was not a pharmacist and a service just providing information as an advisory network I was not breaking any laws regarding the TGA. Understandably my network provided an invaluable asset to these compounding pharmacists because of the position I was in. Sadly to say few came to my rescue in times of financial strife and lack of ongoing funding of my network.

Regardless, doctors were now relaxed, often being inundated by many enthused women, leaving behind information packs, books and tapes. Many women were grateful and relieved as many doctors were prepared to give progesterone a go, often commenting of their reservations.

Now, with doctors and pharmacists on board, there seemed to be a period of flexibility and more choices in natural hormone replacement therapy available. Women were paving the way for other women.

After a few years both had been achieved, (availability of real progesterone cream and cooperative doctors) and women clearly were grasping on quickly that natural progesterone was not the same as Wild Yam Cream and could not be obtained (bought over the counter) without a doctors prescription. Even Naturopaths could not provide progesterone scripts but could sell made up solutions or Wild Yam. Some were however selling progesterone illegally imported or sourced and relabelled as Wild Yam, causing confusion.

Due to product unreliability, with huge variables in preparation, with many inferior compounded creams and unreliable batches, results on progesterone consequently varied also. This proved disasterous as so many women were returning back to their Doctors with short lived results which sadly destroyed a lot of the Doctors faith and confidence, encouraging the doctors to readopt their previous conviction, that progesterone was not of value as hormone therapy. Compounding creams varied so much that some were not as effective as others (as we soon discovered as a group of women comparing our creams). Some women were not getting consistent results, whilst others got worse on these creams.

My home meetings proved beyond doubt that every individual compounding pharmacists cream had its own characteristic in performance. This was the prompting force that led me to fly to WA to seek out and test this manufactured cream that I had heard about called Pro-Feme. As I had resided in WA some 17 years before moving back to Victoria, I had many Doctor contacts, so went about getting scripts and buying Pro-Feme from WA chemists, which several women then trialled on my return.

These women had been coming to my meetings for 7-8 months still with many unsatisfactory results , some remaining or returning symptoms prior to progesterone usage. Within two months on this new cream, all our symptoms had resolved so there was no more need to hold further meetings. It was this clear evidence that proved once and for all that it was the variations in creams that kept us from achieving the results that we were aiming for, promised in the Late Dr John Lee's book "What Your Doctor May Not Tell You About Menopause". Now we were on our way. However now we had to go back to re-educate our Doctors who by now were saying to many of us 'we told you so, we knew you'd be back for HRT and/or natural progesterone was only a placebo etc". We had to now convince them that some of the creams we were using were inferior or in fact were not progesterone (Wild Yam). A few Doctors listened and were willing to register with WA to enable them to prescribe and use the manufactured product Pro-Feme. Whilst many could not see the sense of paying registration fees to legally obtain this product as they no longer had faith or conviction in progesterone. This hormone was now viewed as ineffective, and of little value in treating hormonal imbalance , oestrogen dominance symptoms, menopausal hot flushes and PMS.

There was no evidence and clearly many of the women patients that had already tried progesterone had failed miserably on it, returning back to their previous HRT, or submitting to now using it, as they could not tolerate the symptoms and accompanying discomfort associated with PMS menopause and estrogen dominance in the absence of supporting hormone therapy.

The few that persisted and pioneered through this transition period trialling many unreliable creams on the way proved progesterone to be a successful form of treatment with remarkable results. My book was written to assist women . As time went on a select few of the original compounding pharmacists flew to the USA and studied courses on compounding bio identical hormones and their products continued to improve as did the women's hormonal health and symptoms. It was fine tuning for both and learning days for all. Natural progesterone was regaining popularity and momentum again amongst the women, but now without the support and conviction of mainstream medicine.

The Doctors were more than skeptical and cautious of transdermal therapy and its absorbability and it's claimed benefits. However a few smart compounding pharmacists recognised this resistance and approached many of the prescribing Doctors with better options, supplying and redistributing literature, information and more appealing options, that being, lozenges with doses and combinations in equivalent levels to HRT but with bio identical hormones. These being more appealing, bypassing the liver with fewer adverse side effects and dangers. A lot of Doctors were happy to work with these compounding pharmacists and this form of NHRT treatment. Many clinics sprang up specialising in NHRT. Women flocked to them. Fees were high but the women did not mind as they had Doctors working on their side, and supporting their choices. Lozenges became the name of the day and won over popularity and trends changed as women loved the idea of designer hormones tailored to their individual needs.

Unfortunately in this event, transdermal natural progesterone was fastly being forgotten in the process as more and more open minded Doctors moved into combination creams or troches (lozenges) mixes. Natural progesterone singularly prescribed by these Specialist Doctors was rarely used. My concern and argument was that I felt poor progesterone had never been given its full justice and the lack of knowledge in usage and performance depending on its base and ingredients, was never really fully revealed or mastered and now overshadowed and replaced with natural hormone cocktails. DHEA also became a popular hormone often included in these combinations.

I thought all along, if they really knew how to use progesterone all these combinations mixed together would not be necessary as it was after all , progesterone that was the precursing hormone to all those other hormones(excluding DHEA) . Furthermore these combinations gave women no control over their hormones and made it virtually impossible for dose adjustments.

Those women who chose to stick with natural progesterone continued on isolated and unsupported in a sense but did master usage and dose requirements. They also were able to recognise if they needed additional hormones by determining if progesterone did not go on to building other hormones along the steroid pathway.

My organisation, book, observation and feedback proved invaluable support to so many women 'out there' on this journey, using just transdermal natural progesterone. Those who went to lozenges (troches) (some abandoned progesterone being coerced to do so), were ecstatic. Instantly feeling great and wonderful returning regularly to their Specialising Doctor for blood/saliva tests and tailor dose adjustments. They were on all sorts of combined hormones in one tablet (lozenge) or cream. It was rather fashionable for some, who often skited about their "designer" hormones, indicating creams to be inferior or old fashioned.

Still wary about this and cautious I held strong to my belief that transdermal was the way to go. That this was how hormones were meant to be used in mother nature from our fat cells (stored in lypophilic tissue). Rather than being bombarded with extremely high doses direct to the blood stream via the mouth and some lost to the stomach (swallowed). I felt it was closer to what mother nature intended rather than a trade off of high levels of hormones not of natural levels. Ironically many of these women are now returning to my organisation, distressed, desperate for help with severe hormonal disruption. They have broken through their lozenges effectiveness (I suspect through using too higher doses for too long). It is a similar reaction to coming off HRT in my opinion. The brain becomes conditioned to a high threshold, and receptors can down regulate. These women are back to square one again.

Furthermore many of their Doctors are now not wishing to prescribe these high doses due to the latest medical agenda being issued to Doctors from some insurance companies implying a no cover policy on non legislated script products. This has made them obviously nervous, concerned and rightly so in fear of litigation. This has left many women high and dry and again abandoned, with no alternative options. They are now resorting back to transdermal creams in hope to restore balance again, finding their troches were short lived in some cases.

So now 8 years on, we are back to the drawing board having done a very tedious and hazardous circle in search for co-operation, support and help from our Doctors in our quest for bio identical hormone scripts. It is clear that the rift is widening and it appears that more and more women are experiencing more resistance than ever and finding it difficult to get a prescription for natural transdermal hormone creams, particularly progesterone (there is less resistance for testosterone scripts!)

I receive at least 3-5 phone calls a day now from women seeking out prescribing Doctors in their area because their own Doctor refuses to write a script. They are deflated, frustrated, intimidated and angry. Insurance companies have scared their Doctors off along with the evidence printed on progesterone not protecting against endometrial hyperplasia turning them off the use of this hormone. The article in the Lancet on progesterone not protecting the uterus was the catalyst for Doctors starting to shy away from natural progesterone. No way were Doctors seeing this printed article going to prescribe to their patients with Fibroids or bleeding problems. It would be out right irresponsible from their perspective. Sadly that article was biased. Women have battled and learnt to become devious and deceptive in obtaining their scripts, desperate to use this form of hormone therapy. They have learnt to not declare the full medical history having learnt from the 'rounds' what reactions they are likely to encounter, and what will lead to refusal. In other words they have learnt to reduce or trivialise their symptoms. Women have also learnt that it is easy to go to a bulk billing Doctor or a 'standing in' General Practitioner at a local or weekend clinic and ask for a script for PMS, realising that 'PMS' holds no medical alert dangers in the Doctors minds. Had they mentioned Breast Cancer, history of Fibroids, heavy bleeding, fibrocystic breasts, depression, they would be refused instantly and would walk out with a script for antidepressants and or oestrogens and synthetic progestins.

This is creating a true medical patient Doctor relationship breakdown. Both are doing a disservice to each other and could be both jeopardising each other through lack of honesty, disclosure, trust and rapport. I have witnessed many bad situations occurring through lack of patient disclosure to their Doctor. The patient may be getting a script and using progesterone from one Doctor and being treated by a Specialist (eg Endocrinologist or Rheumatologist) and so may be receiving contraindicated medications for the use of progesterone eg. Cortisone, the oral contraceptive pill, progestins, IVF, drugs for a fertility program. Included is a letter of a women's grief and experience (page114). This is one of the hundreds I receive by email and the constant requests for prescribing Doctors. So what is the answer. *COURAGE*, Honesty and Accountability and a Plan of Action. Firstly we need to understand the reasons for resistance and I have listed a summary of possible reasons why Doctors are reluctant to prescribe.

How do I approach my doctor?
What happens if I am having trouble getting a script?

I suggest women go positively and confidently psychologically prepared with information in hand. Take my book, or The Late Dr John Lee's, information and, if possible, a drug sheet showing contra-indications and indications which can reassure these doctors because they can see that it is a manufactured product which has indications, use, dosage, guidance. Also print off the medical references, off my website provided specifically for this purpose to assist you in your endeavour to obtain a script and provide the Doctor appropriate data. Or if you do not have access to the website please take the book with the references to show your Doctor.

Australian women who previously had difficulty getting their doctors to write a script for natural progesterone can breathe a little easier. Pro-Feme is now listed on their doctor's computer as a recognised prescription drug with dosage clearly defined. What cream you end up purchasing is entirely up to you! It simply means you have fulfilled your legal obligation to obtain a doctor's prescription.

Tell your doctor you have done your research and you would like the opportunity to try this form of hormone replacement therapy. Remember it is hormone replacement therapy - it is not herbal alternatives. Tell them you are aware that it is a form of hormone therapy and that, in some countries, it is acquired without a prescription (which does not apply to Australia and NZ).

In Australia, for example, it is illegal to buy or import for personal use natural progesterone cream without a script. You have done your homework and are not asking for some herbal preparation. You are asking for a bio identical molecular structured progesterone. Be firm in the way you ask but don't TELL him. Doctors can feel threatened and offended being told how a woman expects to be treated. With the right attitude Doctors are happy to work with their patient if they have enough conviction that what the patient is proposing is not dangerous and is it has been well investigated and planned.

Explain how you are fully aware this is not test trialled, that there is little supporting data, and people believe it is only one man's opinion yet to be proved. However, tell him how your research states that because it is a natural occurring molecule in the body it has a huge safety margin and the body does not react as it does to the altered synthetic progestogen version.

The body can assimilate it better because it recognises this molecule as already existing in the body, rather than introducing a foreign derived molecule that has the potential to cause serious side effects, health risks, and is harder on the liver.

Natural progesterone, given topically, is more absorbable, more effective, bypasses the liver, and doesn't have the same metabolic end result as synthetic HRT. This has strong data back-up. You are stating to your doctor the reasons why you would prefer to take this form of progesterone. Perhaps you've had a bad experience on HRT and if you have experienced problems on the Pill or other HRT therapies - Point This Out!

You should point out that you are not referring to wild yam or synthetic progestogens. You are asking for something that will be safer to use and promises better end results than the synthetic variety. If you have, in the past, reacted to the contraceptive Pill, have a family history of blood clots, Breast Cancer or stroke, or HRT has caused you to become depressed, gain weight, retain fluid etc., one would expect your doctor to embrace your decision to trial natural progesterone.

The next approach to take with your doctor is to explain: "I recognise that, as my treating physician you need to err on the side of caution *when there is no listing of this drug in your manual (i.e.applies to WA only).*

However, as your patient, I take full responsibility for this form of treatment and I'm prepared to sign a disclaimer (which some doctors have insisted their patients undertake here in Australia). I would like to involve you in the progress of my treatment, and to that end I'm willing to chart my symptoms and report back to you if there are any problems".

How can they argue when you are taking responsibility and over-ridden all their objections? If the doctor then proceeds to tell you that you don't know what you are talking about or that he wants to prescribe you progestogen for endometrial protection etc., you restate that before you go down that track you want to at least have this opportunity to trial natural progesterone.

That all you are asking for is six to twelve months (of your time), and you will be receptive to synthetic hormone replacement therapy if the proposed natural hormone replacement therapy doesn't go according to plan.

We find that this approach often works. You are a woman on a mission. Your mission is to get your script. Get your doctor to respect your choice and listen to what your needs are, not tell you what you ought to have. A good many women who go in with this expectation walk out with that script and smile. Try to get at least 5 repeats!

If you failed to get your progesterone script and walked out with another doctor's bill wondering what went wrong, I suggest you re-evaluate why you allowed yourself to be (a) intimidated, (b) made to feel insignificant such that your needs were not worthy of acknowledgement, (c) disempowered by your doctor's presumption of knowledge on natural progesterone, and (d) why perhaps the approval of your GP was more important than your right to have a say in what goes into your body.

There are occasions when a woman seeking natural progesterone can be 'out foxed' by her doctor. By asking for progesterone, the doctor may see an opportunity to impose synthetic HRT on you regardless of your request. Because you have stated you need hormone supplements, you've exposed your vulnerability and been cornered.

You have unwittingly strengthened your doctor's position to administer HIS/HER choice of HRT - not yours. I've seen women walk out of the surgery with HRT scripts instead of natural progesterone, submitting to their doctor's wishes - and been billed for it.

Often women will bend to pressure purely because they feel uneducated (comparing themselves to their doctor), wrongly believing they have no right to question their doctor or state their needs. In fact, many women don't even tell their doctors the full story in fear their doctors will think they are hypochondriacs.

Some doctors have absolutely no idea the extent to which these female patients suffer or how many symptoms they actually experience, purely because they modify their list. Often women fail to get their script because they sense their physician will refuse to treat them. Way too many stories of emotional blackmail, particularly involving specialists (Breast Cancer) have been heard.

Women have basically been told that if they elect to take natural progesterone, particularly if they have had mastectomies, they will be encouraging the regrowth of cancer. Any refusal to follow their doctors' recommended treatment justified a discontinuation of his/her services.

Another example of medical practitioners being behind the times is the usage of Tamoxifen. *Evidence can be found in recognised medical journals that* **progesterone actually does confer endometrial protection**, *especially in the usage of the drug Tamoxifen - as Tamoxifen can promote endometrial cancer. Progesterone, on the other hand, offers protection by opposing estrogen activity in the body.*

Here's a copy of a letter NPAN received from Marie, in South Australia who typifies the problems and distressing situations women are faced with.

"...I've just finished reading a book on natural progesterone loaned to me by a friend in New Zealand who, after meeting you, is now using the cream and has had a remarkable improvement in her menopause symptoms.

I must say, the book made interesting reading and if I had had access to the information years ago, I would never have taken synthetic hormone replacement therapy. Why didn't my doctor assess me for hormone and progesterone levels or at least tell me about the cream!!! She put me on Ogen and just over 3 years later (1999) at the age of 57, I was diagnosed with grade III estrogen receptive Breast Cancer requiring 6 doses of chemo and 30 doses of radio. My life was turned upside down as you can well imagine. I don't see that doctor now !!!

My GP has reluctantly given me a prescription for progesterone cream which is hard to obtain and has suggested I speak to my breast surgeon before using it as I am taking Tamoxifen for 5 years, and although there seems to be no information as to whether the cream will affect the benefits of Tamoxifen, I need to be very, very sure. Having had cancer, I am reluctant to take even a headache tablet!

And so I write to you seeking information on the progesterone cream, its benefits and its side effects. At the moment I am struggling with hot flushes, night sweats, memory loss, sore joints, bloating, disturbed sleep, complete loss of libido, and weight gain. Sound familiar? **(Incidentally Tamoxifen can exacerbate hot flushes along with other uncomfortable side effects)**.

I am quite happy to pay for any information and look forward to your reply..." This letter is all too familiar.

I encourage women to do their homework. Be firm. Be sure. Often women fail to get a doctor's prescription purely because they are not quite sure themselves. They allow confusion to reign and their doctors to take control of the situation.

Many women are frightened and not comfortable taking control of their lives, so this is a huge step for some of them. I encourage you to have courage, be persistent and believe in yourself. After all, it is your body and your birthright to become well again.

Walk into your doctor's surgery with a list of suggested guidelines. Once you've got your doctor on side and the script has been written, I suggest you ask your doctor to help you begin charting your progress immediately by ordering tests to establish baselines. These would include for example a blood profile, blood pressure reading, a bone mineral density reading and, if you suspect or have had a history of Cervical Hyperplasia, a pap smear and an ultrasound if you have a history of Endometrial Hyperplasia, Fibroids or Polycystic Ovarian Syndrome. Take these tests and any other tests your doctor may suggest. This is acting intelligently and with your doctor's help and assistance. It is also providing baselines to refer back to.

There is a place for medicine and there is certainly a place for very sophisticated diagnostic tools. I don't say run into your surgery, get your script and run out the door. Rather, be intelligent and be sensible about this. Make the most out of it. Your doctor is not your enemy. He may be just as uneasy as you but hides it behind his/her façade.

Unfortunately we have put doctors on pedestals and made them God. However, doctors often don't feel like Gods because they are very prone to litigation and probably have more to lose than you. (High levels of legal indemnity fees has influenced this attitude).

Medicine is like any profession where you seek out and respect expertise. It's like bringing in a painter to paint your house. You want the best job done but you may want a colour scheme that he doesn't feel suits. Do you allow the tradesman to paint according to what he wants? No, you expect him to follow your instructions if he wants to get paid.

It is the same principle when you go to the doctor and ask for a natural progesterone script. You are allowing him to offer advice, which I hope you listen to and take on board with an open mind, because doctors have a lot to offer. But you are also suggesting that maybe you would like a treatment (which you have thoroughly researched) that meets your needs rather than his.

Women have reported to me that their past honesty and disclosure has been to their own detriment and prescriptions are being more successfully obtained by women who go to:

- Doctors that bulk bill or Doctors that do not regularly practice at these clinics
- Where they trivialise their symptoms and just say they need progesterone for PMS problems
- Where they avoid mentioning depression, Fibroids, Hysterectomies, Breast Cancer or family history of heavy bleeding

- When they emphasise a history of blood clotting, strokes or cardiovascular problems
- When they tell their Doctor of their horrific experiences and side effects experienced on the Pill, patches, combination synthetic HRT, injections and implants.
- Admission to being a smoker

This unfortunately can be to a women's detriment which I later go into but firstly women need to understand why Doctors are being so resistant and that their reluctance to prescribe this hormone is based on their knowledge and information which is different to ours thus their reluctance. Remember they are not doing this deliberately to antagonise you.

Possible reasons why Doctors have become resistant and cautious about writing scripts

Why are Doctors so reluctant to write scripts for natural progesterone?

- Firstly there are no manufactured and registered products federally with the exception of Pro-Feme WA (which is manufactured and state bound within Australia, to date).
- Whilst it is in their drug manual and on their drug computer little information is offered on natural progesterone let alone trials and back up data to substantiate its use.
- As it is a non patented product no drug companies are behind the sale or promotion of natural progesterone. Therefore no drug representatives to educate and promote this product to Doctors.
- They are not taught in depth about progesterone in medical school other than it being for pregnancy.
- They are taught that menopause is estrogen deficiency. Progesterone doesn't come into consideration.
- Many Doctors are of the belief that progesterone is the same as progestins/progestogens. Many Doctors do not realise that progestins have a different molecular structure to natural progesterone which is the exact replica (copy) to the body's real hormone despite both being made in a laboratory derived from the same source. e.g. Diosgenin. This altered configuration delivers different messages. It is not in the Drug Companies best interest to point this out but more so to point out why the synthetic progestigins were designed, benefits and the purpose of which they are used to treat specific symptoms. No drug company has a vested interest in natural progesterone's benefits and purpose (to assist women to get well and hormonally balanced).
- Some Doctors believe that some synthetic HRT does the same as progesterone.
- Some insurance companies do not cover protection for non registered drugs and

products and are making this point very loud and clear to Doctors causing concern.

- Unbalanced information published in medical journals.

- No drug company has designed a natural progesterone deliverance technique as will estrogen and testosterone patches and/or progesterone vaginal gel (Crinone in USA).

- Some Doctors believe progesterone (natural) is dangerous and contains harmful untested plant ingredients and preservatives. This shows a lack of understanding of progesterone products and highlights the misleading propaganda from drug companies.

- Some Doctors believe it is illegal to prescribe progesterone.

- Some Doctors do not understand that they do not need to be registered in W.A. to write a script. They just cannot write 'Pro-Feme'. If they are not registered or reside in W.A. It is not of the Doctors concern or jeopardises them legally, where you obtain your cream from and which compounding pharmacist you choose to use.

- A Doctor is acting within the law (outside W.A.) if he or she does not write a brand name. All that is required by the compounding pharmacist is a script written - progesterone, dose strength and usage. eg progesterone 3.2% to 50gram tube/jar 32mg daily from day 12-26. The local compounding pharmacist will be happy to guide your Doctor. Most Doctors write progesterone 3.2% 6 repeats as per instructions.

With all this in mind it's no wonder they are reluctant to prescribe natural progesterone or do so with caution. It is our job to educate them so they are no longer fearful of prescribing progesterone. This can be a slow process as I have witnessed over the last 8 years. The phone never stops with frustrated women trying to seek out a prescribing Doctor. Gone are the days where I hand out Doctors lists as these were mis used and unfortunately many women were disrespectful in the way they approached their Doctors assuming it was their right to have a script. This attitude only bought resistance from the Doctors and many of them approached my organisation to remove their name from my list. Furthermore many Doctors were being harrassed by some ambitious compounding pharmacists.

My aim in this is to help women to have confidence in approaching their Doctor for a script but of course this process is a two way process and trust is required from both parties.

This letter received from a lady recently is just one of the reasons demonstrating the existing problems women are facing with their Doctors.

Hi Jenny,

After meeting you here at your seminar and talking to you on the phone, I was very excited about natural progesterone and natural testosterone too. I have seen my doctor and she too was interested in reading your book. Unfortunately she (and all other practitioners) have been advised by the AMA that they will not be covered by insurance if they prescribe the progesterone. She said that there is a female testosterone coming available soon but it is not in cream form. She will not prescribe either. I can understand her situation with the AMA (Australian Medical Association). Do you think that this product will ever be approved by the TGA? I am disappointed about the whole lot. I cannot take HRT and rely completely on natural remedies. Fortunately I do not have many symptoms. I only had a full Hysterectomy 18 months ago. Could you tell me how other women get prescriptions and do you think it will ever be made available to all of us. My doctor herself is looking for an alternative as she is nearing menopause and will not take HRT because her mother got Breast Cancer while on HRT.

Look forward to hearing from you. I admire you for what you are doing but at the same time it is getting a lot of women's hopes up, only to be unable to source the products you are promoting.

Regards LS, Queensland Far North

Winning over a working relationship with your Doctor

Now that you can appreciate it from the Doctors perspective it is important to realise the need to understand how to speak his/her language. Doctors are trained to be analytical, structured, methodical, logical, calculating precise careful professional, practical and knowledgeable in their matter of fact treatment and reasons for prescribing - mostly based on test results and facts. Not emotions (Psychiatrists and Psychologists specialise in this!)

I have thought a lot about this subject and the dilemmas we face in acquiring our progesterone prescriptions, so have put together a guideline approach which you can write and formulate in your own words to fit your own personality, beliefs, needs and situations. You can practice this and go prepared. Experience has proven that women who are profoundly 100% sure and adamant about what they want will walk out with their requests being met. They have an air of confidence and diligent approach of self assurance, devoid of any room for doubt or a need to become defensive. (which can become aggressive in response). You too must learn to be practical, non attached to outcome or approval, assertive in your approach but not aggressive. The chances are you may be ridiculed or criticised for your choice so be prepared for a response from your Doctor that may not be what you expect or desire. I can recall my Doctor tried many times to coerce me to take bone building drugs and instilling fear in me that without these my Osteoporosis could only worsen. Suggesting that I give up my hormone options and come to my senses. Especially since I broke my arm in 2003. I reminded her it still was not an option, for bone building medications, it was still early days and that I was not depending on progesterone and testosterone alone to rebuild bones and that I had also adopted a holistic approach. I did comment wittingly 'that at least I didn't break my hip, so things may not be as bad as they seem'. She threw her arms up in the air in exasperation and gave me one of those looks, however I gently reminded her that since I have bouts of Irritable Bowel Syndrome taking bone building drugs for me is out of the question as I did not wish to impede further absorption problems of valuable minerals. She now respects my stance but does not agree but that's okay. This is a demonstration of being able to have a working relationship with your Doctor in your health with some input and being able to be honest without jeopardising medical treatment and both respecting each others opinions and reasons behind various treatment options.

I have included a suggested guideline on how you may wish to approach your Doctor.

Suggested guidelines on how you may wish to approach your Doctor:

YOUR REQUEST:

I am here today to seek your assistance and support and respect as my Doctor. I have been researching natural progesterone and bio identical hormone replacement therapy and I would like to try natural progesterone as an option first to see if this can assist me before I consider using synthetic HRT.

I have a history (or family history) of Heart Disease, blood clots or Breast Cancer.

I could not take the oral contraceptive pill as I have severe reactions and side effects on it in the past.

I also smoke (if you actually do so you may be criticised for wishing to take 'natural' or safer hormone options with this contraindication health hazard! As one lady discovered and was his grounds of refusal based on this logic!)

I recognise that this type of hormone therapy has little supporting evidence in its favour, not being highly trialled. I understand this is probably due to the fact that it is not able to be drug company patented (owned). I also recognise that some of the trials that you have seen in your journals may have been sponsored by companies with other agendas. It is for this reason I have copied a list of trials that have been conducted and would like to leave these with you to read. Medical references and a drug information sheet can be printed off my web site, www.npan.com.au or found in the back of this book.

I would also like to leave you with some contacting phone numbers - one of a manufactured progesterone product in WA. It is a 1800 number and will cost you nothing to speak to the manufacturer of this progesterone product produced under the Code of Good Manufacturing Practice as described by the TGA. Incidently this product is in your drug lists on your computer and listed in your MIMS (drug manual).

Also is a list of, or a 'phone number of my compounding pharmacist, making these bio-identical hormones as you may wish to speak with them personally for further information.

I recognise that Doctors are wary to prescribe a non registered S4 drug product, and I am happy to sign a consent form to free you from any threat of litigation or ramification. I fully take responsibility for my choice and request.

All I am requesting is a hormone that my body should naturally produce upon ovulation. I am not asking for a dangerous listed medication. I am not asking for a synthetic analogue which has more side effects.

I am also asking you to work with me as my Doctor and respect my choices and wishes for treatment.

I am happy to keep you informed with my charting and progress and if this does not prove successful for me, then I am happy to look at other options that you may consider to suggest.

For the moment this is what I wish to do. And as you are my Doctor I want to be open and honest with you rather than sneak off behind your back to another Doctor.

Here are the responses/answers you may get from your Doctor upon request and suggested answers you could reply in a cordial and respectful but firm way.

It does not give endometrial protection or prevent endometrial hyperplasia but HRT does. Therefore it would be far more effective and safer. You wont risk the chances of Fibroids or endometrial cancer etc.

Your reply:

Whilst that may be the proven medical evidence, there is other evidence that suggests natural progesterone can do the same (especially intravaginally or in higher doses). Furthermore it is not going to cause the risk of nasty side effects that we are now reading in the papers. It also should protect me from cancer as it opposes oestrogen and oestrogen proliferation, which promotes cancer.

Doctor, I would prefer to take my chances with natural progesterone, diet management, regular monitoring, rather than use HRT, the OCP, anti-depressants or whatever. Being a natural copy of molecular stucture to my own real progesterone I fail to see how it could be possibly harmful to me. It is what nature intended for me. Not synthetic or altered versions or medications that can be harsh on my liver with many side effects

Your Doctor may wish to put you on hormones that have 'progestogenic benefits'. These are not natural progesterone. They are progestins as is in the synthetic form of HRT. Eg. Deprovera. Livial (whilst this is conveyed to have progesterogenic benefits) this is still not natural bio identical progesterone and will not deliver the same progesterone messages to the body.

Your reply:

Because natural progesterone is in a cream form (or troches/or pessaries/or suppositories) it bypasses the liver so will be less harmful to my liver and will not cause it to become overloaded having to break down the higher required doses administered orally. I am also overweight and do not wish further pressure on my liver.

How will the special tests and my doctor's examination benefit me if I want to use progesterone?

Certain tests will determine whether there is an absence, or presence of any underlying problems. If everything looks good, you can begin progesterone therapy. Certain tests, such as a pap smear, are very advisable. This will detect cancerous or pre-cancerous cells, or changes in cell structure of the cervix. A mammogram can detect early signs of Breast Cancer, lumps or abnormal cell changes (although regular self-examination is encouraged).

A bone mineral density (BMD) test can detect Osteoporosis. A blood count and hormone profile will determine estrogen, progesterone, the follicle stimulating hormone (FSH), testosterone and DHEA levels. Your doctor can order a screening of blood sugar levels, and cholesterol LDL/HDL ratios. Other specific tests such as liver function and thyroid function may be beneficial. Comparisons can be obtained through both blood work and saliva assays.

Abnormalities will indicate any sign of metabolic disorders and, where a woman is in her menopausal, peri menopausal or post menopausal stages, it will also show whether she has an absence of progesterone.

Urinalysis will show signs of any kidney disease, signs of infection, or even detect signs of glucose which indicates diabetes or pre-diabetic conditions.

A pelvic ultrasound will determine diseases of the uterus and the ovaries, and is useful for women where a pelvic examination may be uncomfortable, difficult or inconclusive. It also gives us a good picture of what is happening on the ovaries and also the state of the pelvis in general. A vaginal ultrasound is more informative and will show up the thickness of the uterus, Fibroids and the state of the ovaries more clearly.

Some women also have a bladder function test to determine the amount of urine they can hold, and we have had lots of women who have required bladder hitching surgery, and others, bladder stretching on a regular basis. We believe this is hormonally linked and often women report improved bladder capacity 12-18 months after using progesterone on a regular basis.

The doctor's physical examination should include:

- Blood pressure: detect whether you run any risk of Cardiovascular Disease, hypertension (high blood pressure) and risk of stroke

NOTE: Cardiovascular and high blood pressure is a high contra indication not to use synthetic HRT and be very wary of estrogen administration if offered. Estrogen increases blood clotting particularly if you smoke.

- Weight: determine whether you are underweight or overweight (very indicative of hormone imbalance, particularly estrogen dominance and Syndrome X)
- Thyroid: detect if there is an abnormality, growth, enlargements, lumps; a thyroid function to determine over-activity or under-activity such as hypothyroidism (may require a T3 and T4 Thyroid test and medications).
- Breast examination: check the breast tissues and see that there are no

abnormalities, puckering or presence of lumps or multiple Cysts, changes occurring in texture / colour of tissue or nipple

- Abdomen: check for any tenderness, lumps or swelling / distension particularly over the pelvic area or around the liver area
- Pelvic examination: check your pelvic organs, the condition of your ovaries and whether they are tender or if there is any hardness, lumps, any enlargement, signs of cancer
- Uterus : check whether prolapsed
- Vaginal tissue: signs of atrophy or whether the vaginal tissue is in good order and healthy skin colour and texture, no signs of Thrush or discharge
- Bladder: check whether prolapsed, investigate problems such as discharge, irritation, sensitivity, bladder shrinkage, Stress Incontinence or Cystitis, and other related problems
- Urethra: may be inflamed, doctor may also want to do a pap smear and bladder tests if you repeatedly complain of urethritis or vaginal itching and so forth, which can indicate low grade infection that may need a culture
- Full blood profile: check haemoglobin reading (anaemia), B12 deficiency, cholesterol profile and any others required.
- Ovarian Cancer Blood Test this is available but not listed as a standard procedure as they are not totally reliable.
- Because most GPs appear to be running to a very tight schedule and often under pressure, we recommend women take along their list to remind them of the things they would like checked out to ensure they get value for money, and book a double appointment if you feel you need more time.
- It sounds pretty daunting doesn't it? However, if you go in armed with knowledge, reasonable expectations, and your list, chances are the doctor will take you seriously, and know that you are not there to waste his time. That you have specific needs and requirements of his service to you.
- Get your blood pressure reading and , if due, pap smear, mammogram etc.

Ultimately he will respect you for having done your homework and being a person of clarity. You are there specifically for a purpose, and your doctor is there to help you achieve optimal physical and mental health. Is he or she is not, it's time to change doctors.

I feel guilty using progesterone behind my doctor's back because I know he does not approve of natural progesterone. Is it harmful to withhold this information, being a natural product?

Yes. Natural Progesterone is a hormone even though natural to the body. This must be understood. It is a human hormone existing in our body so it can be safely introduced into the body because it is identical to the progesterone molecule found 'naturally' occurring in your body. Just remember, it is a hormone and *any hormone used incorrectly can create an endocrine disturbance in the body.* All hormones must be imbalance with each other.

It is wise to work with a doctor who knows exactly what you are using otherwise, if he doesn't have the full story, how can he treat you correctly? If your doctor refuses to support you, it may be wise to change to a doctor who will. Ask your doctor for a copy of your complete medical history and test results so that you can take your file along to your new doctor. Some women continue on with their doctor out of obligation, or perhaps because of family / peer pressure.

Over and above being detrimental to your health, withholding information is a disservice to your GP and yourself. Even though natural progesterone is a relatively safe hormone, out of balance or outside physiological dosages it has the potential to disturb the ebb and flow of other hormones. Further, your doctor may prescribe a treatment that is not recommended in conjunction with progesterone therapy. In other words, it may be contra-indicative of your progesterone. This has happened in many, many situations with women.

*For example, your doctor may put you on the contraceptive Pill, contraceptive implant, an IUD, a synthetic progestogen or give you a cortisone injection, all of which basically **negate** the effectiveness of your natural progesterone.*

This has happened many times over, simply because women withheld information. They very quickly discover they have become severely hormonally imbalanced once the actual drug administered negated progesterone's positive impact on the body, and consequently compromised the benefits of progesterone by many months.

Some women, for example, go to the doctor with fluid retention in the first few weeks of progesterone use, not understanding that sodium retention is a result of estrogen build-up/estrogen dominance which can be exacerbated with the reintroduction of progesterone (eventually it should rebalance and subside).

As stated previously, when progesterone is reintroduced into the body, it can actually increase the symptoms of estrogen dominance, purely because it is sensitising estrogen receptor sites. Progesterone wakes up estrogen receptors, encouraging estrogen to work more effectively. Progesterone stimulates estrogen, and estrogen stimulates progesterone. Each hormone is intrinsically linked to the other, but out of balance they can cause havoc in the body.

When estrogen receptors wake up, often women will find they have increased headaches and intracellular edema (sodium moves through the cells into the inner cell, bringing water with it). Your doctor, seeing this problem and not knowing you have just started progesterone, could prescribe a diuretic that can not only create electrolyte imbalances, but also retard progesterone efficiency in the body.

I have seen women prescribed anti-depressants after they became teary-eyed and depressed on progesterone supplementation, not realising that these symptoms are part of estrogen dominant wake up. In prescribing anti-depressants, the doctor has inadvertently retarded the opportunity for progesterone - a mood enhancing hormone

- to relieve hormonally induced depression naturally once the body has had time to adjust, and estrogen dominance has been defeated.

Increasing the progesterone in initial stages if teariness occurs may be all that is required to overcome this rather than resorting to anxiety and antidepressant drugs. I always remind women that the first indication that progesterone is working effectively is the restorative and improved sleep. This usually happens very early and can be corrected within a couple of days of adjustment of doses.

At NPAN I have observed that many women experience increased intensity of joint and muscle pain at some stage of their progesterone therapy. One such case was myself experiencing significant discomfort around the seventh month.

In those early days I understood very little about the side effects of progesterone therapy, I panicked and went racing off to my rheumatologist who wanted to put me on a cortisone-based anti-inflammatory drugs which would have counteracted progesterone benefits long term and perhaps impaired my hormonal health.

It is now believed, based on women's input, that the incidence, or exacerbation of joint and muscle pain while taking progesterone is a result of receptor activity "waking up" in those areas. When women complain of this insidious yet common experience, I encourage them to bear with it because it is an experience a good many women connected to NPAN have gone through.

It occurs on different levels at various stages (7-8 months average), however, more importantly, the incidence of pain and increased discomfort does not appear to be suggestive of progressive degeneration of any pre-existing disease. Rather, my conclusion based on my own and women's experiences is that it is an indication cell receptors are waking up; in most cases, a sign the body is responding favourably. If joint pain continues indefinitely seek further advise.

Many women with arthritic or inflammatory problems find that after about two years on progesterone they are reporting significant joint and muscular mobility, and their pain has dramatically reduced, allowing them to resume physical activities that were once restrictive or beyond them. Intake of essential fatty acids the Omegas 3,6 & 9 play a huge role here also Book 2 Natural Progesterone More Secrets Revealed covers the significance of these essential fatty acids along with other valuable nutritional advise.

NPAN encourages women who are arthritic, battling auto immune problems, or residual joint damage and subsequent long term pain to avoid pain killers that are harsh on the liver. Instead take a premium bone and joint supplementation formula that will nourish joints, bones, cartilage and muscles with essential minerals to compliment progesterone therapy to ensure they derive the full benefits from their hormone balancing. (You may wish to read the chapter on Osteoporosis.)

One case I would like to share with you here. Nancy came to me after being diagnosed with Breast Cancer and her mastectomy was scheduled in 3 weeks time.

Nancy was referred to NPAN by a concerned friend seeking information on natural progesterone. She began progesterone replacement therapy along with nutritional supplementation with her husband's full support .

Progesterone therapy began immediately on prescription from a local GP without her endocrinologist's consent. This was contrary to any advice provided by NPAN. In fact, I suggested she go back to the doctor whom I knew had written the progesterone script and, incidentally, was operating a women's clinic.

It was up to her doctor, in my opinion, to liaise with Nancy's specialist and relay this vital information. This did not happen. And Nancy was too frightened to open her mouth, perhaps intimidated by both doctors.

Prepping herself for surgery, she started applying progesterone in high doses to saturate her body prior to her mastectomy. She had read a medical article supporting the theory that if women ovulated (producing progesterone) prior to surgery that the likelihood of metastases would be reduced. Nancy wanted to cover all her options.

Following surgery she underwent chemotherapy. Her doctor, however, was concerned because her periods had remained cyclic, with no signs of hormonal disruption after completing her course of chemo. This demonstrated to NPAN the positive impact progesterone was having on Nancy's body under extreme conditions, possibly supporting and/or protecting ovarian integrity.

Tragically, to Nancy's detriment, she did not inform her specialist that she was still using progesterone. In response to this unusual occurrence, her specialist scheduled Nancy in for more chemotherapy because, in her opinion, Nancy's periods should have stopped.

Her justification for this decision may have been based on the premise that while Nancy continued to menstruate, her estrogen levels were too high which could jeopardise further risk of cancer. This would have been a high probability without progesterone in the equation to oppose estrogen.

Had Nancy been up front with her specialist, or had the GP who prescribed progesterone (who to this date still continues to treat her with progesterone) informed the endocrinologist that she was treating Nancy in such a manner, then perhaps the second lot of chemo may not have been necessary. And Nancy may not have entered menopause so abruptly.

If this information had been revealed at the onset, perhaps the endocrinologist would have been forced to look at the possibility that the second lot of chemo may not have been warranted. And possibly viewed progesterone's place in Nancy's treatment, recovery and outcome more favourably.

In closing, Nancy is now taking Tamoxifen against her better judgement, and continues with progesterone therapy in secret. Further, Nancy's doctor continues to keep this information from her specialist. Nancy's case demonstrates the plight of women in Australia.

If you are going to go to your doctor and withhold information, make sure you understand the symptoms of estrogen dominance and the progression of progesterone therapy before your doctor starts treating you, if only to avoid unnecessary conflict of interest and unwanted ramifications.

I advise women to undergo any tests your doctor may recommend to rule out anything sinister. (Refer to my Section on 'Stages of Natural Progesterone's Action In The Body' (page 138) and 'How will the special tests and my doctor's examination benefit me if I want to use progesterone'(page 118). Please refer also to saliva assays page 129).

My doctor will not prescribe progesterone on the grounds that I am testing positive to estrogen receptors and progesterone receptors.

From my interpretation of the question posed and that of the information provided in The Late Dr. John Lee's publications, The Late Dr. Lee believed that perhaps doctors may not understand the distinction between these two very different receptors, and two very different hormonal roles in the body. One receptor responds to estrogen, and one responds to progesterone.

Hormones can be likened to chemical keys that turn vitally important metabolic locks in our cells. The turning of these locks stimulates activity within the cells of our brain, intestines, muscles, genital organs and skin. Without the hormonal keys the metabolic locks in our cells remain closed and the full potential of our cells is not realised.

The Late Dr. Lee maintained that the very fact that you have progesterone receptor sites is very positive. *The progesterone receptors carry messages to breast cells to inhibit proliferation, preventing growth of Breast Cancer cells.* Estrogen, on the other hand, promotes cell proliferation, increasing the risk of Breast Cancer.

In a The Late Dr. John Lee medical article (June, 2001) he wrote: "It is clear that unopposed estrogen (especially estradiol) is a causative factor in Breast Cancer. Other studies show that estrogen stimulates breast cell (and Breast Cancer cell) hyperplasia and dysplasia, whereas progesterone inhibits it. Still other studies show that estradiol stimulates the oncogene Bcl-2, whereas progesterone activates gene p53, which increases apoptosis and blocks the Bcl-2 carcinogenic effect.

When the mechanism of action revealed by all these studies are understood, it becomes clear that estrogen dominance is a major factor in increasing the incidence of Breast Cancer, whereas progesterone prevents it.

In 1996, the British Journal of Cancer published a study by Dr. Mohr et al. which found that the 18-year cumulative survival rate after Breast Cancer surgery in **node-positive** *patients was twice as good (64 percent vs. 33 percent) among patients with normal progesterone levels than amongst patients with low progesterone levels on the day of their breast surgery."*

Women approach NPAN so distressed when their doctors tell them they cannot take progesterone because their progesterone receptors have tested 'positive'. This is to imply that progesterone therapy will jeopardise them further. But no one seems to be able to give them an answer as to what this exactly means. Helplessly, all I can do is refer them on to Dr. The Late Dr. John Lee's website and his book "What your Doctor's may not tell you about Breast Cancer'.

This topic is clearly *too controversial* for me to comfortably make any further comments here. But The Late Dr. John Lee does go into detail in various articles in his publication The Late John R. Lee, M.D. Medical Letter where he regularly addressed issues relating to Breast Cancer, treatments, and research.

Other articles that reference this very dilemma can be found in issues dated:

- April 1998 - 'Preventing and Treating Breast Cancer with Progesterone (Part 1)'
- May 1998 - 'Preventing and Treating Breast Cancer with Progesterone (Part 2)'
- May 1998 - 'The Tamoxifen Tangle'
- June 1998 - 'Dr. Lee's Basic Breast Cancer Prevention Program'
- October 1998 - 'New Study Showing Progesterone's Effect on Breast Tissue'
- October 1998 (page 7) - 'That's a Good Question'
- January 1999 - 'When is Breast Cancer not Really Breast Cancer?'
- November 1999 - 'Pesticides Raise Risk of Breast Cancer'
- July 2000 - 'Are Breast Cancer Treatments Working?'
- September 2000 (page 3) - 'Hormone Receptors in Breast Cancer'

Dr Lee is putting the finishing touches on his next book, "What Your Doctor May Not Tell You About Breast Cancer", due for publication January 2002.

The Late Dr John Lee's web site to my knowledge to date is still operating and his newsletters, articles, books and tapes can still be purchased.

How does the doctor know what progesterone dosage to put me on, and when to adjust?

In countries where progesterone is a prescription drug monitored by your doctor, problems arise when your doctor is asked to write a script for a drug she/he knows very little about.

Most GPs err on the side of caution and follow drug indicated usage. Which is what most compounding pharmacists are already recommending with doses of between 16-20mg from Day 12 to 26 if you are menstruating or 25 days on, 5 days off if menopausal.

The truth is, women are going to have to improvise, and hopefully rely on their charts and NPAN observational data to determine their parameters. To tune into their bodies, adjust their doses according to symptoms, initially working with higher doses in the first 6-8 weeks and weaning back to where they are asymptomatic and when they feel comfortable and confident to reduce doses.

I have observed that some doctors who are progesterone 'cautious' have been very quick to reduce a woman's dosage to a physiological dosage well before progesterone has had an opportunity to work effectively in the body, bringing about a rapid return of symptoms or a flare up of a particular disease or condition. Many Doctors panic when they view above normal saliva results. Yes they will possibly be high particularly if you are applying high doses (reflective in your saliva readings proving you are absorbing the progesterone from your cream). However while symptoms rage, a call for higher doses is initially required regardless if the reading goes off the page. So many women have fallen into the trap being guided by saliva readings aiming to achieve the supposedly perfect saliva guideline range. Rather than being guided by their symptoms (and a need for higher doses to address these). I believe saliva assays are more useful in cases of fertility programs or when a women wishes to assess all her hormone levels to get accurate readings of her true bio available progesterone level (and other hormones). You will need to be off your progesterone for a couple of weeks if you wish to get an accurate reading of what your body is producing. ***Do not stop progesterone if you suspect you are pregnant and wish to do your saliva assay.***

It is a fact that NPAN encourages each and every woman to take responsibility themselves during progesterone therapy. My publication includes my opinions and observational data, and what the women have reported to be effective in their own use and experience with progesterone. I impress upon women not to take my information as gospel. They are my truths based on my observations collected through years of my own work, consultancy, phone work case histories and reading the Late Dr John Lee's work using his teachings as a reference point.

Use my information and experiences and tailor it to your own needs and opinions, or not. Many women follow their own intuition, feeling that perhaps a little bit of extra progesterone could help in the initial stages.

Adjustment Guide

If you are having an estrogen dominant 'wake up' crisis, increase your cream to double the strength versus what you're on now, providing it's under 10% or 100mg. If the symptoms subside within 24 hours, then you know you are on the right track and should maintain a level where you are holding your symptoms. Once you settle, start gently reducing. Usually you will see changes either way within 24 to 36 hours. So, if you feel you need to go up a bit, try it for a few days.

Alternatively, if you're feeling worse on a higher level, try going the other way and see if your symptoms get better. Some women actually need to decrease their progesterone in the first eight weeks purely because it is actually reacting in their body, particularly if their liver is not in good working order or their receptors are very slow to wake up and they just can't cope with high levels of if they have reached saturated levels quickly - so start observing around week 6.

These same women may cope with high levels further down the track. NPAN urges women to experiment, but keep in mind that at the end of the day your goal is to work to physiological doses, mimicking nature (equal to ovarian output at ovulation of roughly 16-20mg).

Remember you don't want to end up having an imbalance through too much usage of progesterone. Book 2 covers Estrogen Dominance Wake Up Crisis extensively.

How do I know whether to buy a 1.6% or 3.2% or 10% cream? Which is the one usually recommended?

Firstly, let me explain how to interpret the progesterone content of your jar or tube of cream. Cream said to contain 1.6% progesterone would equate to 16mg per application. 3.2% would mean your cream contains 32mg of progesterone per recommended dose. Just try to keep in mind that a 1% cream would equal 10mg, 2% equals 20mg, 10% equals 100mg, and so on. Incidentally, 16mg is The Late Dr. John Lee's recommended average dose. (Not mine, in my work I go slightly higher - usually in the vicinity of 32mg that is 3%).

Some women, however, opt for the higher concentrations simply because it works out more economical, and they rub on less cream. There are women, particularly the post menopausal group, who find the 32mg an ideal 'maintenance' dosage to balance the symptoms that tend to accompany change of life.

It's important to carefully follow application instructions. Measure your cream according to the dose indicator outlined by the cream manufacturer. For example, if you are using a tube of 1.6% cream the manufacturer might recommend squeezing roughly 2cm of cream onto the skin - 2cm in this case being equal to 16mg of progesterone, 4cm would give you 32mg (refer to 'Drug Information Sheet' Lawley Pharmaceuticals).

Alternatively, some creams measure their applications by a provided plastic measure ruler or teaspoon. Again, you shouldn't have to guess here. All relevant information should come packaged with the cream. If it doesn't, ask for information to be sent to you. It is important that you know how much cream dosage you are using per application.

High progesterone doses within the range of 100mg (10%) per application are usually prescribed as treatment of estrogen-driven conditions such as endometriosis, PCOS, uterine hyperplasia, Fibroids, migraines, severe PMS or severe post natal depression. High dosage typically continues for three or four months (up to 7 months) before women report a turn around and can start weaning back.

NPAN has observed women treating specific conditions with high levels of progesterone beyond six months or more, and it's interesting that they report loss of cream efficiency and their estrogen dominance symptoms reappear. I believe this is due to failure to reduce dosage according to symptom reduction or lack of breaks from cream, leading to receptors 'tuning down'. (Down regulating). Inferior creams have often shown this characteristic and the need to keep increasing, indicates that something is wrong. Change your cream supplier.

Further, increasing dosage and frequency of cream application can lead to progesterone overdosing, which I go into in detail in another chapter.

A good rule of thumb - least is best.

If you have been using high doses of progesterone cream, it is suggested you wean back to levels where you are asymptomatic. If you find your cream has become ineffective for reasons listed above, taking a break from cream altogether for a month or so is another way to enhance cream effectiveness. If you doubt your cream have a break for a month if you can and possibly try a different progesterone cream.

Another tip I have discovered is changing the route of delivery. That is alternating with intravaginal at minimal doses. This will stimulate different receptors and possibly improve cream performance. If you have an Estrogen Dominance Wake Up Crisis you know you are responding differently. Refer to intravaginal use, pages 175,216,217.

Women become caught in a cycle where increased body fat raises estrogen levels, and estrogen increases the tendency to accumulate body fat. If you are significantly estrogen dominant, I suggest you consider losing weight thereby reducing your estrogen dominance.

Progesterone dosage will correlate with your degree of estrogen dominance. The worse the symptoms, the more cream you apply. It follows then that your goal should be to reduce estrogen dominance through lifestyle changes, diet, exercise, and making sure that your liver is doing its job, with a view to reducing the progesterone cream back to its absolute minimum. Slapping more cream to oppose weight gain and increased estrogen dominance, is a band aid effect.

Progesterone is not the answer to every ailment. I cannot emphasise strongly enough a woman's need to look at other big players in her overall hormonal health (e.g. diet, nutritional supplements, lifestyle changes). All too often women read The Late Dr. John Lee's publications and naively expect all their symptoms to vanish with the introduction of progesterone cream. For the record, John clearly stated that hormone imbalance is multi-factorial. That progesterone is not a 'silver bullet'. Chances are you'll have to do more to help yourself than slap on some progesterone cream and wish your symptoms away! We are a quick fix society, condition to swallowing pills and potions to get rid of our problems. Passing the buck and giving our power to drug companies to come up with bigger and better magic potions (a hefty price to pay, eliminating ourselves from responsibility and promoting an attitude of blame). Suing McDonalds for obesity is a classic example of not taking responsibility for our own behaviour and actions. Don't give your power/hormones away and the amazing knowledge of who you are in essence when you are hormonally balanced. Giving up your power to drug companies for synthetic hormones or drugs to cure our hormonal symptoms will cost you dearly as many of us have discovered.

So many women have commented, "But I thought this was going to be easy!" Hormones fluctuate throughout the day, as they do in your lifetime. You need to understand this, and learn to read your body's bio-rhythms.

Refer to questions When Should I use less progesterone? How would I know if I have to use more progesterone? See section on Charting your Symptoms and also in Book 2 Natural Progesterone More Secrets Revealed - usage variations is covered in great depth, including Estrogen Dominance Wake Up Crisis management.

Now that I have my prescription how do I process it?

You have filled your legal obligation by acquiring your script for progesterone. To get your progesterone processed it must be compounded by a pharmacist specialising in bio identical hormone production, not every chemist can do this so be wary. There are many compounding pharmacists so you are free to post your script to the pharmacist of your choice and they can legally post your compounded product back to you if you do not have a compounding pharmacist in your local region. Make sure you choose a compounding pharmacist who has gained years of experience in this specialist field of bio identical hormones.

To assist women source natural progesterone in Australia, I have included a detailed list of available Australian Compounding Pharmacists on page 407

CHAPTER 8

Measuring progesterone with saliva assays versus blood serum

- The Late John R. Lee, M.D. Medical Letter - Saliva Vs Serum or Plasma test for Progesterone
- What a blood test measures
- How progesterone travels in blood
- Absorption of transdermal progesterone
- How to use Saliva Hormone Assay to determine progesterone dosage
- Achieving Balance is the Key
- Progesterone levels and PMS
- Progesterone and Endometriosis
- Progesterone and Estrogen Receptors
- References
- Saliva Hormone Testing as used by Researchers
- Good Evidence Concerning the Absorption of Steroids Through Human Skin
- The Evidence of Red Blood Cell Transport of Progesterone
- Direct Comparison of Plasma and Saliva Levels After Topical Progesterone Application
- Why not do a blood test to check progesterone rather than a saliva test?
- Conversion Formula for Saliva Tables provided by Garth Birdsey, Clinical Pharmacist.

The Late John R. Lee, M.D. Medical Letter - Saliva Vs Serum or Plasma test for Progesterone

(This information on Saliva has been graciously made available by The Late Dr. John Lee to help educate women and their treating doctors. July 1999 Issue.)

Confusion exists among medical professionals and the general public about the question of progesterone absorption. This confusion often hinges on a misunderstanding of the test used to measure progesterone levels in the body. Let me try to clarify the issue.

What a blood test measures

"Blood" tests for progesterone refer to the serum or plasma concentration of progesterone. Plasma is the watery, non cellular portion of the blood from which cellular components such as red blood cells and white blood cells, are excluded. Serum is essentially the same as plasma except that fibrinogen has been removed.

Serum and plasma, being watery, contain water-soluble (hydrophilic) substances such as water-soluble vitamins, carbohydrates, and proteins. Serum and plasma do not contain fat-soluble (lipophilic) substances. For the purposes of this discussion, serum and plasma are interchangeable and I will refer to them as serum.

Sex hormones such as progesterone, estrogen and testosterone are fat-soluble steroids similar to cholesterol. When you have a serum cholesterol measurement, you are measuring cholesterol bound to protein which makes it water-soluble. (Recall that serum cholesterol is described as HDL or LDL cholesterol, referring to the proteins to which it is bound.)

How progesterone travels in blood

The ovary-produced progesterone found in serum is also largely protein-bound. Protein-bound progesterone is not readily bio-available to receptors in target tissues throughout the body. It is on its way to the liver to be excreted in bile. Only 2 to 5 percent of serum progesterone is "free" or non-protein-bound. This is the progesterone available to target tissues and to saliva. Thus, progesterone measured by serum levels is mostly a measure of progesterone that is not going to be used by the body. A serum test can be used to compare one woman's progesterone production to that of another woman, or to test how much progesterone is being made by a woman's ovaries.

When progesterone is given intravenously, 80 percent of it is taken up by red blood cell membranes that are fatty in nature and therefore available to fat-soluble progesterone molecules. Less than 20 percent will be found in serum. It is obvious that serum levels would not detect the great majority of the progesterone added to whole blood.

Absorption of transdermal progesterone

Progesterone is a highly lipophilic (fat loving) molecule that is well absorbed through skin into the underlying fat layer. In fact, it is among the most lipophilic of the steroid hormones. From the fat layer, the progesterone is taken up gradually by red blood cell membranes in capillaries passing through the fat. The progesterone transported by red blood cell membranes is readily available to all target tissues and to saliva. This progesterone is completely bio-available and readily measured by saliva testing. Only a small fraction of it is carried by the watery serum. Obviously, serum testing is not a good way to measure transdermal progesterone absorption.

Yet, many doctors continue to question the skin absorption of progesterone. A recent example is a report in the April 25, 1998 issue of the Lancet that serum levels did not reflect a substantial rise of progesterone after topical application in postmenopausal women. This report is being used to argue that progesterone is not well absorbed. This implication is erroneous.

Rather, it means that the authors did not understand the significant difference between serum and saliva progesterone levels. Some even imply that saliva testing is relatively unknown and its reliability is unproven. This is an odd admission since researchers have been using saliva testing for years and a number of laboratories offer routine saliva hormone testing. A sampling of references supporting all points of importance in this matter can be found at the end of this report.

How to use Saliva Hormone Assay to determine progesterone dosage

Achieving Balance is the Key

The goal of progesterone supplementation is to restore normal physiologic levels of bioavailable progesterone. Progesterone/estrogen balance is the key. When sufficient numbers of normal ovulating women are tested by saliva hormone assay, the typical range of progesterone is found to be 0.3 to 0.5 ng/ml. Under usual circumstances, there should be no reason to exceed that range.

In my experience, the topical dose required to achieve a saliva level of 0.5 ng/ ml is commonly only 12 to 15 mg per day. For creams containing 900 to 1000 mg per 2-oz container, 12-15 mg a day for 24 days would use up only about one-third of a 2-oz container. Larger doses are often used initially to "catch up" on the existing progesterone deficiency state, but the maintenance dose will usually be around 15 mg per day. Since considerable variation in progesterone is well tolerated, a modest elevation of saliva levels to 0.8 to 1.5 ng/ml is acceptable.

Progesterone levels and PMS

Saliva progesterone levels several times higher than 0.5 ng/ml are justified in certain situations. In PMS, for example, stress is often a factor. Stress increases cortisol production. Cortisol blockades some progesterone receptors and thereby prevents progesterone function. To compete with this cortisol blockade, topical progesterone in the range of 30 to 40 mg/day is sometimes initially required to achieve a beneficial effect.

Progesterone and Endometriosis

Likewise, in women with Endometriosis, the goal is to increase progesterone levels to that found in women two months pregnant. This level may require that supplemental topical progesterone be in a range of 30 to 50 mg/day from day 8 to day 26 of the menstrual cycle. (See the July '98 issue of the The Late Dr. John Lee Medical Letter, for a more detailed article on the causes and treatment of Endometriosis.) Progesterone dosage is determined largely by response: the right dose is the amount that results in progressive decrease of Endometriosis pain. When pain is largely gone, levels can be decreased gradually over time to doses necessary to maintain the progesterone benefit.

Progesterone and Estrogen Receptors

In women whose doctors are giving them excessive supplemental estrogen, a different problem must be faced. Excessive estrogen in circumstances of deficient progesterone induces a decrease in receptor sensitivity. One of progesterone's functions is to restore the normal sensitivity of estrogen receptors. When progesterone is restored, estrogen receptor sensitivity is restored, also. It is not surprising that, in these cases, some women develop symptoms of estrogen dominance (water retention, headaches, weight gain, swollen breasts) when progesterone is first supplemented. Obviously, the estrogen dose must be lowered. If this is done too rapidly, however, hot; flushes can occur. The key is to reduce estrogen gradually while progesterone is being restored.

In my experience, estrogen dosage can be reduced 50 percent as soon as progesterone is added. Then, every 2 to 3 months, the estrogen dose can be further decreased gradually. Many women eventually discover they do not need any supplemental estrogen at all: the estrogen normally produced by body fat in postmenopausal women is often sufficient; for its needs once the progesterone is restored.

References
Saliva Hormone Testing as used by Researchers

- Painter-Brick C, Lotstein DS, Ellison PT. Seasonality of reproductive function and weight loss in rural Nepali women. Hum Reprod May 1995; 8 (5): 684-690.

- Ellison PT, Painter-Brick C, Lipson SF, O'Rourke MT. The ecological context of human ovarian function. Hum Reprod Dec 1995; 8 (12): 2248-2258.

- Ellison PT. Measurements of salivary progesterone. Ann NY Acad Sci Sept 20 1993; 694: 161-176.

- Campbell BC, Ellison PT. Menstrual variation in salivary testosterone among regularly cycling women. Horm Res 1992; 37 (4-5): 152-136.

- Lipson SF, Ellison PT. Reference values for luteal "progesterone " measured by salivary radioimmunoassay. Fertility and Sterility May 1994; 61 (3): 448-454.

- Bloom T, Ojanotko-Harri A, Laine M, Huhta-niemi I. Metabolism of progesterone and testosterone in human parotid and submandiblular salivary glands in vitro. J Steroid Biochem Mol Biol Jan 1995; 44 (1): 69-76.

Good Evidence Concerning the Absorption of Steroids Through Human Skin

- Johnson ME, et al. Permeation of steroids through human skin.
J Pharmaceutical Sci 1995; 84: 1144-1146.

The Evidence of Red Blood Cell Transport of Progesterone

- Devenuto F, et al. Human erythrocyte membrane: Uptake of progesterone and chemical alterations. Biochim Biophys Acta, 1969;193:36-
- Koefoed P, Brahm J. Permeability of human red cell membrane to steroid sex hormones. Biochim. Biophys Acta 1994; 1195: 55-62.

Direct Comparison of Plasma and Saliva Levels After Topical Progesterone Application

Dollbaum CM, Duwe GF. Absorption of progesterone after topical application: plasma and saliva levels. Presented at the 7th Annual Meeting of the American Menopause Society, 1997. The last reference is particularly revealing.

Creams with varying concentrations of progesterone were applied to menopausal women after which both plasma and saliva levels were measured. The results are illustrated below.

Pg Cream	Plasma	Saliva
(daily dose)	(ng/ml)	(ng/ml)
0 mg	0.36 ± 0.06	0.03 ± 0.006
0.34 mg	0.50 ± 0.09	0.152 ± 0.025
30 mg	1.8 ± 0.3	8.7 ± 3.5

As can be seen, in these menopausal women given the placebo topical cream, the plasma level was more than 10 times greater than saliva level. This indicates how little of their blood progesterone was of the non-protein-bound, bio-available kind.

When only 0.34 mg of progesterone was applied topically, the plasma level rose 39 percent, whereas saliva level rose 5-fold. This indicates that only a small portion of the added progesterone entered the plasma, whereas the saliva clearly showed a hefty increase of bio-available progesterone. When an 88-fold larger dose was applied topically, the plasma level rose only 3.6-fold while the simultaneous saliva level rose 57-fold. This indicates that only the saliva reflected the great increase in absorbed bio-available progesterone. The progesterone found in the saliva obviously was blood-borne, but it should be clear that the portion of the blood carrying the progesterone was not the plasma (serum) but, rather, was via red blood cells.

In all situations, however, it should be clear that plasma progesterone levels are not indicative of the true level of bio-available progesterone such as is obtained from topical application. Saliva levels are far more appropriate for this purpose.

(This concludes The Late Dr. John Lee's information sheet on Saliva.)

Why not do a blood test to check progesterone rather than a saliva test?

A lot of women want saliva assays to determine that they are on track and it is a very good idea to do your saliva from time to time to check your hormonal composition but a lot of doctors offer a blood test and that is not going to give the true readings. This is because the progesterone is protein bound and it is not carried on the watery part of the blood. When you do a blood test they test the serum which is that water part which doesn't show the true bio-availability of the progesterone. Therefore it is not an accurate reading.

Conversion Formula for Saliva Tables provided by Garth Birdsey *Bpharm Grad dip hos.pharm* , *Clinical Pharmacist.*

There is evidence and reference ranges for progesterone and saliva, have reference ranges in blood. We know that we can match saliva levels with an effect. With these levels we know whether you need to increase your dose or decrease your dose. However your doctors are more used to using blood levels, because this is how they are trained and this is how the vast majority of drugs are monitored. The problem is that to date we do not have a proven reference range of drug levels for progesterone in peri-menopause or menopause. Until we do we cannot suggest monitoring with blood levels.

In the fertility field we do have reference ranges for progesterone in blood, but that is for specialist fertility clinics not menopause. We will list the reference ranges and conversion methods below, however we do need to state that the reference ranges listed in your laboratory results are those of women not using progesterone. These ranges often confuse women because they are comparing ranges with non progesterone transdermal users. That means for example a menopausal woman will show low reference ranges if she is not ovulating.

When I got my first saliva assays result back and nearly freaked out thinking I'd overdosed on progesterone because it was way above the reference range guide. Until my husband, Garth, a qualified pharmacist and lecturer, sat down with me and explained that my ranges were 'spot on' when he worked the conversation and did a comparison. It also served to confirm that my dose of 32mg almost equivalent to the saliva results, indicating effective absorption and bio-availability. Unfortunately, I didn't arrange a hormone blood profile to determine what progesterone serum results would look like.

Women are feeling stranded when it comes to getting their doctors to interpret saliva assay results with confidence largely because, as stated above, their doctors have no comparative reference ranges to work from, as they do with blood serum results. Women were wasting their money ordering saliva tests as these tests are not recognised by their GPs. This meant they relied on information from overseas or contacted NPAN for advice which, until now, we were unable to provide.

For this reason, Garth has put together this Saliva Formula Table to assist you in conversion, probably only relevant if you live in Australia or NZ and get your results from overseas. This will also assist you if you are referencing The Late Dr. John Lee's recommended saliva ranges.

Since this conversion table was designed and supplied by Garth in 2001, for user friendly purposes it has been noted saliva assays and reference ranges are far more comprehensive and continually evolved as more and more Doctors are embracing and learning about saliva assays. I've seen several saliva results over the years and all not being my area of expertise and when it comes to figures/freeze out as do a lot of women, I suggest you allow the laboratories to analyse and simplify it for you on your behalf. Now like most tests I advise the results are deciphered accompanying comments for the Doctor to read very quickly, indicating too high and low or not enough.

We all have the same problems in hormonal imbalances and we share progesterone products and its benefits globally, but when it comes to treatment we're worlds apart.

Conversion Table	International Units	United States Units
Post Menopause	<125 pmol/L	0.04ng/ml
On Treatment with Progesterone Cream	2540 - 4750 pmol/L	0.8 - 1.5 ng/ml
Luteal Phase	250-800pmol/L	0.08-0.25ng/ml (up to 0.5 ng/ml)
If aiming for Luteal Phase Levels	320 - 1800 pmol/L	0.1 - 0.55 ng/ml

Conversion Factors

From pmol/L to ng/m   pmol/L X 0.0003145 = ng/ml
From ng/ml to pmol/L   ng/ml / 0.0003145 = pmol/L

CHAPTER 9

Cream Usage & Guidelines

- Where does NPAN stand on progesterone dosage.
- Stages of Natural Progesterone action in the body
- Guidelines to cream application
- Why do women expect progesterone to fix all their problems?
- I've started taking progesterone and I feel awful. I want to stop using the cream. Should I?
- What happens if I am allergic to the cream, e.g. rash?
- When is the best time to apply the cream and when do I start the cream?
- What do you do now that you have your cream?
- Where do I rub the cream?
- Some tips myself and women have found useful in cream application:
- What is the right dose for me?
- When do I have a break from my cream?
- Barometers that may indicate progesterone overuse and the need to adjust dosage:
- Breast changes
- Other physical barometers of overuse or under use
- When should I use less progesterone?
- How would I know if I have to use more progesterone?
- What can cause progesterone shortage?
- Are there any side effects using natural progesterone?
- I have been on progesterone and it is not working. Why would this be?
- I feel nauseous on progesterone, why is this?
- Why is the liver important for hormone balancing?
- Can I treat hormonal imbalance with nutritional and diet plan strategies alone?
- If using your cream without nutrition or supplementation.

Where does NPAN stand on progesterone dosage.

Over time, in my work and organisation NPAN , I along with the women began to identify the need to individualise dosage according to each woman's unique hormonal profile to treat her symptoms. This came about by my observation, women's feedback and my consultancy case studies and phone work.

Women concluded that a physiological dose of 15-20mg was an unrealistic 'maintenance' dose for most of the women working within my Network. Nearing 8 years work in progesterone usage, I am still of this opinion that 15-20mg is unrealistic maintenance dose (to remain asymptomatic) as suggested by the Late Dr John Lee. Perhaps this is because we are now living in a sea of estrogens (more pollutants of this century) and that we are 25 plus years on from when the Late Dr John Lee began his work in natural progesterone in his own practice.

The only two categories that fall into the 15-20mg maintenance dose are the elderly taking progesterone for Osteoporosis and suffer no symptoms of hormone imbalance, and the younger women that appear to have relatively healthy functioning ovaries. Interestingly, these younger women may or may not need to remain on progesterone once they achieve balance.

Our working range has been from 20mg (2%) to a maximum of 100mg (10%), and found no reason to go beyond this range **EXCEPT** with the rare exceptions of doses ranging from 200mg to 400mg for the categories of women suffering migraines, Fibroids and heavy bleeding. This is an exception to the rule and it often requires specialised administration.

Could it be I am only seeing those women who experience considerable health issues like Endometriosis, PCOS, Breast Cancer, Fibroids, Osteoporosis, menopausal, PMS? I do not have the experience of women and their physiological maintenance dosage in other countries such as in the USA, Canada, UK, Europe, New Zealand, South Africa, and around the globe who suffer these same conditions. I do not have the evidence that they are managing to maintain hormone harmony with physiological doses of 15-20mg? Perhaps they're not?

Having addressed ALL other factors that may contribute to hormone imbalance, our women clearly do best on an average maintenance dose of 32mg once they have achieved balance. Are the every-increasing xenoestrogens in our environment coupled with our very overweight population major players here? I believe so!

Evidence suggests, from our neck of the woods anyway, that there's a growing epidemic of hormone imbalance emerging with the post-war baby boomer generation and their off-spring and apparent Ovarian Dysfunction.

I acknowledge there are probably thousands, upon thousands of women who use progesterone very successfully without the need for direction or guidance. However, there IS a need (upon which NPAN was founded) to address the group of women out there floundering and in need of support, information, direction and comprehensive guidance outlined in my books.

It is through the networking of thousands of women, my publications evolved. Their experiences battling major health and hormonal concerns, and the incorporation of progesterone as an alternative therapy was the genesis of ('Natural Progesterone – The World's Best Kept Secret' and now Book 2 Natural Progesterone More Secrets Revealed).

Stages of Natural Progesterone action in the body Created and developed by Jenny Birdsey©.

These stages have been formulated and recorded as a result of my work and observations. This information has not been obtained from anyone else's work or data and has been supplied to assist women as a general guideline to the stages of progesterone usage.

When can I expect to see results from using the cream? From 1-8 weeks , 4 months, 7 months, 12 and 18 months?

Progesterone seems to work at various stages and at various levels. These changes occur for the majority of women (I have observed) in the first 10 days, 6-8 weeks, then there is a change at 4 months, another at 7 months, a further change around 12 months, and finally another roughly at 18 months, based on the individual and her specific condition.

For example, many women suffering chronic fatigue, diabetes, fluid retention, lymphatic sluggishness exhibit a delayed response, and their phases may kick in weeks later than the average woman. These stages of natural progesterone's action in the body have been too consistent to be dismissed.

During these different stages that occur along the journey, slight adjustments are often required to maximise progesterone's effectiveness. If you are not aware of these stages, you may misinterpret the signs as progesterone losing its effect, when in actual fact it can represent the opposite.

Overall summary of Progesterone's behaviour and characteristic bodily response

First 10 days - Estrogen Dominance Wake Up Crisis

Because you are reintroducing progesterone back into your body thereby sensitising and stimulating the estrogen receptor sites, there are the immediate, and long term benefits and side effects (estrogen dominance wakeup crisis).

From observation, I have found the immediate benefits which generally occur within the first 10 days of usage range from instant calming, clearer thinking, feeling more grounded, an awareness that you are able to cope with stress better, reduction or elimination of headaches, a deeper, more restorative sleep pattern that draws comments like, "best night's sleep I've had in years!". (This incidentally can kick in on the first night!)

You may find you will shift body fluid as a result because progesterone acts as a natural diuretic. Breast tenderness, PMS and other symptoms may reduce dramatically, and many women comment that their face glows and looks healthy.

There have been reports of women feeling very euphoric such that some have experienced orgasms in their sleep, and the return of colourful, happy dreams. These are but some of the many reported benefits that women experience with the reintroduction of their essence hormone - progesterone.

On the other side of the coin, as a consequence of bringing progesterone back into the body and waking up estrogen receptor sites, women can actually go through a roller coaster of symptoms that can be quite frightening and debilitating unless they understand the reasons, and how to overcome these problems of estrogen dominance 'wake up'. I term this Estrogen Dominance Wake Up Crisis.

And that is why I suggest the usage of a very good phytoestrogen formulation throughout and to tone down the wake up crisis. There are many premium products on the market (see section on Phytoestrogens). By using a good phytoestrogen (not in cream form) it helps to tone down and reduce estrogen dominance wakeup and associated symptoms.

Some of the more common symptoms reported can be increased PMS, breakthrough bleeding (spotting) or the onset of a very heavy non-cyclic period, increased tenderness of the breast, headaches ranging from unrelenting dull headaches to severe migraines, uncontrollable hot flushes, fluid retention, anxiety, teariness, depression, anxiety, aggravation, irritability and aggression, panic attacks, increased joint and muscle pain, exacerbation of Thrush, impetigo, acne, weight gain, lethargy, palpitations, heartburn, constipation the list can be endless.

These wake up symptoms are intrinsically connected to the waking up of the high levels of estrogen already in the body that have become dulled (toned down) due to the absence of progesterone up until now. I remind women that *estrogen and progesterone are a pigeon pair*, each requiring the other to stimulate its activity in the body. That's why it's so important to maintain the correct balance (ratio) between these two hormones. Once they are on par together and estrogen dominance is over-ridden, symptoms settle or subside. (See Estrogen Dominance Wake Up Crisis in Book 2).

Because of this severe wakeup in the body where the symptoms of estrogen dominance are exaggerated, I often recommend women double their recommended dose for the **first** 6-8 weeks continual use in conjunction with a phytoestrogen supplementation to over-ride this phase.

For a smaller number of women, estrogen dominance crisis may occur weeks to months down the track (delayed response). I believe this is due to a sluggish cell receptor response. In other words the progesterone is not being utilised effectively. It is almost as if the cells and the chemical messages are partially asleep and non responsive. Additional nutritional supplementation often enables the body to have a more efficient response to progesterone and assist chemical conversion. Selenium helps nutritional enzyme transportation to the nucleus of each cell (mitochondria) where many hormones are made. Magnesium also will assist chemical communication.

1-8 Weeks - Reaching Saturation

During this period, double doses are well tolerated because the body is busy soaking up the hormone it has probably been deprived of for years. And being a fat-soluble hormone, whilst the body will get some benefits from progesterone, considerable amounts will find its way to fat cells. My observation is that around 6-8 weeks the body reaches a saturation level at which point dosage can require adjustment (gradual reduction) depending on the individual and her symptoms.

Because many women have high levels of estrogen dominance wakeup and have not reached saturation, *I often suggest they* **do not** *take a break in the first 8 weeks.* (In other words continue application through one true period, not a break through one, and take the first break on the second period or where it is due). By a continuing progesterone through the first period it will not interfere with your normal cycle or compromise hormonal balance and health.

Note, your normal period will still come on time (if there is a cycle) while you remain estrogen dominant. However, I strongly advocate that only in the first 8 weeks can all rules be broken while the hormone is reaching saturation point but, thereafter, **strict adherence to cyclic breaks must be followed**, and dosage tailored to where you are asymptomatic.

Women are very reluctant to take a break from cream for fear of symptoms returning. But they fail to realise that if they don't start taking their breaks, estrogen dominance may eventually return either because their receptors have down-regulated and render progesterone ineffective or progesterone goes on enthusiastically making more estrogen down the steroid pathway (see hormone cascade diagram).

Further, the failure to take breaks and fluctuate hormone levels from month to month, mimicking nature, may possibly throw cycles out of sync.

In simplistic terms, once you have topped up your progesterone reserves it then settles, and progesterone can be used more effectively for other roles now that the body is no longer depleted of this hormone. And this represents the baseline for women to establish their physiological dose.

You can test your own level of reserves during breaks from cream by testing how long you can go without feeling deprived. When your reserves are maximised, your body will comfortably tolerate up to a two week break before you start missing progesterone. (Not in a menopausal woman).

At this point, don't be too anxious if you can only tolerate small breaks each month within the first year because reserve levels can fluctuate depending on how you are utilising progesterone. The body is going to be busy taking advantage of the renewed levels of progesterone to perform multi-factorial jobs within the body.

It is important at this stage, that you start having **regular breaks (no less than 3 days monthly)** from the cream to prevent down-regulation of cell receptors.

If you do not rest the sites, by taking breaks and allow them to freshen up, *progesterone will become ineffective*. Once the initial saturation process has taken place, subsequent resaturation, which can vary from month to month, is quickly achieved. Some women saturate very quickly and can maintain their reserves, while others use their progesterone very rapidly and don't appear to have the ability to maintain saturation levels. I go into this later in Dose Administration when to increase and decrease your progesterone dosage.

Other women have extremely high saturation levels (in saliva readings) but appear not to be assimilating progesterone or deriving any benefits. To comfortably maintain balance, it's really a case of learning to read your body, understanding when your stores are depleted, and comprehending how your body uses progesterone in relation to things that are happening in your life, and the internal/external demands (refer to Charting). Your monthly score sheet will determine how effectively your progesterone is working in relation to addressing symptoms. Be active in this process, it pays off.

4 months - Stabilising & Settling

It appears a four month period/cycle is required before the body really falls into synchronisation. Up until now progesterone has performed numerous jobs that result in many benefits throughout the body. But the greater results are evident around the fourth month or fourth period where women actually feel the deeper benefits of treating longstanding, hormone-related conditions. The body now starts to settle and is now more aligned with this hormone.

Women report they are no longer clotting or bleeding as heavily, periods are showing signs of regulating, ovulation is often re-established, PMS is well under control, fibro-cystic breasts diminished, the pain and trauma associated with Endometriosis is dramatically reduced, and migraines become, for the first time, manageable. *Libido if it is going to respond to progesterone will usually have returned by now.*

At this point, the body appears to have well and truly settled and is very relaxed. Often women are not consciously feeling the benefits of progesterone because levels have been restored and homeostasis has been achieved. Progesterone, like any of the steroid hormones, works its magic silently in the body, and only when it is absent do we realise it's not providing the balance which we often take for granted. The absence or diminished supply of progesterone won't usually show up until the second period or month.

This hormonal balance (as nature intended) can be very foreign to some women. And because their body has plateaued and they are asymptomatic without the euphoric highs and sense of wellbeing they reached when using progesterone for the first time, they often interpret this absence of intensity or euphoria as a sign that progesterone is no longer working. Wrong!

And in an effort to revisit these wonderful early 'highs', they begin to slap on high doses which can perpetuate estrogen dominance (because progesterone will go into making more estrogen along the steroid pathway). A vicious cycle is then established, of which women are none the wiser.

On the other hand, many women fall into the trap of believing they no longer need progesterone supplementation and/or adopt a careless approach to their dosage and usage. I have seen extremes where women have stopped progesterone cream altogether because their symptoms have disappeared. Or applied progesterone only when they remember, which can bring about a re-emergence of symptoms and/or irregular periods which usually won't show up immediately - perhaps four to six weeks later or on the second period (thus the connection isn't made). A slap dash approach will inevitably bring slap dash results long term.

I caution women to respect that progesterone IS a hormone. That once you reach the plateau between 4-7 months you adhere to physiological doses, regular application, and appropriate breaks if you want to reap the long term benefits that come with hormonal balance. Note: It may take 12 months for you to establish what is your physiological (minimum) baseline to work from. Whilst progesterone is addressing symptoms you can be assured higher doses are well tolerated. So do not be to frightened in overdosing in the first 7-9 months even up to 12 months. I liken it to a pregnant women and what mother nature provides. In pregnancy progesterone is in the body uninterrupted for 9 months (this does not mean you can have 9 months without a break!) This indicates the body has a huge dose capacity to this natural hormone, as in the last trimester of pregnancy the placenta is producing up to 400mg a day. Not only fascinating but indicates a range between ovulation of 16-20mg to 400mg in pregnancy. The body is designed to accept huge variables in dosage of this hormone. (Its friend and supporter in maintaining life and multifactorial benefits).

7-12 months - Estrogen Dominance "Wake up" Revisited

Estrogen dominance wakeup can recur or unusual symptoms appear between 7-12 months but not in the case of every woman. Symptoms can range from increased muscle and joint pain, periods can become erratic and may be associated with heavy bleeding and clotting, Polycystic Ovarian Disease can become exacerbated, depression may occur, often libido may flag, and unexplained weight gain is commonly reported.

There are several reasons why this phase may surface. A genuine drop in hormone production may be a contributing factor. High estrogen levels as a result of increased weight gain - a by-product of a dysfunctional liver, that has disrupted all hormone levels rendering the existing dosage ineffective.

High levels of external /internal stress, such as pain, anxiety or illness, will take progesterone down the corticosteroid pathway to produce cortisol - the survival hormone - which negates the action of progesterone in the body (because progesterone is being converted into another hormone that competes for the same receptor).

Another factor can be the change from HRT to natural progesterone, and the time it takes stubborn synthetic progestogens to move off the progesterone receptor sites thus freeing them up for natural progesterone activity for the first time, or estrogen/progesterone imbalance begins to resurface as stores are now depleted as a result of estrogen therapy ceasing some months before.

I cannot say whether this phase is the result of estrogen sensitivity, overdosing with progesterone unnecessarily or failure to break and/or down regulating or receptors or progesterone deficiency. It can also be as a result of progesterone working at a deeper level, affecting perhaps for the first time, receptors that are only now responding to the presence of progesterone. In other words once progesterone addresses many initial symptoms it then goes on to deeper levels to attend to other tasks - all because of years of deprivation. Imagine like all the dominos falling over once the first domino is righted the body continues to correct the next domino and on it goes.

At this stage of your journey the body may require an increase in dosage to facilitate the demand for progesterone to oppose and address these problems and/or accommodate the body's need for extra progesterone working on this level. Check on what else might be happening in your life at the moment with family, diet, lifestyle, perhaps personal trauma or stress, all of which can draw on progesterone reserves and contribute to hormone depletion.

Too many women are reporting similar activity at this stage for it to be termed non-specific. I encourage women to maintain their journals, increase their dosage temporarily according to symptom relief supporting the body's demands for higher levels, and work through this phase, because additional benefits of their progesterone therapy are ultimately achieved.

In most cases, any unusual physiological activity that is not life-threatening, is a good sign that progesterone continues to work in your body. Just remember it took many years for progesterone deficiency to compound in the body and it will take time (often years) to reverse.

In fixing one problem, it often gives rise to another that will need to be resolved. This is why using progesterone cream over many years can be so beneficial.

18 months - Fine Tuning

IMPORTANT TO DO YOUR SCORE SHEET AT THIS PERIOD AND COMPARE WITH YOUR INITIAL SCORE SHEET SYMPTOMS.

Women have found their physiological maintenance dose to be very effective but suddenly may find themselves presenting with estrogen dominance symptoms despite following all the rules and nutritional supplementation. Most women in this category are nearing menopause and experiencing dramatic hormone fluctuations, therefore levels are more difficult to control. The way to test whether more cream dosage is required or less is simple. Ask yourself do I feel better or worse on my break? If better time to reduce and back off this hormone gradually if worse time to increase for awhile until symptoms resettle and abate. You may find that your physiological baseline dose has slightly increased. I recommend if any increase is required always assess your response in 24-36 hours and this will give you a guideline answer. If you have become progesterone deficient over a period it may take a month to restore your balance and to start to feel the benefits again.

This is where I suggest vaginal application can be of value, rapidly elevating and sustaining progesterone levels, while offering a more direct absorption route and targeting different receptors (one that I believe has additional benefits) Vaginal use is only one option and does not suit everyone and it must be adhered to strictly and done under your Doctors supervision if you wish to adopt this method of administration. Please also refer to vaginal administration route and other routes of application addressed in both books I have written on progesterone usage.

Some women alternate transdermal and vaginal application. This offers the body a cross section of deliverance and has been found to be very effective. Note: Vaginal application daily could build up too high levels and therefore needs to be monitored, that is why I suggest two to three days only vaginally if you are a woman who builds up reserves quickly. (From my own experience and my observation).

A small number of women have managed to successfully control their Fibroids Endrometriosis and Polycystic Ovarian Disease with progesterone, and have at approximately 18 months experienced a remission-like stage. Then, out of nowhere, it appears something has triggered estrogen activity and a flare up. Stress and personal grief, fatty liver and other factors need to be considered here.

Nonetheless, I am beginning to form an opinion from these reports that perhaps no less than a 4% cream level should be used as a baseline dose (40mg). However the average maintenance stable dose appears to be between 5 and 6% (50 - 60mg) for Fibroids, Endometriosis, and Polycystic Ovarian Diseases. Some fibroid cases have had to work with exceptionally high levels to control and shrink Fibroids. On a baseline physiological dose of around 40mg, if a flare up occurs higher doses have been administered by women with success particularly with the vaginal route option.

Whilst 4% may be a maintenance dose for women who have stabilised their condition, observation indicates that this dosage does not allow for any buffer in times of stress, thereby not giving additional backup. It is important to recognise your base level and your additional requirements at these times, as a minute variation can make all the difference.

Once re-stabilised, reassess your symptoms and determine whether you need to return to your baseline. I strongly urge women to undertake regular ultrasounds to monitor the stages of their Fibroids and/or endometrial thickening, and to determine the success of their progesterone dosage. Saliva assays would be helpful to draw a baseline of all hormones. However the "perfect within range" saliva results does not necessarily mean being asymptomatic.

Around the 12-18 month phase, I invariably hear back from women who have gradually moved away from the principles NPAN has found to work for women to maximise progesterone usage.

These ladies believe they have a handle on progesterone based on the fact they've had great results, not yet realising the importance of incorporating the correct diet and nutritional supplements in adjunct to progesterone. They haven't made the correlation between the two. Far too often one of the keys is their abandonment of daily usage of phytoestrogens and magnesium and supplementation and neglect of the liver.

If progesterone has carried them up to this point, in the absence of nutritional support and other principles, symptoms will insidiously creep up and hormone imbalance will resurface. Adopting and complying to the hormone balancing principles dealt with in both books will again restore the imbalance within a couple of months.

Guidelines to cream application

I am constantly learning about progesterone dosage and its usage. In summary, here are some simple guidelines to follow: In the beginning you can comfortably double your dose uninterrupted for 6-8 weeks (usually around 64mg -100mg is found to be a comfortable dose to oppose estrogen dominance. Then cyclic breaks according to these guidelines, to aim for:

Menopausal - start straight away, cream usage 3 weeks on 1 week off. (3-5 days minimum break if 7 days is too long).

For cyclic women: In the beginning you can start straight away uninterrupted breaking on 2nd real period or cycle, then adhere to your cycles.

Cyclic (regular periods, 28 day cycle) - start day 12 - 26. The first day of bleed is counted as day 1.

Cyclic (regular periods, 30 day cycle) - start day 14 - 28. The first day of bleed is counted as day 1.

Non-cyclic (no regular period is established) - start immediately. In the beginning 6-8 weeks on then follow pattern 2 weeks on cream and 2 weeks off. This will mimic a cyclic pattern, day 12 - 26, whether you are having a period or not. If a cyclic period emerges, adjust your breaks to fall into line when bleeding starts, resuming day 12 - 26. Periods will synchronise if the body is attempting regularity and then you can rely on your breaks according to where the pattern has been established. (Vitex may help promote this).

Elderly - start immediately, 5 day break each month or, if this is going to prove difficult such as in nursing homes, simply break from cream every weekend where possible. (I have many elderly women one 94 years of age enjoying the benefits from progesterone).

NOTE: Always consult with your medical practitioner particularly if you have bleeding concerns that extend beyond 4 months into progesterone therapy. In other words if the body has not settled. A handy checking point here is to have your iron levels and stores tested. Also an ultrasound (vaginal) to eliminate any potential problems such as Fibroids.

Why do women expect progesterone to fix all their problems?

I have listed many of the benefits of progesterone, so therefore it is only natural that women would expect progesterone to fix all their estrogen dominant symptoms. In the equation one must ask the question, why are they estrogen dominant in the first place and or progesterone deficient or both?

Hormonal imbalances masquerading in many problems such as estrogen dominance and/or progesterone deficiency may take many accumulative years to manifest and present themselves, often in insidious ways. As it took time to arrive at this point, it will take time to improve, reverse and eliminate many of these problems.

I have found that if women only have mild estrogen dominant symptoms, or have been estrogen dominant for only a short period of time, their likelihood of response to progesterone is going to be much faster than for someone who has been estrogen dominant over a number of years, or who may have other medical conditions, including over weight and auto-immune diseases.

Many women despair that the cream hasn't fixed them instantly and this is where persistence and commitment need to be embraced. Over the years I have found that many woman do not understand the functioning of their own bodies, let alone understand their hormonal and reproductive health. But intuitively they have sensed the inner answers and know there is a missing link to their hormonal health and wellbeing. Once they have discovered progesterone and started using it, it resonates with their body and it feels right.

Sadly, this is where I pick up the casualties. Women realise they have discovered their missing health links but do not know how to carry it through because of lack of education, understanding of their own bodies, and how to use progesterone successfully. You might also like to read my section on 'Why is the liver so important in hormone balancing?' and the use of nutritional supplementation explained in Book 2 Natural Progesterone More Secrets Revealed along with many strategies outlined in this book.

I've started taking progesterone and I feel awful. I want to stop using the cream.
Should I?

Progesterone therapy is complex. Not every woman reacts in the same way. Every woman's biochemistry and ability to absorb and use cream is different. Most, however, fall into two categories.

Those who experience an incredible response almost immediately - they feel fantastic and cannot get enough progesterone cream.

Then there are those who feel absolutely dreadful and believe the cream is actually making their condition worse. My introduction to this hormone, although I intuitively knew it was right, my experiences were horrific as I was experiencing Estrogen Dominance Wake Up Crisis and did not know about this. I spent a week in bed feeling like a beached whale, very fluid retentive and migrainal. No one had told me about the wake-up crisis and how to over-ride it and I experienced it full on. I bluffed my way through it to save face with my very distressed and concerned husband, who called into my lounge room two Doctors who were involved with my Hysterectomy to try and bring me back to my senses with this ludicrous "left field approach" changing directions and self treatment. Because the estrogen dominance crisis is such an unpleasant experience it gave me incentive to learn how to avoid or minimise those following in my foot steps. Thus the introduction of phytoestrogens and higher initial doses in the first 2 months. This is where I have adopted my principle that the first 8 weeks uninterrupted with higher doses can be of great value in the journey. Fortunately I was on a very premium cream which I obtained prior to it being removed from the market called "Renewed Balance". Because it was in a good strength it demonstrated how women could cope with higher capacities of doses in the first 8 weeks. This cream was used by many of the women with great success before our supplies dried up and legality took over our ability to purchase this cream.

Recognising the role phytoestrogens played in opposing estrogen dominance this is how I eventually came into association with Dr Sandra Cabot and her product Femme Phase, then in a powder form. Our group of women at my lounge room meetings trialled and tried nearly every phytoestrogen on the market and 90% of us could not surpass the ingredients contained in this product and the response we were achieving from using it. A chapter has been written specifically on estrogen dominance crisis and causes primary and secondary in Book 2 Natural Progesterone More Secrets Revealed. This deals with all aspects and management when estrogen dominance arises.

There are those that experience feelings of euphoria, however this will begin to taper off once your body has adjusted to the higher than usual progesterone levels in your body. Conversely, progesterone can actually 'wake up' your estrogen receptors, initially exacerbating various degrees of estrogen dominance (reports of feeling like a "beached whale", foggy, throbbing head, unable to get going).

Be mindful that progesterone and estrogen are a 'pigeon pair'. One compliments the other. Remove progesterone from the equation and you leave estrogen to dominate the hormonal environment. Eventually your estrogen receptors will compensate by 'tuning down'. But will continue to do havoc in your body unopposed.

This blunted response to estrogen is heightened when progesterone is added back into the body. Progesterone restores estrogen sensitivity resulting in what appears to be exacerbated estrogen dominance symptoms (NPAN refers to this activity as Estrogen Dominance Wake Up Crisis). This is perfectly normal, a good sign in fact that hormone imbalance is being treated. There is no need to suffer like we did in our ignorance. Increase your phytoestrogen and progesterone dosage.

Unusual things can happen when you start using progesterone and I suggest you journal it. Take notes because these signs and symptoms will be *idiosyncratic to your hormonal profile*. There have been various reports of itchy ears, sinusitis, breakthrough bleeding, tingling nipples, sore breasts, headaches, fluid retention, heavy periods, sore sinuses, phlegmy throat, increased diuresis (urinating), restorative sleeps to colour dreams. Some women have lost 1/2 a stone in a week mainly being fluid when they started progesterone.

Anything is possible when progesterone levels are being restored to normal physiological levels. Even accelerated aches and pains can indicate estrogen receptor wake-up symptoms. Give it at least ten days for the symptoms to subside. It can take some women two to three months to restore receptor sensitivity. Be warned that every woman has her own unique receptor 'wake-up' episode. You might be one of the lucky ones who suffers very little. If, however, the whole experience is becoming quite trying, hang in there. You'll turn the corner very soon ... and your body will definitely thank you for it in a few months time and years to come if this hormone is for you.

Another reason why women may feel awful on the cream is because many women fall into the trap of stopping their cream because they feel great and/or they forget to take it. They then find themselves back with the recurring symptoms because they haven't taken their cream consistently nor have they incorporated precautionary or maintenance steps to control their environmental estrogens and reduce their own estrogen impact on their body.

To maintain themselves on a stabilised level they need to continue to take their cream on physiological doses according to nature and cyclic events as nature intended, so they have progesterone always in their body to get the full benefits. Otherwise they end up with inconsistent levels and progesterone deficiency eventually reoccurs.

There are certain aspects we can't control such as the impact of our environment. We can, however, control our dose and application of progesterone. Stopping and starting, or random dosage is not the way you use this hormone. It will confuse the body, and may make you feel awful or just not give you the full mileage.

Another reason for progesterone ineffectiveness is some women stop every time they menstruate (could be twice a month) thus ending up deficient and following the menstrual cycle further out of synchronisation. Periods, if more than once a month should be ignored and progesterone usage continued right through to the break time or where the real period is due. These irregularities of periods are often what I refer to as the premenopausal dance. All the attempts to regulate a period will fail if the periods are not to be regulated, by this I mean menopause is nearing. The dance of these irregular unpredictable periods may go on for 12-18 months in some cases. So you can see breaking where the period dances are too frequent, can render you deficient or if you haven't had a period for some months you are over saturated with progesterone. Just keep a regular cyclic break happening regardless of the lengthening or shortening menses cycles (periods).

This needed to be *clarified* as some many women have been confused as to where to take a break knowing it should be in the bleeding time. (When mother nature does not have progesterone in the body). Bleeding irregularities has been dealt with extensively in Book 2 Natural Progesterone More Secrets Revealed.

Hormone imbalance is not about adding more progesterone and more estrogen. It is about balancing the hormones as nature intended. I am referring to physiological doses here. If your body already has high estrogen levels then you need to address your estrogen dominance separately to the issue of progesterone deficiency.

In many cases, women are already ovulating and producing normal physiological progesterone levels that would be enough to keep them well ... if they weren't estrogen dominant! Simply adding more cream can sometimes be a copout for taking some personal responsibility.

What happens if I am allergic to the cream, e.g. rash?

Some women have experienced a reaction to the cream ingredients (eg herbs, essential oils, nuts), but, if the cream is a pure micronised progesterone, the body will not react adversely, because it is a bio-identical molecule which is familiar and recognisable to the body.

That's why it is very important when you start the cream that you test the base, and apply to skin areas that are not sun altered (e.g. face, neck) or normally sensitive to chemicals.

Also don't put it on areas that are open to wounds or are prone to rashes, particularly the face if you have got acne or a tendency to butterfly mask etc.

Start off using it on areas that are unaffected and test your skin. If you continue to have a rash, stop the cream and question the ingredients. If you know you have an allergy to nuts, check on the contents that the oil used is not that particular nut oil (some creams have a Macadamia base). If you suspect it does, test the cream on a small area of skin on the inside of your wrist.

Please, do not apply to your throat as an adverse reaction could potentially lead to constriction of the airway (if you discover you are allergic to a particular ingredient in the cream base).

When is the best time to apply the cream and when do I start the cream?

What do you do now that you have your cream?

You can start your cream straight away in other words that morning or that night. This is if you are going to follow the program that a lot of the women have adopted when they first start progesterone therapy, which is using the cream uninterrupted for the first 6-8 weeks. In other words missing the first cycle (period) and taking a break on the second period or when it is due if you are not cyclic. This is covered in great depth in "Bleeding Irregularities" in Book 2 Natural Progesterone More Secrets Revealed.

Or you can start according to instructions usually this is from Day 12-26 or from what your medical practitioner has advised.

When you first start the cream it is best to **split the dose** to allow for approximately 24 hr progesterone coverage. The cream has, based on my observation, about an 8-11 hr influence on the body, therefore, if you split the dose into a morning and night application you are maximising the benefits of progesterone with a more even deliverance over 24 hours. The cream is best applied directly after showering when the pores are open.

Hormones are needed throughout the day and the night to do various jobs.

It is better to make your evening dose larger than your morning dose to facilitate a good night's sleep, and allow for maximum absorption during your resting phase. Some women find this 'relaxing' sensation slows them down too much during the day whilst others find it increases their energy levels.

There are those women who prefer a single morning dose claiming it assists them with stress management. So it's important to experiment and discover what levels work for you and when you prefer to take your cream.

As you become physiologically balanced and feeling more comfortable, having built up your progesterone reserves, you may wish to change your split dose (by now considerably lower) back to a single evening dose for more convenience (and sleep).

NATURAL PROGESTERONE-THE WORLD'S BEST KEPT SECRET

Where do I rub the cream?

For optimal results, the cream is rubbed onto thin skinned areas where blood vessels are closest to the skin's surface, rotating application around the body. This allows for optimal uptake and gets the progesterone into your blood stream quickly. *Avoid fat areas such as the stomach* as it will take longer for the cream to reach its sites of action. Breast tissue is not a fatty tissue but a very absorbable route as it is full of capillaries and rich blood supply.

The least effective areas will be the fatty areas of the buttocks, stomach (unless thin), outer thighs and generally where there is a store of fat, cellulite or poor blood circulation.

Why is this? It is a fat loving hormone, and being lipophilic it will go into the fat tissue and be stored until the blood vessels collect the hormone, sweeping it along and taking it to the progesterone receptors to deliver the messages. (See 'What is a Progesterone Receptor' in chapter 4, page 82).

If a woman has poor circulation, or poor lymphatic drainage, or is overweight where there may be low capillary density, the hormone's effectiveness is slowed down. For this reason, it is important to apply the cream closest to the blood vessels where it can be transported around the body to latch itself onto receptors to work more effectively. Soles of feet, hands, temples, vagina and breasts are fast absorption areas.

I have had women who have applied to their buttocks and fatty abdomen and have experienced delayed results with progesterone for months on end, simply because this fat-loving hormone sat in fat tissue, or their very sluggish circulation delayed the uptake. Be aware that areas where you tend to 'store' body fat is not an ideal location for cream application. Where you can see blood vessels - perfect!

I advise that you rotate your progesterone application around the body, alternating different locations daily. The larger the area of skin the cream is spread on, the greater the absorption. Rotation allows for rejuvenation of the receptor sites, thus obtaining optimal benefits. It also nourishes the skin usually because it has Vitamin E in it.

There are areas that are particularly good such as the palms of the hands, soles of the feet, inside of the arms (not the armpit), inside of the thighs, neck, chest and breast where tissue has a high capillary density allowing for efficient absorption. Any area that tends to 'flush' indicates blood vessels are close to the surface.

Other very receptive areas that respond to progesterone are directly over the ovaries, behind the knees, on the temples, back of the neck, back pelvic ligaments, joints and inside of wrists. Save a little extra and apply to areas of pain (except during breaks). A little dab under the eyes for gritty, dry eyes will work wonders. You will be amazed how it will help with pain management, particularly joints, knees, headaches, and stress points also some over varicose veins.

Do not wash the skin for at least an hour after applying, even though a good cream should allow the micronised molecule to absorb through the base and through the skin pores and into the blood within minutes.

Some tips myself and women have found useful in cream application:

- Applying cream just before bedtime and taking some Magnesium supplements will induce a very deep and restful sleep.

- For fibrocystic breasts and tenderness rub some cream over breasts twice a day (not during your breaks) until pain subsides and breast tissue softens and returns to normal.

- It pays to carry a spare tube or jar in your handbag for management of stress, hot flushes, anxiety, or headaches. Dab on temples or back of neck hourly.

- If you're suffering joint or muscle pain, or tender varicose veins, apply cream to that area causing you discomfort.

- For ovarian pain, a little dab over the ovaries can provide relief, (try hourly, may need a few applications).

- For period pain and the dragging down feeling of the back ligaments apply cream regularly to these sites, especially if you have Endometriosis.

- For sore soles of feet in the morning and Restless Leg Syndrome apply to soles of feet on bedtime.

The women continue to discover new ways and means of maximising progesterone application.

What is the right dose for me?

Ideally, the least amount of progesterone cream needed to resolve your estrogen dominance symptoms is your correct dose. It's up to you to figure out how you're going to achieve your monthly dosing goal. Just remember, even if you don't match the daily doses exactly, your body will continue to steadily release progesterone into the bloodstream. So breathe easy ... the sky isn't going to fall if you fail to get it right every time.

But it is important to know how much progesterone is contained in your tub or tube of cream. If you don't know, it is important that you find out from your supplier. Application and Instructions should be included with your container of progesterone.

Instructions should include the strength (mg or %) that is being delivered per application. Only with this information can you make sense of the recommendations/ observations.

Just remember, you can have too much progesterone in your body! Balance is the key. Charting and score sheets will guide you in your response and dosage requirements, according to your symptoms, thus enabling you to determine whether you require an increase or a reduction. Please note this is not a medical book it is the opinion of myself and other women using progesterone.

(Refer back to Stages of Natural Progesterone's Action in the Body page 138)

When do I have a break from my cream?

In the first 2 months a woman can actually go through without a break as the body is usually very deprived of progesterone, and a majority of the hormone is being soaked up into fat tissue. This is also the reason why a higher dose is well tolerated.

Not breaking from cream in the first 6-8 weeks will not, from observation, adversely affect your periods. You will continue to get your period with possibly a break through bleed or period as well. And it's likely, during this time, you will still be estrogen dominant. In fact, double doses help negate the estrogen wake-up promoted by the introduction of progesterone back into the body which stimulates the estrogen already present in your body and may exacerbate your symptoms.

After 8 weeks, it is advisable to establish a rhythmic pattern back into your body. So it's important you begin taking a break from cream (as saturation has most likely been achieved around this time). This is also the time when weaning back to physiological doses can be initiated, as determined by symptom relief and charting. *Don't be too anxious to wean back too fast, this process may take 7-12 months,* but remember you cannot stay on high doses indefinitely as the receptors will down regulate.

A break from cream must now be taken to fall into line with your menstrual cycles, i.e., a menopausal woman would follow a calendar pattern of 3 weeks on, 1 week off; a cycling woman would follow a program of 2 weeks on cream, 2 weeks off according to her period.

This is the aim - to achieve balance using progesterone on physiological doses ('least is best' principle) such that symptoms are relieved. However, be mindful of the fact you could take many months to a year to achieve hormone balance and maintain the appropriate breaks from cream without feeling the absence and/or deprivation of progesterone.

Remember it is so important to have at least a 3 day break in order to restore receptor sensitivity. To do otherwise is to risk losing the full effectiveness of your progesterone cream (down-regulates).

If you cannot achieve lengthy breaks when you first start progesterone therapy, work towards increasing the breaks each month. When a woman is 'progesterone balanced' she can take 1-2 weeks break without discomfort. (Refer to Stages of Natural Progesterone Action in the Body). With recent hysterectomised and tubal ligations procedures 3-5 days break may be as much as can be tolerated and even with women suffering from severe hot flushes.

Barometers that may indicate progesterone overuse and the need to adjust dosage:

Some of the 'hormonal' barometers reported by women indicating the need to make adjustments are listed below. But of course every woman is unique and will have her own hormonal template once she starts charting. The breast is a good example of how to monitor dosage as I will explain:

Breast changes

Breasts are a fantastic barometer to guide you with your hormonal balancing. In fact, many women use their breasts to assess their progesterone dosage. If women are using too much progesterone after they have had a period of balance, they may experience itching, tingling, or soreness of the nipples.

Breast engorgement, a feeling of fullness, a dull ache, or general breast tenderness appears to be the first indication to women to reduce their dosage. If symptoms are relieved upon reduction of dosage after 2 days, then you know you're on the right track. Don't confuse these symptoms and reduce progesterone if your period is due.

Clearly, your breasts are extremely responsive to hormone fluctuations, some more than others. If you're one of these women, allow your breast messages to help you fine-tune your hormones. Learn to listen to your body.

Other physical barometers of overuse or under use

- Period changes - ranging from heavy, or sign of clotting, slight spotting.
- Sinusitis - women complain of sinus or hay fever-like symptoms, often indicating the re-emergence of estrogen dominance.
- Return of headaches - fogginess, tight band around the head, scalp tension
- Fluid retention - puffy ankles
- Re-emergence of sleep disorders - waking at 2am - 4am very common
- Hot flushing
- Vertigo
- Unexplained muscle/joint pain
- Sense of uneasiness - apprehension, anxiety, panic attacks, quick to tears, slight depression

Other things to be aware of:

From observation, because of the need to address so many problems with **progesterone, overdosing inside 7 months is rarely experienced providing there is a genuine need for progesterone supplementation.**

Generally, it takes about 12 months for a woman to really master her hormonal profile and achieve balance. For this reason, I urge women to not pre-judge their results on progesterone inside this timeframe.

When I talk about the need to reduce dosage, this usually applies to women who've been on progesterone at high levels for more than 7 months and may not have adjusted dosage according to the reduction of their estrogen dominance symptoms. High doses tend to frighten some women in their initial stages of progesterone, and subsequently their dosage is inadequate. Most instructions recommend 25-30mg so it is understandable that when in the initial stages of using progesterone women can be frightened to go any higher in dosage and often around about 64mg dose is required in the first couple of months to override Estrogen Dominance Wake Up Crisis. Women tolerate quite comfortably 100-200mg in the earlier stages for instance if they are suffers of migraines, Fibroids and heavy bleeding.

If you are on minimal doses in the initial stages for example physiological recommended doses of 16-20mg you may find that this is not enough to get initial benefits and it may take months to arrive at a point where your progesterone is working to its optimum. It also may be a dose that is inadequate for the level of your estrogen dominance but enough to tease and aggravate the estrogen receptors.

When should I use less progesterone?

Now that you've been on the cream for at least 4-7 months, reassess your charts and your symptoms will determine your dosage. As symptoms are relieved, your dosage should be reduced, working towards the 'least is best' principle. Reduction should be according to the condition you are treating and how you respond. Use your monthly score sheet to monitor dosage reduction according to reduction of symptoms. (Print off charts from the website.) Refer to charts on pages 327, 328.

If women do not adjust dosage accordingly upon symptom relief but instead maintain a high dose regardless, then the benefits of progesterone may actually wear off and symptoms possibly creep back in and estrogen dominant crisis which may reoccur which I address at great length in Book 2 Natural Progesterone More Secrets Revealed.

For the uninformed woman, her automatic response might be to increase dosage seeking to reclaim that initial euphoric state she first experienced on progesterone. Or by not adjusting progesterone accordingly she has either accidentally down-regulated her progesterone receptors or stimulated more estrogen production pushing her body back into estrogen dominance.

Once you are asymptomatic, I recommend you use the LEAST amount of progesterone possible to keep your symptoms under control. I personally believe the optimum dose for women falling into the non cyclic and not in the fertility/ovulation category, it is more effective to work on a comfortable minimum base dose and take shorter breaks, (minimum 3 days), rather than larger doses and longer breaks.

How would I know if I have to use more progesterone?

To understand and appreciate the full context of this question, you need to read the above question "When Should I Use Less Progesterone".

If reducing dosage doesn't help or perhaps increases discomfort, then it indicates the need to increase your progesterone dosage, and pay particular attention to increasing your intake of phytoestrogens to oppose estrogen dominance crisis.

This situation of estrogen wakeup often follows an episode of stress which would account for the shortage of progesterone and the increase of estrogen levels. Drop progesterone back to your previous dose once balance has been achieved and symptoms have subsided.

To summarise both questions, when to use more and when to use less, you have to address why you require dosage adjustments. Are you becoming more estrogen dominant or hormonally imbalanced from over use or under use?

SUMMARY OF DOSE ADJUSTMENTS:

General rule: to test if you have too much progesterone or not enough?

Estrogen dominance as a result of too much progesterone is if a women has had months of no symptoms (asymptomatic) and is on a higher than required maintenance dose and symptoms re-emerge. She also could have failed to have taken her regular cyclic breaks. If this is the case of these two examples and symptoms are starting to re-emerge this is what I classify as Estrogen Dominance Wake Up Crisis. To test this out reduce dose dramatically for 24-36 hours and if symptoms start reducing, you know you need to reduce your dose. It also may pay you to have a 7-12 day break when due to clean out the reserves in your body and freshen up the receptors.

Progesterone Deficiency this is when there is too little progesterone and a need to increase, again if you feel worse with the reduction 24-36 hour testing points. If this is the case increase your dosage over the next 24-36 hours to saturate your body and assess. The calming plateau will be the right dose.

What can cause progesterone shortage?

One of the biggest players in robbing progesterone supplies and creating hormone imbalance can be STRESS, pulling progesterone into another steroid pathway to create the 'survival' hormones - cortisol and adrenalin.

If there has been stress, high pain levels, shock, trauma, surgery, illness, or unresolved emotional issues, chances are there is a progesterone deficiency in the body requiring higher levels of progesterone cream to help compensate temporarily.

When high cortisol is present in the body (our anti-inflammatory hormones) there is a competition between progesterone and cortisol for the same receptor's sites, so higher-than-usual levels of progesterone are required, to compete for these same receptors.

Progesterone has a calmative effect and anti-stressor influence thus helping to address the stress itself, reducing the need for continued high cortisol production. Reducing stress allows the opportunity for progesterone to work its benefits in the body once again.

You can apply more cream until you reach an emotional equilibrium, that place where you begin to feel an inner sense of wellbeing and calmness, in spite of your physical symptoms (that could take a few days to settle, even a month).

But, of course, the most reliable way to ascertain whether you need more or less progesterone is to do a hormonal saliva assay. Particularly if you are struggling to re-establish balance with dosage versus symptoms. Check if your low levels match symptoms.

I include here for your benefit an email addressed to NPAN that I believe typifies the scenario we commonly face. It highlights many issues.

"... think the burning sensation is flushes, they settled down for a little while when I first started taking progesterone (13 months ago) they happen if I'm stressed, hurrying or concentrating hard, and always if I have a drink.

I usually have anywhere between 18 and 24 day cycles, used to start the cream around day 11 but have started lately around day 7 or 8 so I get enough days in with the cream. I use between 1 and 1.5 cm per day at night. I originally used a little more but used to get teary and emotional and sore boobs, so cut it back a bit. (1.5cm in this case equivalent to 16-24mg.)

Decided estriol cream would be the go, because after doing some reading it seems the *other 2 estrogens are more likely to cause cancers*, and from what I can understand **estriol doesn't** and it also has some cancer protection, so I thought that since estrogen is supposed to stop the flushes, (which it seems to for other women) maybe I might be a bit estrogen-deficient and that it would be the safest one to take, if that makes any sense!

So if that was the way to see if it would help, I was wondering if you knew where to get a cream that wasn't synthetic, Dr ... has tubes of estrodiol, but I don't really want to use that, because I'm not sure if my problem is that I am estrogen-deficient.

Diet hasn't changed much, only that I have given up milk in my numerous cups of tea that I usually drink each day and have limited the amount of cheese and butter to very little - over last few weeks - but the red/purple face has really been an on-going thing for 4-5 years, just become very frequent and severe lately.

I am 48. *Tubes tied*. Never taken pill. Same soap. Skin not itchy, has always been a bit dry. Hormonal health, much better since going on the progesterone, don't have the PMT and long sleepless nights like I used to ... Julie"

Firstly, 'Julie' does not understand 'hot flushes', she hasn't mastered the use of progesterone nor has she completely understood the role of progesterone in her body. Julie probably doesn't realise that progesterone therapy works in stages, and often needs reassessing at 12 months to re-evaluate dosage according to symptoms. Given that Julie is 48 years old with a history of tubal ligation and PMS, in my opinion I believe she needs to increase her dose because clearly 16-20mg (1.0-1.5cm) is not addressing and settling her hormone fluctuations.

I don't believe Julie has incorporated phytoestrogens into her diet which would help stimulate estrogenic benefits and sensitise progesterone receptors. She has attempted to reduce saturated fats from her diet (dairy products) but has not, to my knowledge, increased her intake of essential oils (Omega 3-6).

In the past, Julie's experience of estrogen dominance symptoms such as tears, emotional and sore boobs led her to believe she should reduce her dosage. While this may have worked in the past, the dose level is obviously not holding her any longer. She needs to increase her dose, and be prepared to work through the estrogen dominance wake-up barrier until her symptoms abate. Her tubal ligation is now taking its toll as her hormones are being severally compromised as her ovaries are flagging with age.

By incorporating nutritional supplements in conjunction with liver work, she will go a long way to restoring hormone balance and fine-tuning her cream dosage to suit her individual profile. Julie can become more aware of these subtle hormonal changes through charting and comparison.

I wouldn't recommend estrogen supplementation until Julie has maximised the benefits of progesterone and, if there is a deficiency confirmed by blood tests and saliva assays and continued hot flushes in spite of progesterone increase, then and only then consider estrogen supplementation. Clearly the doctor prescribing and supplying cream has very little understanding and, through lack of support, has left Julie no choice but to self-medicate and seek out answers elsewhere.

I suggest you refer to 'NPAN's Formula for Hormone Harmony'.

Are there any side effects using natural progesterone?

The Drug Information Sheet (Chapter 15) for natural progesterone reads: "Adverse Reactions ... because progesterone creams contain the hormone identical to that produced by the human ovary, side effects are usually minimal.

If experienced these may include breast tenderness and swelling, fluid retention or slight vaginal bleeding. Dizziness, nausea, fatigue, headaches and light headedness have been reported occasionally and usually disappear with adjustment of dose..."

NPAN, whilst aware of this information, rarely sees cases where there is not a logical explanation for the abovementioned side effects. Most of these symptoms are interpreted as Estrogen Dominance Wake Up Crisis where the introduction of progesterone is 'waking up' and stimulating the estrogen receptors exacerbating the estrogen effects in the body and symptoms do subside in most cases. In the presence of both hormones the ratio difference variants is reduced, enabling a more balanced body with less symptoms and of course reducing estrogen having the dominant control.

However these side effects may occur in cases of long-term use at high doses when not indicated and where breaks from cream have not been adhered to, or where inferior creams have been used. I talk about this throughout my books, and provide techniques for overcoming estrogen dominance with the use of progesterone.

Like any drug it has side effects, good and bad. However, 'bad' in the case of progesterone does not indicate 'dangerous'. Progesterone, being bio-identical, has a huge safety margin in the body with which to work within.

For argument's sake, a woman could apply a dose of 400mg progesterone (similar to levels of a pregnant woman in her last trimester), and perhaps experience a state of relaxation and drowsiness. This dosage would not represent a risk to her health even though the recommended physiological dose is 15-20mg, imitating the output of the ovaries at ovulation.

This demonstrates the enormous flexibility of drug dosage levels, and its relative safety factor. I do not recommend that you slap on 400mg of progesterone cream, but simply pointing out that should extra cream be necessary to treat your symptoms, it's not going to harm or jeopardise your health, particularly when your body is using the progesterone you are applying.

In Australia, regardless of its good safety record and extremely low toxicity, and being used for years in women's cosmetics, progesterone is still classified an 'S4 poison' because of the category it falls under rather than its drug characteristics.

As previously mentioned it has a huge safety margin, therefore, if you were to overdose you would probably go to sleep. In earlier years they used to use progesterone intravenously to control epilepsy with children so we know it has natural sedation effect.

Long periods of progesterone use without breaks can actually tone down the receptors and make the progesterone sites ineffective, creating estrogen dominant symptoms again. If the situation has occurred where progesterone has become ineffective, a break may be advisable for a month or two to restore and freshen up (up regulate) the receptor sites. (Or change your route of administration)

When you first start using Natural Progesterone cream you can start getting estrogen dominant symptoms (e.g. headaches, breakthrough bleeding because it is waking up the estrogen receptor sites). These will usually pass once your dosage initially opposes this "wake up" stage.

So don't worry too much if that happens the first month or two. It is your body re-acquainting itself with progesterone. It is also stimulating the estrogen. Even though you have the estrogen in your body, it is making you aware of the activity - it is more pronounced. The simple way of understanding this is to imagine your body has just become deafened to estrogen and progesterone wakes it up.

I suggest this is a time to take a lot of phytoestrogens to counteract the estrogen wake-up period. This also can happen when you have had a break. It is a good sign that things are working, that the estrogen has been stimulated again and that progesterone is taking some effect on your body.

I again remind you that progesterone and estrogen sensitise each other thereby maximising their impact on the body. Either hormone out of balance will cause the other to tone down. They need to act like a partnership and needs each others presence to be effective in a positive way.

I have been on progesterone and it is not working. Why would this be?

- The cream may not contain progesterone at all
- Poor quality cream or in the wrong base
- Unrealistic expectations of progesterone as a magic bullet
- Inconsistent usage

- Failure to take breaks to avoid down regulation of receptors
- Unrealistic timing
- Lack of knowledge or information
- Incorrect usage and dosage
- Certain drugs which inhibit or are counteracting the effects of progesterone
- A dysfunctional liver / fatty liver / overweight/Syndrome X
- Not specifically tailored to address chronic long-standing conditions like FMS, CFS, Endometriosis, Diabetes, PCOS, chronic stress
- Very tired adrenals (adrenal exhaustion) or malfunctioning thyroid
- Inability to absorb (inappropriate cream base, poor skin absorption)
- Insidious factors unknown impeding assimulation/performance/utilisation
- Diseases with unknown interaction to progesterone therapy
- You may not require progesterone replacement therapy
- Poor circulation, sluggish lymphatic drainage, non cellular response
- Lack of appropriate vitamin and mineral supplementation and essential fatty acids
- Lack of adequate use of phytoestrogens, poor diet/malnourishment
- Lack of estrogen if genuine deficiency - as maybe the case with very thin women

I feel nauseous on progesterone, why is this?

The experience reported is likened to morning sickness commonly experienced in the early stages of pregnancy. The reintroduction of progesterone creating hormone fluctuation can bring on this nauseous feeling, particularly in the first few days. If so, cut dosage right back and gently use small amounts until the feeling passes. Then increase as your body adjusts. Usually the feeling of nausea subsides within 10 days. In my experience with my consultancy about 1 in 100 women experience this phenomena when starting progesterone. The onset is rapid. They also may feel very queasy.

Experiences of nausea, nearly always indicates liver dysfunction, or a history of Liver Disease such as hepatitis. A minor few may not have either nor have experienced morning sickness whilst pregnant. Whatever the reasons it indicates a high priority and the need to support this organ. The dysfunctional liver cannot tolerate and cope too well with the introduction of a new hormone (even one that is natural to the body). These women usually react quite violently to HRT. Please read next question.

Observation confirms that these women suffering poor liver function are candidates for progesterone supplementation after years of deficiency, problems which compound into conditions like FMS, CFS, chronic Endometriosis, adrenal exhaustion, other auto-immune problems.

Use progesterone in these cases with sensitivity and a program that incorporates steady increases in dosage over time. I suggest you start with very small doses (less than 10mg). You can expect to experience in 2-3 weeks time an estrogen dominance wakeup.

The liver should cope now to higher doses. This is when you may need to increase or double your dose to override wakeup symptoms. The receptors would have been stimulated slowly and have taken their time to response (usually because the conditions stated above often have slow, sluggish cell receptablity).

The small doses have been enough to tickle and tease the estrogen receptors to wake them up but the progesterone doses (tolerated) have not been adequate enough to oppose and over-ride estrogen levels and this hormone's effects in the body.

Some women who have experienced levels of nausea on progesterone are nervous and reluctant to increase their dose.

Nonetheless, it is important to emphasise that the dose they are currently sitting on is actually creating estrogen dominance problems like headaches, fluid retention, feelings of PMS. Contrary to what one lady was told, nausea is NOT caused by using cream through a period (she was only 3 weeks into her program suffering from Endometriosis).

Favourable outcomes result from going beyond this barrier of estrogen dominance. It is suggested from other women's feedback you try an extra 1-2% dose and assess how you feel. But pull back if you experience extreme nausea. The objective at the end of the day is to treat your symptoms with progesterone.

If low doses aren't resolving your health issues, you need to push forward onto a high dose. With a good liver program in place, women are surprised how well they can now tolerate appropriate doses to treat their problems (achieve saturation) before pulling back to physiological doses.

Please see why the liver is an integral part of hormone balancing in 'I have been on a diet and cannot lose weight. Why would this be?' and also read 'Stages of Natural Progesterone's Action In The Body'. It is my experience and observation that people with liver dysfunction and sluggish metabolism experience delayed stages. Refer also to 'Cleansing & Detoxification' - Resources. (The Body Shaping Diet Book, Dr. Sandra Cabot and the Liver Cleansing Diet Book). In Book 2 Natural Progesterone More Secrets Revealed - Liver Tonics in the Nutritional section and strategies are dealt with.

Why is the liver important for hormone balancing?

The liver is where the body makes the building blocks for your hormones (from cholesterol), which it gets from foods rich in essential fatty acids Omega 3,6 & 9. That is why they are called essential fats. See the diagram of the steroid pathway on page 79.

The liver is also the organ that breaks down the excess hormones as part of the body's balancing of the hormonal (endocrine) systems.

These detoxifying systems in the liver are easily overloaded. If you have excess of synthetic hormones, or hormone-like compounds (e.g. xenoestrogens) in your body, then the natural balancing of your hormonal system is lost. Fat soluble toxins such as xenoestrogens if not eliminated accumulate in fatty organs e.g. endocrine glands, resulting in symptoms of hormonal imbalances such as estrogen dominance, Infertility, sexual dysfunction, breast pain, menstrual disturbances, adrenal gland exhaustion and early menopause.

It is vital you maintain your liver's health, so that it can adequately cope with the metabolism that your body needs it to do. The healthier your liver, the easier your rebalancing of your hormones (thereby reducing estrogen dominance and weight problems) associated with hormone imbalance.

In summary, the liver helps make and metabolise your hormones and maintain them in a state of balance. If your liver is dysfunctional so are your hormones, not to mention your possible weight problems.

A woman with a fatty, dysfunctional liver will require far greater dosages of progesterone perhaps with minimal benefits. She may also be intolerant to progesterone initially and may feel quite nauseous. (See above question).

Many women fall into the trap of believing that taking Silybum Marianum (St Mary's Thistle) and Taurine supplements are adequate to detox a sluggish liver.

NPAN always advises women to get their hands on a premium formulation that contains the necessary vitamins, herbs and essential nutrients to facilitate removal of toxins and the burning of fat from the liver itself. I recommend Health Directions Liver Tone Plus which the women have found to be beneficial perhaps due to the high quality and exceptional ingredients that are required to perform the phase 1 and phase 2 detoxification pathway.

(Books I recommend to read "The Liver Cleansing Diet", "The Body Shaping Diet" & "The Healthy Liver & Bowel" books by Dr. Sandra Cabot) Please visit www.liverdoctor.com website.

Can I treat hormonal imbalance with nutritional and diet plan strategies alone?

There are three scenarios to consider:

1. If using your cream without nutrition or supplementation.

I have always tried to present progesterone with balance and acknowledge that progesterone is not a silver bullet. It is not the answer to every health issue and problem a woman might encounter. Some women mistakenly think that using progesterone will resolve all their health issues without the need to do anything else other than apply the cream.

I have always emphasised to women that progesterone in itself will not work effectively or to its maximum benefits without the support of some nutrition fundamentals and a good eating plan in place.

However, if a woman is truly progesterone deficient she may still derive benefits from progesterone alone, given the numerous roles it plays throughout the body. It just won't perform to maximum capacity and potential.

If a woman is estrogen dominant by virtue of the fact she is overweight and/or exposed to xenoestrogen in her environment progesterone will have some benefit, but she will not realise sustained improvement - largely because progesterone cannot negate obesity or constant exposure to foreign estrogens without attention to these existing problems and the state of the liver.

2. If using nutrition and diet without using progesterone.

If a woman is reluctant to use hormone supplementation and instead tackles hormone imbalance with phytoestrogens, a Wild Yam cream, a good diet and health plan, exercise regimes, a liver support & detoxification program, etc., she will possibly achieve hormonal harmony without progesterone. Incorporation of herbs such as Vitex or Macca have proved to be very beneficial in substitution of progesterone in some women, restoring hormone function.

Women who may not require progesterone therapy.

Healthy women who are ovulating women that are not in adrenal exhaustion who exercise and are not overweight, and women who do not display estrogen dominant, progesterone deficient symptoms.

I often suggest that women who are considered low risk and possibly do not require hormone replacement therapy try this strategy first before introducing hormones into their body because there's a likelihood their hormonal function is perhaps toned down. Their adrenals might be exhausted, and with the right nutrition and eating plan the body can crank up itself and hormone balance be restored, along with improved overall metabolism. Omega 3,6 & 9 in ratio balance are also vital plus rest, sleep and liver work.

3.Women using progesterone with nutritional supplementation.

I have, however, observed a common thread throughout all these different types of scenarios: that progesterone works brilliantly with a good eating plan and nutritional program, outweighing progesterone usage, or nutrition on its own.

Conversely, it is not uncommon to speak with women who have incorporated nutrition, diet, stress relief, exercise and so forth searching for that elusive feeling of wellbeing, only to discover that, for these women, the missing link is actually progesterone. Is this perhaps because it's our 'essence' hormone? Many women find their way to me after years under a Naturopath or Nutritionalist because they have not had the progesterone link to complete the totality of their well-being.

For those of you who have been very frightened, put off, or in the past disgruntled about using nutritional products purely because you felt it was a marketing con, it had not proved beneficial, or perhaps you hadn't seen the results, please don't give up or abandon the idea completely. Chances are you didn't have the missing piece to the jigsaw. I didn't!

Yes, progesterone can work without nutritional support. However, if you want the best mileage out of your progesterone cream, incorporate nutritional supplements, exercise and a balanced diet.

For some women a good diet, lifestyle modifications and nutritional supplements can be enough to rebalance their body and keep them symptom free. After all, natural hormone replacement therapy may not be for everyone.

I always err on the side of caution with young teenagers in hormonal disarray. All avenues must be explored before progesterone therapy is administered in my opinion.

See: Women who are considered low risk and possibly do not require hormone replacement therapy, page 350.

CHAPTER 10

Contra indications with progesterone and the most asked questions with other medications and treatment.

- *What drugs are not compatible with progesterone supplementation (or contra-indicated)?*

- *Caution /consideration when using medications in conjunction with progesterone*

- *Most Asked Questions in relation to other medical treatments*

- *Will progesterone increase my blood pressure and interfere with my blood pressure tablets?*

- *Can I take progesterone while I'm on my anti-depressant drugs?*

- *Can I take progesterone while I'm on thyroid medication?*

- *Can I take Tamoxifen and progesterone at the same time?*

- *Can I take progesterone through chemotherapy treatment?*

- *Can I take my bone building drugs such as Fosamax and Raloxifine (Evista) with progesterone?*

What drugs are not compatible with progesterone supplementation (or contra-indicated)?

Contraception (Refer page 346)**:**

Conventional hormone contraceptives that contain the progestins/progestogens:
Levonorgestrel
Norethisterone
Cyproterone

Mini Pill
Levonorgestrel (Microlut/Microval)
Norethisterone (Micronor/Noriday)

Progestin Depots
Medroxyprogesterone (Depo-Provera/ Depo-Ralovera)
Etonogestrel (Implanon)
Levonorgestrel (Mirena) a hormone releasing IUD

Emergency Contraception
Levonorgestrel (Postinor)

Hormone Replacement Therapy (Refer page 347)
Medroxyprogesterone (Provera/ Ralovera)
Norethisterone (Primolut N)
Estrogen/ Progestin combinations
Equine estrogens with progestins
Estrogen patches with progestins
Dydrogesterone (Duphaston)
Tibolone (Livial)

Other Steroid compounds
Prednisolone
Prednisone
Cortisone Acetate
Cortisone based analgesics or injections

Synthetic progestogens/progestins compete with natural progesterone for the same progesterone receptor site, negating progesterone benefits. This also includes estrogen/progestogen combinations. *Estrogen patches on their own can be used with natural progesterone.* Refer to sections on Estrogen.(Chapters 16 & 17, and page 347). However if estrogen is being administered higher levels of progesterone are required.

Some of the women in our group on Natural Progesterone cream have resorted to using the Morning After Pill. It has been observed that women experience a huge backwards step as a result of the high levels of progestogens introduced into the body, short term. I personally would prefer this, to continual use of the pill. This has enabled women to use progesterone and derive benefits despite a small setback.

The effects have varied with each woman. I cannot determine how long it takes for the progestogens to move off the receptor sites to allow progesterone access once again. Women have asked me if they should stop progesterone when using The Morning After Pill, and I suggest they continue on with progesterone supplementation as usual, otherwise it could cause a greater disruption to their cycles. You might like to refer to the section on 'Fertility / Infertility / Contraception / Postnatal Depression', on pages 225, 283, 306 and 'Side effects of HRT and O.C.P.' on page 346.

Caution /consideration when using medications in conjunction with progesterone

Some medications may interfere with the progesterone effect. To date, I don't have sufficient information to determine the level of interaction with these medications. Women frequently ask if their medication can be taken in conjunction with progesterone. This is why it is imperative you refer back to your GP and the list above.

I am not a medical professional and this information came from various sources in my own observation and my husband's knowledgeable input on drugs. It is for information purposes only and is not a prescription for your particular needs. Consult with your health care professional if in doubt or if you have questions. I do not diagnose or try to overrule the advice of your health care professional.

Most Asked Questions in relation to other medical treatments

Will progesterone increase my blood pressure and interfere with my blood pressure tablets?

Progesterone can be used with your anti-hypertensive drugs but must be done with strict supervision of your doctor and regular check ups and regular blood pressure testing. Again, progesterone helps to eliminate the fluid retention aspect of the body because it is actually negating the estrogenic effects of sodium retention.

Too much estrogen will cause fluid to be retained in the body. With the addition of progesterone, it reduces the amount of estrogen and the effects of retention, thereby often reducing the blood pressure in the body (progesterone also exerts an anti-spasmodic influence of blood vessels).

It is emphasised that blood pressure changes may be due to physiological effects or other reasons and not to self medicate because of high blood pressure. Reports have indicated that the reduction of anti-hypertensive drugs have been necessary over a period of time under the doctor's supervision purely because their blood pressure has been restored to normal. Do not take yourself off your medication. Work with your Doctor.

Addition to hypertension: There is a potential interaction with progesterone and the group of medications known as BETA BLOCKERS. This interaction may cause an increase in the resistance to blood flow in the hands and feet. The result may be an increase in the side effects of the beta blocker, especially the cold hands and feet. I stress that there have NOT been reports of this effect as yet, but the potential is there. You are referred to the **Mercuro article** in our 'Medical References' pages 420-423. For more information, Book 2 covers anti hypertensives that actually increase hot flushing and other options.

I suggest also that you work seriously on your liver and weight (if over) to assist reduction of blood pressure, cholesterol and also look at the possibility of Syndrome X.

Can I take progesterone while I'm on my anti-depressant drugs?

Yes you can. Again I emphasise that anyone on any form of medication and using progesterone should be under the supervision and the monitoring of their doctor.

Many women have found after seven months on progesterone they feel the inclination to start weaning off their anti-depressants over a period of a few months, under the supervision of their doctor, and have had excellent results in maintaining a state of anti-depression. For others, if they qualify, testosterone has helped tremendously in cases of depression.

They also have found that once coming off their anti-depressant drugs, often their libido and sex drive have also improved because a lot of the anti-depressants have also suppressed a lot of their libido and/or an ability to be sexually aroused or orgasm. Not all anti-depressants have done this, but overall a lot have had this common denominator.

Some anti-depressants may impair the functioning of the limbic brain including the hypothalamus which may affect the menstrual cycle. One of our ladies who had been on progesterone for several months, having achieved wonderful results, began to experience anxiety of unknown origin. Her doctor put her on low doses of an anti-depressant drug which completely destroyed her libido and was unable to experience sexual stimulation and orgasm and her hot flushes returned with a vengeance.

One and a half weeks into the medication, she experienced migraines for 3 days, constant nausea, her breasts became swollen, night sweats, break through bleeding, and she started neglecting herself. This lady has a history of severe liver damage from substance abuse.

Hormone balance had been achieved through the use of natural progesterone, complimentary nutritional supplementation and diet. Clearly, her body could not cope with any form of medication that would put workload back on her liver, throwing out her finely tuned hormone balance. Within a week of stopping medication, her progesterone kicked back in and hormone balance was restored.

Can I take progesterone while I'm on thyroid medication?

If you have been diagnosed with a thyroid problem, and you are on thyroid medication, and now want to incorporate natural progesterone into your regime, there's no reason why you can't providing you do so under the strict supervision of your treating physician.

Progesterone may increase the effects of thyroxine leading to hyperthyroidism. Normal T3 and T4 levels with elevated TSH suggests impaired thyroid hormone activity rather than insufficiency. Periodical TSH testing should be adopted on initiation or progesterone treatment in these patients.

Please do not stop your thyroid medication because you have read that progesterone helps thyroid function. Your thyroid dosage, however, may require regular adjustment as progesterone exerts an influence upon the thyroid gland. Correcting estrogen dominance may not correct your thyroid function. Estrogen is believed to protein bound the thyroxine thus rendering it unavailable for the body to use appropriately thus the cold hands, feet experienced by hormonally imbalanced women.

The thyroid gland function can be improved with trace minerals such as selenium, iodine, zinc and manganese. (I recommend a synergistic formulation).

If you are unsure whether your thyroid is functioning optimally that can be characterised by an inability to lose weight, puffy and swollen body appearance, lethargy, muscle weakness, dry skin, hair loss and constipation, I suggest BEFORE resorting to progesterone to fix these problems you might be well advised to ask your doctor to order the appropriate tests. This includes blood profile to measure the levels of both thyroid hormones, T4 and T3, and also TSH (Thyroid Stimulating Hormone).

A shortage of T4 would be administered in the form of thyroxine tablets (T3 medication may also be required). In the USA, thyroid replacement therapy is available in cream form by way of natural thyroid hormone replacement using bio-identical hormones. See Dr Sandra Cabot's USA website address in chapter 22, page 408.

Can I take Tamoxifen and progesterone at the same time?

Tamoxifen is prescribed to women for the treatment of Breast Cancer. Tamoxifen is sufficiently estrogenic to cause endometrial hyperplasia as the action of Tamoxifen specifically targets to block specific estrogen effects on breast tissue. As such, progesterone will block this effect.

Women report some terrible side effects while taking Tamoxifen such as hot flushes, and get great results once they go on progesterone therapy, which takes about 4 months to take full effect.

Don't forget to make sure your doctor orders regular pelvic ultrasounds to check that your endometrial lining isn't thickening too much. And make sure your doctor knows you are taking progesterone.

Evidence to date shows Tamoxifen will increase the risk of Breast Cancer reoccurrence if estrogen is prescribed to treat hot flushes (one of Tamoxifen's side effects). See Medical Reference section, page 420.

Many women come to me for this problem unable to control their debilitating hot flushes and lack of sleep as they are unable to take estrogen, looking for alternatives to solve this problem. The usage of progesterone combined with phytoestrogens, diet and lifestyle changes has been successful in many on Tamoxifen.

Can I take progesterone through chemotherapy treatment?

I don't know medically if there is a reason why you can't, except that the endocrinologists may be very adamant about no other form of treatment. Some even frown on taking vitamins.

Yet some women have reported initiating progesterone replacement therapy because they've asked their doctor if they can take natural things throughout their treatment and the doctor has indicated that it's fine. Nonetheless, I remind women that this is a hormone and not a vitamin. If you do elect to do this, make sure it is not a Wild Yam cream that you are using (which is a phytoestrogen not a hormone) if you want progesterone benefits. Phytoestrogen usage is also very beneficial.

Throughout surgery, many women have continued to take their progesterone prior to, and directly after surgery as it appears to assist their body with the stresses and the corticosteroid pathway. The body may be in shock and traumatised, so progesterone being the mother hormone, can actually help build other vital steroid hormones and enhance healing.

I personally know for a fact when the body is stressed, whether it be mental, emotional or chemical, it will actually use more progesterone as it transforms it into cortisol. Often women will suffer the next month as a result with period problems or heavier bleeding, or headaches and signs of estrogen dominance. This is purely because progesterone levels that would normally sustain the body are just not enough under stress.

Surgery is therefore one of those qualifying periods where I say to women, if you can't take progesterone during surgery, certainly increase your dose prior to, and resume progesterone application directly afterwards where possible, particularly if used cyclically. You need to try and follow those cycles as closely as you can, otherwise you may be throwing the rhythm of the body out.

Can I take my bone building drugs such as Fosamax and Raloxifine (Evista) with progesterone?

Yes, you can. Fosamax will not effect progesterone benefits for other uses in the body, however, if you are using progesterone for bone building it will be severely compromised, if not rendered ineffective for this purpose.

There is no clear data to support other than what I have learnt from the Late Dr John Lee. But I do know from my clients, men (included). Fosamax has a detrimental effect on the gut for those prone to problems such as constipation, heart burn, history of ulcers and IBS to name a few. Elderly are prescribed once a week administration of Fosamax ! Many of these elderly people are not eating 3 meals a day, suffering digestive disorder and gastric discomfort so it is prescribed with caution to prevent further gastrointestinal complications. So many daughters have bought their elderly mothers to me. These poor dear old souls with skin dried, thin skeletal problems and digestive disorders and bowel problems. Clearly the Fosamax is disagreeing with them and causing them discomfort, providing little pain coverage for their bones. With the co-operation of the Doctor offering them progesterone assists these people in gaining a good sleep and balance again. Some of these clearly are on mood altering medications such as heavy drowsy inducing medication (sleeping tablets), which in fact increases their changes of falling over thus risking higher incidences of fractures. It makes Fosamax look ridiculous in the bigger picture.

I suggest you consider why you are taking the bone building drugs in the first place and decide for yourself whether it is bone delay that you are seeking or bone building. Because the bone building drugs are not forming new bone, they are actually stopping and delaying the resorption of old bone. Age has to come into accountability too. There are many things you can do to build bone rather than to depend on bone building drugs or medication alone. Bone building is a holistic approach.

By taking bone building drugs these can actually block off the action of absorbing old, brittle bone, prevents progesterone moving in to build new bone in place of the old. On X-ray, bone building drugs look fantastic as the bone appears dense, but in actual fact may be quite weak and brittle because the X-ray is depicting 'old' bone that should have been removed and replaced with new.

Slowing bone resorption doesn't necessarily make your bones stronger. As explained above, there are two different actions involved in bone formation, that is taking away old bone and rebuilding new bone.

I cannot make the *decision for you* but I strongly urge you to seek out options, information, and do drug research. Ask your doctor for full disclosure of side effects, benefits, and the test trials, then look at these seriously because at the end of the day, it is your health, your decision, and your body. You might like to visit the Late Dr. John's website to learn his view on bone builders. Articles on his website on particular issues can be still ordered. The late Dr John Lee's books outline the disadvantages of using bone building medications.

There is some evidence suggesting that dietary plant phytoestrogens perhaps have a higher role in bone protection and that dairy is not as conducive as a source of calcium intake as we have been led to believe. Visit www.notmilk.com

CHAPTER 11

What to be aware of with your Natural Progesterone and the different deliverance systems

- *What to be aware of with your Natural Progesterone and the different deliverance systems*
- *Oral (not available in Australia):*
- *Creams Used Topically:*
- *Intra-Vaginal: Intra-vaginal application of creams*
- *Lozenges / Troches:*
- *Pessaries/Vaginal Suppositories/Vaginal Gel:*
- *Anal Suppositories:*

What to be aware of with your Natural Progesterone and the different deliverance systems

Oral (not available in Australia):

Research has shown that progesterone is most effectively absorbed and utilised by the human body when applied transdermally as a cream. It is not as effective when taken in capsule form because the liver breaks it down before it can exert an effect in the body.

For example, you would need to ingest 100mg of natural progesterone in capsule form (not available in Australia) to get the equivalent dosage of 10mg topically. The remaining 90% is rendered inactive by the liver and excreted in the bile. Alternatively, *direct transdermal application is taken up immediately by the body and used before being excreted through the liver.*

Please note: If you live in Australia and are taking 'oral progesterone', it may be a synthetic progestogen (unless you have ordered it yourself from overseas and have a guarantee of your product). Homeopathic progesterone drops do not have high levels of progesterone if you are attempting to seek physiological required doses for the body.

Creams Used Topically:

Progesterone cream is applied directly onto the skin surface where it is absorbed and taken up by the blood vessels. This also bypasses the liver.

There is *NO patch to date that contains natural progesterone*, possibly due in part because research has shown that natural progesterone is most effectively absorbed and utilised by the human body when applied as a cream. Blood assays do not convince/prove to the medical fraternity of absorption, whilst estrogen and testosterone patches do!

Intravaginal/Vaginal: Intravaginal application of creams

Not a standard procedure unless you are using Crinone Gel. It must be fully understood as side effects can be experienced using transdermal progesterone cream intravaginally and must be done under the supervision of your Doctor. In my organisation women have voluntarily adopted the use of transdermal progesterone cream delivered vaginally (internally - i.e. intravaginally). Transdermal creams have not been designed for this deliverance route yet. (Other than Crinone Gel USA).

So Warning, *I personally have only used Pro-Feme so cannot guarantee other creams and their ingredients for safety or usage. My observation with other women has been on using Pro-Feme.*

The manufacturer of this product *will not endorse* this procedure and *it was not designed for this purpose.* It has been assured however that the ingredients contained within have no additives that may be potentially dangerous, being macadamia and Vitamin E base. **Crinone vaginal gel was specifically designed for fertility use**. The drawback in this deliverance system is it is possibly very sticky and gooey.

While there has been scattered evidence that vaginal absorption with creams has been very effective, there is no drug company endorsement of this unique approach to cream application as opposed to gel and suppositories. Most creams will have instructions for EXTERNAL USE ONLY.

If you choose to work with natural progesterone cream applied vaginally, this is strictly a personal choice and one you must be prepared to take full responsibility for, and err on the side of caution. You must consult with your medical practitioner.

I am NOT making reference to the product 'Crinone Gel' which is for vaginal use. My studies and observation have used Pro-Feme which has not been designed for vaginal use. I am not in a position to make comment on any other creams attempted to be used this way.

Disclaimer: I am not a Medical Practitioner and this information came from various sources in my own research. It is for information purposes only and is not a prescription for your particular needs. Consult with your health care professional if in doubt or if you have questions. I do not diagnose or try to overrule the advice of health care professionals. Refer to Medical References on vaginal use.

Common guidelines to adhere to for vaginal application:

- Ensure the cream is of the highest quality.
- Vaginal tissue is very delicate and sensitive, and can be thin, dry and atrophied, particularly for postmenopausal women. So check with your cream manufacturer or compounding pharmacist that there are no irritants or ingredients that contra-indicate this form of usage. Be very gentle using an applicator as it may traumatise vaginal tissue because of the above reasons.
- Always insert with a clean, sterile applicator. Many market products come with reusable applicators such as the anti-fungal creams and estrogen vaginal creams.
- If you do not have an applicator, massaging cream up into the vagina with finger insertion will also have some good results and may be more effective than topical application, but certainly will not have the impact of a deep vaginal deliverance. This is often a good way to start using progesterone (vaginally) to test sensitivity and skin irritation.
- Do not use before sexual activity. Best results are achieved at night-time because you are relaxed, lying still and the cream has time to be well absorbed.
- Insertion of cream vaginally may cause a slight burning sensation or internal throbbing. Smile, grin and bear it because it's usually short-lived. I frequently use estriol estrogen cream 1mg. (Ovestin) and have found that by putting just a dab of Ovestin on top of the applicator after measuring out my progesterone dosage in the applicator it actually stops the burning sensation.
- I have had a Hysterectomy, am 8 years into surgically induced menopause and am prone to vaginal atrophy and bladder infections and sensitivity. I have found this delivery system to be exceptionally successful, long-lasting, more consistent and has helped maintain mucosal tissue, vaginal and bladder integrity.
- Sensation of vaginal burning seems to correlate with the time of the month, amount of vaginal secretions and mucosal health which usually is particularly pronounced in the latter stage of your cycle.
- Because of it's effective route of absorption, vaginal application should be very gradual (small dosage to start with, and alternate your days).

- Suggested dosage should be no more than 10-15mg of progesterone vaginally. (This is equivalent to 20-45mg transdermal - remember the vaginal absorption route provides for double absorption therefore less cream is required on application.

- I usually suggest 5mgs (= to 10mg transdermal) for the initial dose so you can assess your body's reaction. If you're getting a favourable response, I suggest you apply cream once or twice a week, building up to alternate days and, if need be progress to daily doses.

Various options can be adopted in using this route.

Some women prefer to alternate between vaginal and transdermal delivery for optimal site receptivity. Some women find once a week is all they need with this method to enhance their progesterone effectiveness and levels.

Some women do both together ie a little vaginally and the remainder topically for some days when more boosts are required eg. If on 30mg daily an example here would be 5mg intra vaginally (which = 10mg) and the balance of 20mg transdermally = 30mg total.

Advantages of this route:

- When cream renders ineffective and women reach a plateau and cream becomes ineffective, vaginal application has worked very well where topical delivery has rendered the progesterone therapy ineffective. These women have followed all the rules, taken their appropriate breaks from cream, but progesterone stopped delivering results. Because of the conditions they are trying to treat / control with progesterone, that may require higher levels of progesterone dosage and transdermal maintenance.

- It is more economical to use less cream and derive the same dosage as that of a topical application.

- Cell receptivity can be severely compromised because of chronic illness, malnourishment, auto-immune disorders, dysfunctional liver, poor skin absorption, increased body fat (overweight), poor or sluggish circulation, etc. The list is extensive. It's in these cases, that the vaginal route has proved a successful way of getting around such health issues and maximising progesterone performance.

- Interestingly, this unique approach to progesterone application seems to have a greater impact (in some cases) on the specific conditions such as Endometriosis, Fibroids, Cervical Hyperplasia, (thickening of the uterus), and Polycystic Ovarian Syndrome. This is because it appears to target tissue in these areas, as well as being systemically available via the blood. It is known for a fact that when a woman suffering Fibrocystic Breasts rubs progesterone cream on her breast tissue, the body responds favourably and very quickly to this direct application approach. So I apply the same principle for vaginal application when attempting to address conditions relating to organs within the pelvic cavity. Women need to discern for themselves and discuss this with their doctor as I am not a medical practitioner.

- Other benefits reported by women using cream this way is halting migraines,
- Improving bladder function such a Stress Incontinence, Thrush, normalising vaginal pH levels, secretions and vaginal dryness. Some women still need to use progesterone in conjunction with estriol cream but they may find they need less estriol over time to maintain healthy tissue and even less progesterone.

Some of the reported feedback SIDE EFFECTS

From women using this delivery of progesterone include; severe heavy bleeding; severe Estrogen Dominance Wake Up; (e.g. onset of a headache, migraine or bleeding) even after being stabilised using topical delivery but not having optimal effects. My observation is that I feel it delivers higher levels of progesterone and turns on more receptors thus stimulating Estrogen Dominance Wake Up. Read pages 216 and 217.

Vaginal application can bring on

- Estrogen Dominance Wake Up Crises and *endometrial activity resulting in a period usually within 24 hours,* (a clean out due to stimulation of these receptors in my opinion), unusual discharge (similar to ovulation discharge), colour (not offensive in smell), shedding of fibrous matter, are other things that have been reported by women with Fibroids.
- Pelvic pain within 12-24 hours. Leg pains (groin area) bearing down feeling.
- Headaches and even migraines can result, breast tenderness, severe PMS and associated symptoms can be some of the other side effects.
- If this is the case, stop. Resort back to phytoestrogens and topical application until it settles and then try again on a lesser dose. *The body needs to be slowly prepared for this technique of application.*

IF IN DOUBT, DON'T SELF MEDICATE, SEEK APPROPRIATE TESTS TO ENSURE THERE ARE NO UNDERLYING PROBLEMS.

PLEASE DO NOT ATTEMPT THIS APPROACH WITHOUT FULL KNOWLEDGE OF YOUR CONDITION, PARTICULARLY IF IT'S OF A BLEEDING NATURE. OR IF YOU HAVE NOT UNDERGONE A RECENT MEDICAL CHECK-UP THAT INCLUDED AN INTERNAL EXAMINATION OR ULTRASOUND.

Indications when NOT to use cream vaginally:

- Recent surgery
- Signs of infection
- Active Thrush (optional)
- Cystitis (optional)
- You suspect you are pregnant
- History of STDs
- Unexplained bleeding or any condition that is being treated by a doctor.

Note: This form of usage may result in a change of vaginal lubrication and discharge (usually within 24 hrs). You may notice vaginal secretions to be somewhat similar to that of ovulation - thick, sticky, odourless, clear to slightly yellow in appearance. This discharge IS NOT always present after cream application. Check and make sure you DO NOT mistake this discharge for ovulation. Over a period of time, this discharge will not always appear after an intravaginal application. When I revisit this route after a break from cream usage, I see this once or twice then it settles. It may be due to the fact that I do not have a cervix (and usual secretory glands) and progesterone increases secretory stimulation and expulsion of remaining non absorbed base component.

In summary, advantages of intravaginal application include:

- Doubles the absorption rate i.e. 1mg intravaginally is equivalent to at least 2mg topically. (More cost effective because you use less)
- Stimulates different receptors, influencing higher levels of progesterone receptivity and longer lasting effects
- Ability to raise progesterone levels quickly, particularly in times of stress or an impending migraine, or where reserves are not there
- An alternative when topical absorption appears to be poor or women appear to not assimilate their cream effectively
- Has been reported by some to shrink Fibroids, reduce heavy bleeding and Migraines
- Observation with this method of use appears to be received well with minimal disruption or side effects (severe estrogen dominance 'wake up') with women who have had a Hysterectomy and those in menopause, however for elderly women this can be an awkward method of application.
- Lymphatic body types, overweight, diabetics and chronic fatigue suffers have reported a better response than topical use.

Please note, this overview of vaginal usage of progesterone cream has uniquely evolved out of women's experimentation and providing their feedback to myself at NPAN using one specific manufactured cream. (Pro-Feme manufactured by Lawley Pharmaceuticals).

Prior to pursuing this form of progesterone therapy I did contact the manufacturer asking if there was any ingredient that might be harmful if applied vaginally. His horrified response was, "Not that I'm aware of, but it was not designed to be used that way".

Being the woman that I am, and having come across articles supporting vaginal delivery, I endeavoured to experiment with my body once again. Results to date have been very encouraging for myself and others.

Please refer to 'Medical References' section on Vaginal Progesterone Absorption. All these articles give evidence that vaginally administered progesterone is well absorbed, possibly better than transdermal. It also gives evidence that for those women who feel they must use an estrogen supplement, vaginal progesterone, in adequate doses will protect their endometrium from the estrogenic effects. Dr Sandra Cabot in her hormonal books also promotes intravaginal use and practices it as a medical practitioner.

I personally believe this method and route of application holds incredible possibility in hormone treatment and effectiveness in treating many problems. I am confident that the frontiers that I, amongst other women are crossing is opening the way for future prospects for other women. From my own experience, I have not suffered any untoward side effects or complications, in the years of use so far. It is my preferred choice of administration for many reasons. You may wish to read about stress, incontinence and libido in Book 2 'Natural Progesterone More Secrets Revealed'.

Lozenges / Troches:

Dissolved buccaly (between the teeth and the cheek), these are similar to the topical route in that it bypasses the liver, making it immediately available to the body. It will give you higher doses more quickly but might increase the side effects (break-through bleeding). The down shot of these in my opinion is a loss to the stomach (swallowed) and hormones were not designed to be in the stomach. Because of this loss higher doses are often required and they also require regular dose adjustments and monitoring which can render a lot of expense with Doctor's visits and tests.

Pessaries/Vaginal Suppositories/Vaginal Gel:

The amount absorbed is double that of transdermal delivery. This also bypasses the liver, and results are rapid. Australian pessaries, used predominantly in higher dosage for fertility purposes, are wax-coated and may compromise the delivery as opposed to cream or gel. To date, Crinone gel is not accessible to our Network so we cannot comment on its usage and performance, but we are looking forward to the opportunity.

Anal Suppositories:

Another form of deliverance, one that very few women adopt.

CHAPTER 11

Recommended Cream Dosage for Specific Problems

Recommended Cream Dosage for Specific Problems

The use of progesterone is not the only form of treatment for the following conditions and must be used in conjunction with medical supervision. Progesterone often kick starts other treatments, but has to be worked in with diet, vitamins, stress management and other environmental aspects.

These are the dosages I have observed to be effective. It is unfair to put too much emphasis on progesterone as a miracle hormone to fix everything. Progesterone used intelligently has brought wonderful results for many women providing it is embraced holistically and diligently.

Uterine Fibroids / Heavy bleeding:

Initially NPAN and my work with women with fibroid complaints was recommending conservative doses between 32-64mg. However, over the years it was obvious that these doses were not enough to control, shrink or abate Fibroids. Many doctors have been prescribing more in the form of lozenges with far better results. Whilst other Doctors have been prescribing conservative doses which have been obviously insignificant for the fibroid disease. Women have elected from their own experience of lesser doses with no apparent results to use higher doses in transdermal cream. Greater results have been seen between 100mg-200mg for 4-7 months under supervision of their Doctors. There have been a few women that have required to use between 200mg-400mg for 4-7 months to achieve control. Overall, an average of 7 months on these ranges of higher levels seems to be an effective time frame to get some measure of control. Initially in the beginning there was a reluctance to exceed 100mg, my views have now changed. It is advisable while using higher doses in the initial stages to get regular ultra sounds to assess effectiveness of this form of treatment.

Your barometer is reduced bleeding, reduced clotting and shrinkage of Fibroids along with other symptoms such as more regulated cycles (that may not have been present). Adjust dosage accordingly.

Some women have elected to use high doses 100-200mg (suppositories) under strict medical supervision gradually reducing over a few months with successful outcomes (documented in literature). However, NPAN and my work does not have much experience with the use of suppositories.

I find that women with a history of Fibroids tend to sit on a maintenance average dose between 60mg-100mg rather than risk Fibroids returning, regrowing/enlarging and once in control and stabilised, use the cream 2.5-3 weeks on, 1 week off or 2 weeks on, and 2 weeks off. (This depends on your perimenopausal stage and/or nearing menopause). The reason being in some cases a 12 day break is too long, and needs to be adjusted. I have observed in most cases 12 days break is far too long even for the younger fibroid women as it allows estrogen dominance to reign thus promoting fibroid activity. It is important to adhere to estrogen dominant reduction strategies and incorporate the use of a good phytoestrogen. Bleeding irregularities is covered extensively in Book 2 Natural Progesterone More Secrets Revealed, and Fibroids is covered extensively in this Book 1 Natural Progesterone the Worlds Best Kept Secret.

The depletion of progesterone reserves (be it through stress or imbalance) will not be detected until the second month / second menstrual period, indicating a need to increase dosage temporarily until symptoms settle.

When treating Uterine Fibroids, it's imperative that you master estrogen dominance as fibroid growth is influenced by estrogen. To appreciate this refer to chapter 17 'Estrogen, Phytoestrogen and Xenoestrogens', the section on 'How can I reduce my estrogen dominance naturally', page 363.

Also refer to chapter 14 'Questions and Comments in Relation to Specific Problems' for more information on Fibroids, pages 298, 299 and bleeding concerns pages 250-260.

Over the years with my work on Fibroids and progesterone administration it appears that progesterone does not work with some women suffering from this very common problem. Whilst some women have had great success in shrinking Fibroids, some haven't and have ended up requiring Fibroids to be removed as a preference to a total Hysterectomy. If the uterus can be left intact along with ovaries and cervix this is a far greater option than a complete Hysterectomy however, some surgeons do not have the skills or the understanding of a women's desire to retain her organs. In some cases a Hysterectomy has been necessary due to the inaccessibility of the Fibroids however, it is best to always seek a second opinion if a Hysterectomy is suggested.

Other women have undertaken microwave surgery with great success I am not up to speed with this procedure. Sorry. But it has stopped heavy bleeding and the outcome has been very satisfactory for some.

The up shot of progesterone therapy in treating Fibroids is not always predictable every woman is different in her response. Fibroids are stubborn and have a tendency to do their own thing and appear to manufacture their own estrogen factories, thus promoting the growth, some grow uncontrollably and some don't.

A minority of women have elected to experiment with intra vaginal dosing and have had exceptional results using between 100-200mg. (Equivalent to 50mg-100mg transdermal). Remember the intra vaginal route is a more potent and direct absorption route and appears to be able to target more specifically to this problem. Always halve your dose. Refer to pages 171-175.

Fibroid treatment is multifactorial and the key is to reduce and oppose the estrogen influence that Fibroids depend on for growth. Other strategies must be adopted the body type must be taken into account e.g. The Gynaeoid Body Type has a tendency to lower body weight and storage of estrogen and is prone to estrogen dominance. Other things to take into account high fibre diet, avoid stress, reduce weight, reduce exposure to xenoestrogens, reduce excess estrogen through liver cleansing and increase eating estrogen rich foods (benign plant estrogens) refer to Nutrition for the importance of antioxidants, Omega 3, 6 & 9 oils increasing prostraglandens which balance the thrombotic anti inflammatory process and the use of herbs such as Vitex and the avoidance of dairy products. Nutrition is dealt with extensively in the Book 2 Natural Progesterone More Secrets Revealed.

Caution on Maca - whilst Maca can modulate and balance assisting fertility it has also been observed that it appears to promote more estrogen production in some women.

Endometriosis:

At commencement of progesterone therapy, initial doses of high levels between 6-10% is often required, usually to compete with high cortisol and pain levels created by this disease. The body is also very deprived of progesterone. It may take 4 menstrual cycles until symptoms begin to abate. Then reduce dose according to pain management.

The average maintenance seems to hover around 54mg (5>%) between 4-7 months.

Average out to 54mg, and reduce according to pain levels. Additionally rub extra cream regularly (i.e. daily) if necessary over the ovaries and pelvic ligaments. This often helps pain reduction. A good response is regular and less painful periods. If you are finding that you are bleeding heavily, possibly suffering Anaemia, make sure that you work closely with your doctor. All heavy, non-cyclic bleeding should be investigated. Start day 5-26 then increase to day 8-26.

These women don't cope well with long breaks from cream. But ideally, for the younger women with early diagnosed Endometriosis, the goal is to mimic nature and aim for a 12-26 day cycle using cream (when asymptomatic / pain free). And eventually return to a 'least is best' dosage.

For a young teenager/woman suffering Endometriosis, a maintenance dose would range from 2-4% and often she can wean off progesterone altogether for months on end supplementing with herbs, vitamins and minerals. Women with more established Endometriosis appear to sit between 4-6% maintenance dose for at least a year, then lower doses may be tolerated as healing progresses.

Your barometer of treatment is reduction of pain, a return to regular, pain-free periods, and associated Endometriosis symptoms. If pain re emerges increase your dose by 30-50mg for that cycle and also incorporate the pain management hints.

PAIN MANAGEMENT HINTS:

High levels of magnesium 600-800mg daily for some is well tolerated - use one with four types of magnesium in it

- Avoid Codeine based medication (will interfere with your bowels)
- Gentle exercise
- High fibre diet.
- Vitex has assisted many
- Incorporate antioxidants and phytoestrogens
- Lots of essential fatty acids in balance ratio to exert anti inflammatory and pain

control management and to increase the manufacturing of the prostaglandins You may wish to refer to Ruth Trickeys supplied chart on the pathways of the Omega 3, 6 & 9 pathway production. With a diagram on the essential fatty acid pathways taken with permission from Ruth's incredible book covering herbal medical solutions from adolescence to menopause. Book Title : 'Hormones and The Menstrual Cycle'. This is found in my Book 2 'Natural Progesterone More Secrets Revealed'.

Also refer to chapter 14 'Questions and Comments in Relation to Specific Problems' page 302 for more detailed information on Endometriosis.

Migraines / PMS:

Starting from approximately 32mg from day 10-12, gradually increasing to larger doses (up to 10% if necessary) toward the end of the cycle.

This gradual increase of progesterone levels peaking at around day 26 will usually control the onset of Migraine and PMS. Rub onto your temples, neck, and back at hourly intervals to dislodge the headache or onset of anxiety or mood swings. You will probably find that one or two doses will be enough.

For severe PMS and Migraines, up to 10% levels are well tolerated in initial stages, although some women have gone up to 200mg in the first 3-4 months using these doses prior to the onset of a Migraine.

The maintenance dose appears to be around 32mg-64mg however this may take many months to arrive at. Your barometer being symptoms relief. PMS and Migraines may take months to settle, and usually disappear if managed correctly.

Severe Migraines may take up to 12 months to control, with higher doses for approximately 7 months but with each cycle, severity, duration and debilitation lessens. PSM is slightly easier to conquer, usually over 4-7 months.

PMS does not require elevated doses compared to women who suffer migraines (usually does not exceed 100mg), unless they have PMS with Migraines. Women find that if they start on a lower dose and increase mid cycle when PMS starts to kick in working on higher doses up to 100mg will be able to control PMS. As estrogen dominance is conquered PMS symptoms will subside and lesser doses will be required in the months to come. But it is advisable not to start on the higher dose at the beginning of the cycle but allow for that variable mid cycle on if required.

Refer to chapter 14 'Questions and Comments in Relation to Specific Problems' pages 198-205, 211, 215-217 for more detailed information on Migraines, PMS and management. Also refer to page 174.

Cervical Dysplasia:

The normal dose would be 20-32mg for 4 months and usually positive changes are observed in this time frame, confirmed with another pap smear. For a quicker result *progesterone pessaries or lesser dose via intravaginal application may be of benefit.*

I would highly recommend that you are under the care of a physician and all other tests have been performed to eliminate likely causes such as cancer, STDs, etc. Progesterone is not the only factor here. Nutrition and attention to hygiene needs addressing. You might also consider moving away from tampons (bleaching chemicals) during your treatment.

Any cell change needs to be monitored because they can be a prelude to cancer.

Progesterone has been reported to correct abnormal cervical cells (atypical) where a pap smear reading indicates the need for further investigation and possible surgery. Get a second opinion and consecutive pap smears following 2-3 months on progesterone therapy.

Also refer to 'Questions and Comments in Relation to Specific Problems' for more information on Cancer Concerns and Book 2- More Secrets Revealed.

Adrenal Gland Exhaustion:

This range depends on the degree of your condition. Begin at 32mg and assess your progress. High levels of 64mg are often required for the initial 8 weeks or more to compete with the cortisol output because there will be competition for the same receptors and progesterone has to work harder under these conditions. Reduce as your symptoms improve.

Absorption and assimilation of progesterone has been observed to be very poor in these women, particularly when associated with Chronic Fatigue or Fibromyalgia.   The adrenals need to be supported with additional supplementation, minerals and particularly, Vitamin B complex and SLEEP (in order for the adrenals to repair).

Intra-vaginal application very gradually has proved far more effective in conjunction with nutritional supplementation aimed at rebuilding their immunity.

These women often qualify for additional steroid hormones. This is why a saliva assay is imperative to assess possible depletion of other hormones too, and fine tune levels. The incorporation of **Natural Testosterone** may be beneficial (or DHEA).

Also refer to 'Questions and Comments in Relation to Specific Problems' and Book 2 'Natural Progesterone More Secrets Revealed' for more detailed information on Stress.

Polycystic Ovary Syndrome (PCOS):

The average dose that most women with PCOS seem to be asymptomatic at is around 54mg of progesterone cream daily from day 12-26 of your cycle (adjust accordingly) for at least the first 7 months if there is a regular cycle.

In the initial few months, however, a lot of women take 64-100mg of progesterone cream from day 5-26 to address extreme progesterone deficiency and estrogen dominance symptoms. And after your body has settled down, you may wish to wean back to a lesser dose or to extend breaks to fall into line with a day 12-26 cycle. This technique will also in many cases induce ovary activity and Cysts may begin to burst (pop) also *be aware that on a program of 5-26 days on, on higher doses then coming back to day 12-26 when symptoms are in control, can induce high territory for fertility as the ovaries start to resurge especially if they have been rested.* Alternatively many women in this time may start to experience some bleeding irregularity. If ovaries are popping Cysts just adhere to your cyclic pattern breaks. The periods should re align again. When Cysts burst it can be traumatising and painful (deep pelvic pain like appendicitis) dab cream over area of pain hourly until it settles. The 2 week on 2 week off regime opens up the possibilities of regular ovulation by now.

Get as close as you can to a 'least is best' dosage, long term, and remain asymptomatic. Some women have reduced dosage levels as low as 2-3%, day 12-26, or 14-28 on a longer cycle, and enjoy optimal health.

Gentle Summary Reminder in PCOS treatment using progesterone:

It's important that you have regular ultrasounds to assess the condition of your ovaries, and an indicator of treatment progression. So if you are using a regime day 5-26 in the first 4-7 months until symptoms settle and then returning back to 2 week on 2 week off (day 12-26) on lesser doses you are working with a program that has been highly successful for fertility so if you do not wish to get pregnant (not recommended for at least 6 months on high nutrition and weight loss) please practice safe contraception and DO NOT USE THE PILL. There have been quite a few resultant pregnancies using this program. However a few of these women had been on far higher doses in the first 7 months due to multiple estrogen dominance symptoms, PMS and migraines.

Dosage barometer would be improvement of symptoms such as reduced facial and body hair, no further weight increase, clearer looking skin if suffering acne, less cravings for sugars and refined carbohydrates, regular cycles, absence of ovulatory pain, elimination of PMS and other estrogen dominance symptoms.

Also refer to 'Chapter 14 - Questions and Comments in Relation to Specific Problems' for section on PCOS, pages 206-210.

Nursing Mothers - Postnatal depression:

To treat severe depression, doses >64mg uninterrupted for 4 months have been used successfully (depending on the degree of depression), then wean back gradually to 15-20mg physiological dose. Once their period returns, these women have adopted a cyclic 12-26 day regime to maintain hormone balance.

The advisable dose of 15-20mg, based on observation, hasn't affected prolactin levels. If this dose is inadequate, increase gradually until you arrive at a level where you feel relaxed, getting a sound sleep at night, general improved sense of wellbeing and not feeling depressed. Refer to page 229.

If you wish to use high levels and feel it is necessary, the barometer is your absence of symptoms. *If your milk production is affected, it is an indication that progesterone may be interfering with the hormone prolactin* (responsible for producing milk). We have not had any reports of this, even at 6% (60mg) short term use. *If this dosage is affecting milk supply you need to cut your dose back but there have been no reported cases (up to 100mg).*

Also refer to 'Questions and Comments in Relation to Specific Problems' for more detailed information on Fertility, Infertility, Contraception, Postnatal Depression. Fertility has been dealt with in greater depth in Book 2 Natural Progesterone More Secrets Revealed.

Fibrocystic Breasts:

Physiological dose of 15-20mg, *rubbing some cream on to the breast tissue daily* and the remainder of cream for that dosage rotated around the body. Your breasts will respond favourably to this dose regardless of what else you do. You can remain on this dose indefinitely (with regular breaks) to maintain breast tissue softness and cyst-free breasts.

Barometer would be diminished Cysts, pain and restoration of soft breast tissue. Success of treatment is usually seen within a few months but in some cases a few weeks. Women with chronic Fibrocystic Breasts have reported the disappearance of breast lumps (non cancer) after a few years on progesterone. Women who are highly stressed, or who have a high intake of caffeine may take longer to respond.

If other symptoms are evident as well as Fibrocystic Breasts higher doses (64mg) may be required to address these initial problems, weaning back to physiological baseline doses for women in their 30's around 32mg. PMS often coincides with breast lumps, soreness, fluid retention and breast tenderness, particularly mid cycle when estrogen is surging at its highest point.

Also refer to chapter 14 'Questions and Comments in Relation to Specific Problems' page 265 for more detailed information on Breasts Concerns.

Fertility:

Whilst my work has not had a lot of experience in fertility as it is complex I have had some hands-on personal experience with fertility in the last few years as more and more women are seeking me out as a last resort. So my knowledge within in this field is starting to expand and it is apparent that progesterone usage has a great role. See Kate's Story (Testimonial) in Book 2 Natural Progesterone More Secrets Revealed. Due to the demand of women wanting more information I have elected to share as much as I know on this subject in my second book as well as incorporating a Nutritional Program.

Fertility specialists in America are currently working with a natural progesterone product called 'Crinone Gel 8%'. There may be similar products available in Australia, however, I am unable to name any at this time. Interestingly Crinone Gel, I believe, is now 4% strength and is still not available in Australia.

As a general guide, The Late Dr. Lee recommended using *20mg of progesterone from day 5-26 for 3 months to rest the ovaries (turn off ovulation). Then the next month which is the fourth cycle use 20mg from day 12-26 or 14-28 if you are on a longer cycle.* **Should you become pregnant continue to use the cream increasing dosage to 30-40mg in the first month, after which increase dose to 60-80mg.**

If you fall pregnant and are already on higher doses than the above mentioned **do not decrease your dose or stop.** This can bring on a miscarriage you need to stay on the dosage that you are on until the 13th week gradually reducing thereafter (2nd trimester) under your Doctor's supervision. And if you are uncomfortable about stopping the progesterone, continue until one week before delivery. *If you are going to stop the progesterone* **never stop suddenly.** If you stop using progesterone at any stage of the pregnancy the *reason why you may stop using progesterone by the third month of the pregnancy is because the placenta takes over making progesterone.* But it is always wise to get your progesterone levels checked to ensure the placenta is manufacturing adequate levels of progesterone to maintain the pregnancy. Having more progesterone is not going to hurt the baby as progesterone is the gestation hormone (in the third trimester progesterone levels are in the vicinity of 300mg-400mg). It is better to have little bit more progesterone coverage for piece of mind than not to have enough. But of course you must work with your Gynecologist.

If you stop using progesterone suddenly it could trigger a miscarriage.

Also refer to 'Polycystic Ovary Syndrome', ' Cream Usage' and 'Questions and Comments in Relation to Specific Problems' for more detailed information on Fertility, Infertility, Contraception, Postnatal Depression. Contraception is covered in greater depth in Book 2 Natural Progesterone More Secrets Revealed.

Refer to Katharina Dalton's work - she specialised and pioneered progesterone usage extensively.

Liver function:

If the liver is not functioning properly chances are you will feel very nauseous with progesterone usage in the initial stages. This is the only time I recommend minute amounts of cream (maybe as small as 5mg), gradually increasing as tolerated.

Start supporting your liver function with a premium liver formulation and detox regime (visit 'Liver Doctor' website in Resource page). Also, if progesterone is not helping you for various problems, one must wonder what other factors are at play here. A liver assay would be advisable in this situation. Such as medical history of hepatitis, heavy substance and medication abuse (analgesics, sedatives, antidepressants, anticholesterols long term.) The oral contraceptive pill can also take its toll on the liver. *Even a fatty and dysfunctional liver does not necessarily mean a diseased liver, thus will not show up abnormal liver enzymes however* **will impede on hormone balancing,** manufacturing cholesterol production and progesterone's performance in the body.

It is important that this organ is performing to its maximum capacity to do all the jobs that are required in detoxification and elimination of unwanted toxins and products including ALL the hormones after the body has utilised them. The liver is also where synthetic HRT is metabolised making it available for the body to use. Natural, bio-identical hormones bypass the liver and gut and are taken directly into the blood stream.

NOTE: If you are suffering nausea when you commence progesterone it is an indication that your liver is not coping and that you need to do liver work. However continue your cream use gradually increasing daily as the morning sickness like feeling does subside as the liver adjusts to the reaquaintance of this hormone.

Many cross references to strategies on liver support, diet and management have been covered in both books. Book 2 however delves into this subject in greater depth.

Osteoporosis:

This is fairly controversial with The Late Dr. Lee recommending a more physiological dose, three weeks on, one week off if post menopausal, and if perimenopausal a physiological dose 12-14 days if asymptomatic.

As there are no firm studies to date, except The Late Dr. John Lee's work with his own patients of 20 years practice, I can only use his guidelines.

However, for the first 8 weeks if you are estrogen dominant work on the principal of saturation up to 64mg. If you are postmenopausal you can go for 8 weeks without a break and then come back to physiological doses between 15-20mg as a maintenance dose if asymptomatic. Some people prefer and feel more stable on 32mg. (Men need less.)

A lot of menopausal women do not show signs of estrogen dominant symptoms, but still need to have high doses initially because the body is so deprived of progesterone. If women are perimenopausal, still menstruating and have Osteoporosis, then the principle of saturation and pulling back to maintenance doses 15-32mg for bone building, depending on their estrogen dominance and other symptoms. Arriving at a physiological dose where you are symptom-free other than treating Osteoporosis may take months in conjunction with the diet, nutrition, phytoestrogens, etc.

Dr Lee emphasised more progesterone dosage does not make more bone, in fact, he claimed it can retard the benefits of bone building, because it can down regulate if it's used in high dosages for long periods of time unnecessarily. Higher than physiological doses of progesterone is only beneficial to the body when it is addressing problems at hand (excluding Osteoporosis).

In summary, if you are post menopausal and have Osteoporosis you are not going to see immediate results and may not see results for quite a few years. Adopting a 'least is best' approach will still have the same favourable outcome as opposed to high or random dosage.

Barometer is improvement of Bone Mineral Density (BMD) reading - 3 to 4 year comparison of results, using the same machine.

Also refer to chapter 14 'Questions and Comments in Relation to Specific Problems' pages 267-281 for more detailed information on Osteoporosis, which covers the multifactorial causes and holistic treatment to this disease.

You may also wish to visit the usage of Fosamax, page 168 and Nutritional Supplements in detail including testosterone and bone building which is covered in Book 2 Natural Progesterone More Secrets Revealed.

Hot Flushes:

From my research and understanding, these are really a marker for estrogen and progesterone deficiency. This results in a huge ratio difference between the estrogen and progesterone levels, sending the body's biofeedback mechanism into 'overdrive' to prompt ovulation (wake up the ovaries). The drop of estrogens results in women experiencing Hot Flushes because it sends messages to the brain relay station which causes the body to panic that the ovaries are flagging and its attempting to wake them up, to produce more estrogen. This drop causes the ratio variation and influences vasodilation of the blood vessels.

Initially you can use high levels of progesterone between 6-10% in the first 6-8 weeks (uninterrupted) or longer, depending on severity and occurrence of night sweats and/or flushing. The body will settle once it understands progesterone is in the body to stay and the body adjusts to the estrogen drops (which only drop 40-60%, so women are never totally estrogen depleted). It may take 7-12 months to get Hot Flushes in control but over each month the intensity and duration should lessen.

Using the principle of saturation seems to help to override estrogen dominance wakeup crisis quicker. Severe flushes usually indicate radical fluctuation of estrogen so it's *important to stabilise the ratio between estrogen and progesterone*. This can be achieved by incorporating phytoestrogens ('tricking' estrogens) which are imperative in addressing Hot Flushes successfully. For more detailed information visit the chapter on Estrogen, Phytoestrogens and Xenoestrogens in Book 1 Natural Progesterone the Worlds Best Kept Secret and the Nutritional program incorporated in treating menopausal strategies and Nutrition in Book 2 Natural Progesterone More Secrets Revealed.

Hot Flushes can range from seconds to minutes, and vary in intensity and characteristic with every individual and can be very debilitating. Women find that often regular doses throughout the day and night delivers a more consistent message to the brain and evens out ratio imbalance. Consistent doses are far more effective in the initial stages than a day and night application.

It is important to keep your fluids up, as this helps prevent dehydration from excessive sweating. Continue with this approach and the Hot Flushes will gradually subside as the body adjusts to the progesterone input into the body. Once the Hot Flushes subside, reduce this dose accordingly, working back to asymptomatic doses.

The average dosage most effective to control hot flushing, menopausal or perimenopausal state, is approximately 32mg, usually achieved around the fourth month up to 7 months.

If Hot Flushes haven't subsided within 4-7 months on progesterone *there may be a call for administration of some estrogen, particularly if you have used estrogen replacement therapy in the past.* It is suggested that you read 'What is the safest form of estrogen to use if I have to use an estrogen?' (page 358) and also you need to be aware that ***if you have been on estrogen therapy a weaning process usually needs to be adhered to.*** If you have gone cold turkey in the first 4-7 months and your Hot Flushes have worsened after a few months on progesterone you need to bring a little bit of estrogen back in to stabilise and then to gradually wean back off it.

Also refer to chapter 14 'Questions and Comments in Relation to Specific Problems' page 230 in section on Menopause and Hot Flushes/Flashes. Plus chapters 16 & 17 will give you a broader perspective and an appreciation of options available. Many specific scenarios are considered and addressed in Book 2 'Natural Progesterone More Secrets Revealed'.

CHAPTER 13

Golden Rules For Natural Progesterone Cream

- *Know Golden Rules - General Summary and Guidelines of natural progesterone cream usage*

- *Be Familiar with your Natural Progesterone Cream*

- *Introducing natural progesterone back into your body*

- *Correct application of cream*

- *Cyclic Use*

- *Capturing Your Data*

- *Be active in your choices to maximise progesterone's performance*

- *Progesterone versus Wild Yam cream usage*

- *NPAN's Formula for Hormone Harmony*

Know Golden Rules - General Summary of your natural progesterone cream as formulated by Jenny Birdsey©
Be Familiar with your Natural Progesterone Cream

- Check that your cream contains Pure Progesterone Micronised BP. Alternatively, your cream might contain what is referred to as USP (United States Pharmacopoeia) grade Progesterone.

- Check Cream Ingredients. Make sure you know how much natural progesterone is contained in your jar or tube. And whether you are getting the correct deliverance per dosage.

- Check Correct Cream Base for maximum absorption. **Creams containing mineral oils (paraffin, aqueous cream) will not deliver** progesterone to the body because the progesterone is more soluble in the mineral oil, and as it stays in the mineral oil, it will not adequately absorb through the skin.

- Make Sure It's Not a Wild Yam Extract Cream Containing 'Diosgenin'. Diosgenin found in Wild Yam is a phytoestrogen — a plant compound that has beneficial, hormone-like effects in the body. It's a common mistake for women to think that Wild Yam constituents are converted into progesterone by the body. *Wild Yam, soy, diosegenin* **is not** *natural progesterone.*

- Tightly Close Your Jar or tube of natural progesterone after opening - oxygen breaks down progesterone. And always store in a cool, dry, dark place (70-75 °F; 20.1-23.8 ℃).

- If you are using a jar split the cream and store half the contents so it doesn't loose efficacy as every time you open the jar to use it, it is exposed to oxygen.

- A Good Cream Stored Correctly Will Not Go Off Quickly. Creams stored in the right conditions that have manufactured correctly can last up to 2 years unopened.

- Creams without preservatives in them will go off very quickly, and also creams can go off with preservatives but it takes longer.

- Always Check Expiry Date.

- Preservatives does not necessary denote these natural progesterone creams are harmful or dangerous or unnatural to the body as many marketing ploys insinuate. Many so called natural plant derived cream bases still contain preservatives. Check the selling motives behind such arguments.

- Check ingredients with manufacturers.

- Ingredients by law should be listed in Australia with Batch Number.

- If allergic to cream - eg. Rash, stop chances are it is something in the ingredients you are reacting to. Change to another cream.

- If cream smells rancid or feels gritty suspect quality. Could be off or incorrectly formulated.

Introducing natural progesterone back into your body

The first 10-14 days can be a roller-coaster. From severe estrogen dominance 'wake up' (heightened estrogen receptor sensitivity) to a total euphoric state. Some women, however, experience a delayed response over a number of months. There are many factors determining why these extremes occur. Read 'Stages' pages 138-144.

Always allow 6-8 weeks on natural progesterone therapy to reach saturation levels, adjusting dosage according to symptom relief. A break from cream may or may not be necessary during this time depending on symptoms and individual response. Of course, given each woman's physiological uniqueness, there'll be exceptions. **After the first 8 weeks uninterrupted, PERIODIC BREAKS must be taken.** This is essential and a key rule to abide by.

During the initial 8 weeks of therapy, high doses are well tolerated. I liken it to jumping into the deep end of a swimming pool and working your way back down to the shallow end ... until you reach your unique physiological dosage of achieving your maintenance (minimum) dose, in most cases around 32mg. May take 7-12 months to achieve, your baseline dose. Charting will assist you in recognising when you have reached your optimal levels.

Initial high doses help override estrogen dominance 'wake up'. This allows for the lipophilic activity (soaking up progesterone into the fat cells) before it becomes fully effective in the body. High doses are well tolerated initially because the body is so deprived of progesterone it stores much of it in fat cells. Many women have had years or progesterone deficiency and the body will literally soak it up like a sponge.

During initial therapy, your body will uptake much of the progesterone supplementation and store it in fat cells - lipophilic action. Expect your body to adjust to natural progesterone therapy over 4 menstrual cycles, or calendar months if menopausal. Remaining on high doses for this time, if addressing heaps of symptoms is not usually an issue providing after 2 periods or 8 weeks uninterrupted breaks are taken monthly.

Because progesterone is a fat-soluble hormone, this is why it is not carried around in the watery (serum) part of the blood but instead is transported around the body on the back of red blood cells. The body will access this hormone from the fat stores for usage carrying it via the blood to the appropriate receptors to then deliver messages to perform specific tasks. Receptors are like relay stations.

Refer to section on - Measuring Progesterone with Saliva Assays versus Blood Serum, page 129 to learn more about how progesterone travels in blood.

Understand typical short & long term physiological changes that occur during on-going natural progesterone therapy. (Refer to Charting page 327 and Estrogen Dominance Symptoms page 84.

Recognise progesterone characteristics versus problems that need to be investigated with your GP.

Don't forget to use a premium phytoestrogen and magnesium particularly in this introduction period.

Correct application of cream

- Rotate the cream around your body and apply it to thin skinned areas where blood vessels are close to the surface. (Pulses are a good indication).

- Spilt your dose into morning and evening applications in the initial stages when higher doses are being used to maintain a 24 hr coverage.

- Areas on your body to be avoided (are fatty areas and where fat deposits e.g. stomach). The reasons why this approach is adopted is because progesterone is a lipophilic hormone (stores in fat) and applying cream to fatty tissue areas will delay performance. Advantages of site-specific application are generally associated with the problem you are attempting to treat. One example would be hormonal headaches. Try rubbing natural progesterone cream on the temples hourly to relieve pain, over and above your normal dose.

- *Contra-indications* (indicators that you should NOT be using progesterone), include for example, you might be taking the contraceptive pill or cortisone. Over-dosing of natural progesterone can and does occur. (However not usually in the early months of progesterone therapy).

- Do not swim or shower for an hour after application.

- Do not use cream if it is gritty or smells rancid. Your cream may have gone off.

- Rotate sites around the body for optimal effect and you may use cream to assist in pain management e.g. Over ovaries or to the temples for headaches.

- Aim to work to physiological doses, or achievable doses when you are symptom free.

- Query cream if you're not getting effective results and are following the NPAN's guidelines on hormone balancing. If you change your cream, try taking a month's break before switching to another cream.

- Check absorption levels via Saliva Assays. Do not panic if they are extremely high readings as it will be reflective of high progesterone dose usage which means you are absorbing the cream well.

- Providing you are getting symptoms addressed and benefits by high progesterone doses use this as more of a guideline than a perfect saliva reading. A within range salvia reading does not necessarily mean you are free of all symptoms as most women have found trying to align their dosages to their saliva readings rather than to their symptoms.

- We have found too many Doctors have reduced dosages far too quickly panicking with over the top (higher range) saliva readings. For instance if a women is using 100mg her reading will not be in the range of 16-20mg of an ovarian output.

- Saliva assay tests offer a great baseline prior to progesterone therapy to view the hormone profile. If progesterone is building down the steroid building pathway it will be manufacturing other hormones and this can be checked up in a few months time with another saliva reading. Which could indicate you need other hormones introduced if in shortage.

- Reducing dosages before all the symptoms are addressed will not sufficiently over-ride estrogen dominance. You need to point this out to your Doctor that high doses are not long term. Providing breaks are taken, you should not down regulate your receptors and progesterone benefits.
- Chart your symptoms and progress. You can reduce dosage once stabilised and symptoms have been eliminated. Your charts will be your guideline and a good indication of how your body is utilising this hormone and give you a clear idea on the functioning of the other hormones, aiming for a balance and synchronisation between all of them.

Cyclic Use

- Always follow cyclic usage to avoid menstrual irregularity & problems, and down-regulation of receptors which will render progesterone "ineffective". Down regulation is another way of saying rendering inefficient or deafening of the receptors. They become non responsive (stale).
- Always take a break from natural progesterone therapy on your true menstrual cycle.
- Don't break on the false period as it will throw your body into confusion and chances are may lead to insufficient progesterone. Thereby too much estrogen.
- Ignore breakthrough spotting that may occur in between your normal period. This will assist synchronisation of your body's natural cycle. If you are in menopause, take a break from cream at the same time each month.

But ALWAYS check out any consistent breakthrough bleeding problems.

Capturing Your Data

- Graphically chart and/or journalise your symptoms & dosage to determine trends, recognise over or under-dosing, understand & control symptoms.
- Learn your hormonal barometers, idiosyncrasies, and triggers.
- In cases of estrogen dominance, I recommend introducing *progesterone therapy in conjunction with phytoestrogens*. Natural estrogen therapy has its place when estrogen supplementation is required. They are a pigeon-pair and stimulate the other's action upon the body. Always try using plant estrogens before resorting to real estrogen such as estradiol and estrone to achieve estrogenic benefits in the body and hormone estrogen progesterone ratio balance.

Be Active In Your Choices to maximise Progesterone's performance

- Understand your choices. *Know the difference between* **Natural Hormone Replacement Therapy (NHRT)** as opposed to synthetic Hormone Replacement Therapy (HRT). Give consideration to NHRT over synthetic HRT to regulate hormone imbalance (bio-identical hormones applied topically bypass the liver and gut). NHRT also has less dangerous unpleasant side effects to synthetic HRT.

- Learn how to maximise your body's ability to uptake natural progesterone cream effectively. I endorse a holistic approach, ever mindful that hormone imbalance is multi-factorial.
- Do not under-estimate the value of Phytoestrogens, and vitamin and mineral usage in conjunction with natural progesterone.
- Also learn the importance of the liver - in balancing hormones and reducing estrogen dominance.
- Learn what diagnostic tests are invaluable in the monitoring of hormone balance and assessing effectiveness of treatment. I suggest employing blood serum AND saliva assay profiles to more accurately capture changes in your hormone levels. Example One: Use pap smear results to monitor the treatment of cervical hyperplasia during natural progesterone therapy. Example Two: Use ultrasounds to monitor the progress or regression of uterine Fibroids and ovarian Cysts.
- The intolerance / ineffectiveness of natural progesterone therapy needs to be addressed. Examples would be dysfunctional liver, exhausted adrenals, thyroid problems presence of other diseases and certain medications. Check out all possibilities.
- Develop strategies & techniques for reducing estrogen dominance as a way of life. Learn how to eat correctly to maximise your metabolism and hormonal constitution.
- Incorrect eating and gastrointestinal problems impede nutritional mineral vitamin assimilation thus the utilisation and/or production of hormones.
- Incorporate diet and formula high in plant sterols to induce estrogenic benefits and maximise progesterone performance in the body without increasing estrogen dominance.
- Drink heaps of pure water everyday (2 litres). Flushes out toxins.
- Empower yourself through information. Become more responsible for your hormonal health ... so that when you next visit your healthcare professional you can make an 'informed' choice.

Progesterone versus Wild Yam cream usage

Be aware that instructions on how to use progesterone cream may be similar to those accompanying Wild Yam creams. This is of no real concern other than the need to be aware of the distinction between a herbal preparation and a cream containing a human hormone.

NPAN's Formula for Hormone Harmony as formulated by Jenny Birdsey©

- Get onto a reliable natural progesterone cream
- Use cream as indicated to remain symptom-free

- Take cyclic breaks to enhance cream performance (even if you are no longer menstruating)
- Use a premium phytoestrogen formula to support estrogenic benefits and stimulate progesterone (both work in partnership and enhance each other's performance).
- Reduce your exposure to toxins and xenoestrogen products (environment)
- Chart regularly to monitor fluctuations and to detect patterns / triggers
- Regularly 'spring clean' your liver to enhance immunity, hormone health and metabolism
- Maintain gastrointestinal integrity and efficient bowel elimination
- Identify & control stress levels - exercise, recreation, sun, laughter, sex
- Maintain a healthy weight-to-height ratio
- Avoid foods estrogen laden i.e. non organic chicken
- Eat organic food where possible
- Avoid refined sugars and processed foods
- Increase your essential fatty acids (Omega Oils 3-6), eliminate saturated & polyunsaturated fats - bad fats kill ... good fats heal
- Include premium nutritional supplements, particularly if you're over 40
- Drink at least 2 litres filtered water a day
- Avoid fizzy drinks, alcohol and caffeine where possible
- Get into the habit of exercising regularly
- Learn how to relax through recreation and correct breathing techniques
- Acknowledge changes in your life and address them
- Have annual check-ups and appropriate tests
- Have regular hormone readings and saliva assays - check that hormones are in balance with your stage of life
- Trust yourself - your intuition & instincts
- Love and accept your body
- Recognise your body type and its unique hormonal & metabolic constitution
- Learn to eat correctly and lose weight naturally
- Regularly consume fresh vegetable juice
- Don't over burden your body with heavy anaelgesic use - pain killers, particularly codeine based products
- Try not to overuse antibiotics unnecessarily
- Check your medication and dosage regularly with your Doctor, eliminating or reducing under supervision if require.
- Chart your progress monthly
- Use appropriate nutritional supplementation
- Follow liver cleansing principles as a way of life for optimal liver health and maintenance.

CHAPTER 14

Questions & Comments in Relation to Specific Problems

- Premenstrual Syndrome/Tension (PMS/PMT)
- Polycystic Ovary Syndrome (PCOS)
- Migraines / Headaches
- Fibromyalgia/Chronic Fatigue Syndrome
- What causes FMS?
- Fertility/Infertility/Contraception/Postnatal Depression
- Menopause
- Hot Flushes (Flashes)
- What is the alternative treatment to menopausal symptoms other than conventional estrogen replacement therapy or HRT?
- What is meant by peri-menopause?
- What is meant by pre-menopause?
- Can natural progesterone replace synthetic progestogens at menopause if I'm on HRT?
- Vaginal Dryness
- Bladder Problems (Stress Incontinence)
- Urinary Problems
- Hysterectomy

- *Bleeding Concerns & Menstrual Cycles*
- *Cancer Concerns*
- *Breast Concerns*
- *Osteoporosis*
- *What is a bone density test?*
- *My doctor wants me to take Fosamax but I don't want to. I want to improve my bones naturally. What is the best plan of attack?*
- *Can I take my bone building drugs such as Fosamax and Raloxifine (Evista) with progesterone?*
- *Are there other ways of increasing my daily intake of calcium without using dairy products?*
- *Ageing Concerns*
- *Should my mother or my grandmother use Natural Progesterone?*
- *Thrush, Cystitis, Vaginal & Bladder Concerns*
- *Skin & Hair*
- *Nails*
- *Will my varicose veins worsen or my broken blood vessels on my face get worse with the use of progesterone?*
- *Weight Issues*
- *Stress*
- *Symptoms of Adrenal Gland Exhaustion*
- *Thyroid Concerns*
- *Fibroids*
- *Heavy Bleeding*
- *Endometriosis*
- *Chronic Endometriosis*
- *Tubal Ligation*
- *Memory Loss / Mental Faculty*
- *Musculoskeletal*
- *Will progesterone help with my arthritic problems?*

Premenstrual Syndrome/Tension (PMS/PMT)
What is PMS?

PMS is a term which means Premenstrual Syndrome, sometimes referred to as Premenstrual Tension (PMT). It refers to a constellation of symptoms that, when combined, form the basis of this diagnostic term.

It's a medical term used to describe associated mental and physical problems that occur usually during the second half of the menstrual cycle, although PMS has been observed in many women throughout their cycle.

The main clue in diagnosing PMS is not so much the nature, but the cyclic timing of these symptoms. Symptoms appear around Day 12-14 right through to your period. Some women can display PMS symptoms unabated, even after their period has passed, though a majority will find relief after menstruation commences.

Typical PMS symptoms can include some or all of the following (there are many others, see Estrogen Dominance Symptoms List often associated with menopausal symptoms):

- Irritability
- Migraine / headaches
- Loss of libido
- Fatigue
- Mood swings
- Bloating / fluid retention
- Depression
- Backache
- Lumpy and/or sore breasts
- Weight gain

Many women displaying symptoms of PMS are displaying symptoms of estrogen dominance brought about by a lack of (or diminished) progesterone production. Emotional mood swings and irregular bleeding are commonly associated with anovulatory cycles (where no ovulation takes place). If no ovulation occurs during that month, PMS symptoms are usually more severe as there is no progesterone to oppose the estrogen build up (see diagrams next page). There are a number of factors contributing to estrogen dominance and causes for insufficient or no progesterone as a result of failed ovulation. Excessive estrogen build up in the body creates an imbalance between these two partners (estrogen and progesterone) too much estrogen can be a result of:

Other aggravating factors compounding PMS:
- Exposure and impact from xenoestrogens in our environment
- From our food source estrogen laden foods such as grain feed chickens and stock.

- Overweight - particularly women who store lower body weight - tummy, hips and thighs (the Gynaeoid body type). These pear shaped women are renowned for being estrogen dominant or prone to. Lower body fat stores estrogen in body fat using a hormone to convert this. Progesterone on the other hand does the opposite as seen in pregnancy using body fat to convert to energy, again using a hormone for conversion.

- Stress robs the progesterone to make the stress hormones (corticosteroids). PMS creates more stress so a vicious cycle sets up. Progesterone helps oppose stress by its calming effect and also by supplying and supporting the corticosteroid pathway (progesterone is the precursor to cortisone). Extra progesterone applied during PMS helps compete for the same receptors that the corticosteroids occupy. Eventually progesterone can do its work thus reducing stress and reducing the need for the body to produce the survival stress hormone. This is why progesterone is a wonderful antistressor, controlling the mood swings and stress associated with PMS.

- Bowel problems - constipation, sluggish bowels and Leaky Gut Syndrome create toxicity to the body, circulating back to the liver blood toxins and more xenoestrogens.

  -diarrhoea and diets too high in fibre interfere with hormones and electrolyte imbalance.

- Fatty or dysfunctional liver creates and inability for toxins and excess estrogens to be correctly eliminated and impedes good estrogen production.

- Diet - eating incorrectly too much sugar and carbohydrates can aggravate and compound PMS and fluid retention.

- Lack of Magnesium - high sugar cravings usually indicate low magnesium levels and high estrogen dominance. Magnesium assists in controlling sugar cravings and insulin resistance,

HORMONES AND THE MENSTRUAL CYCLE

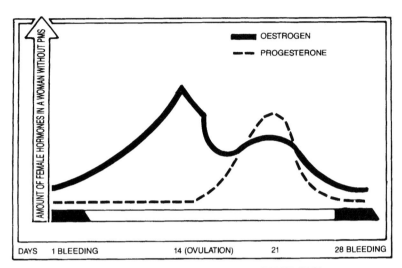

NORMAL MENSTRUAL CYCLE — WITHOUT PMS

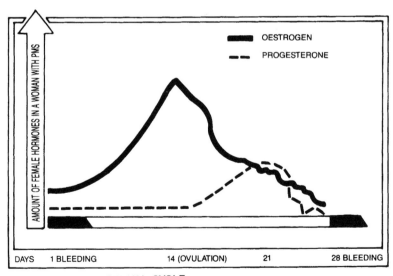

PMS MENSTRUAL CYCLE   PMS ZONE

Supplied & printed with permission specifically for Jenny Birdsey's use from Dr.Sandra Cabot's Book 'Don't Let Your Hormones Ruin Your Life'.

PMS controversy

There appears to be a general misinterpretation of what these symptoms represent. Doctors should consider making way for progesterone (pro-gestation).

For this reason PMS is often treated with estrogen replacement therapy and/or the oral Contraceptive Pill, and viewed as an estrogen deficient condition.

Doctors are assuming that your progesterone levels will surge during the last two weeks of a your cycle. But if you fail to ovulate that month, or produce sufficient levels of progesterone to balance the estrogen, then you will, in fact, be progesterone deficient and the term estrogen dominant.

That's where PMS kicks in. And you may fail to ovulate ... even at a very tender age. You'd be surprised how many women of all ages fail to ovulate every month. (They assume they are because they have regular cycles). Some women ovulate but not every month and other women ovulate monthly but may not have adequate amounts in the last 12 days of their cycle. Ovulation is the appearance of a white mucous discharge (that is egg like in colour) it is stringy in texture and distinct.

This might explain why many women respond beautifully to progesterone supplementation. Certainly, it reinforces the theory that maybe, just maybe PMS is an estrogen dominant disease consequent to inadequate progesterone levels. Women report an easing of symptoms with the flow of their period, that their PMS subsides only to gradually build again next month.

How is progesterone used to treat PMS?

The treatment approach to PMS is to address estrogen dominance before it sets in. Some women find it necessary to commence progesterone earlier than day 12 purely to overcome the build-up of tension and associated symptoms.

In theory and in practice, the best way to treat PMS with progesterone is to work from day 12 to 26 if your have a 28 day cycle, or day 14 to 28/30 if your have a 30/32 day cycle. If you build up your progesterone levels from day 12, increasing gradually prior to your period, you will take control of your PMS very, very quickly. Response to progesterone for PMS is usually effective and perhaps one of the easiest conditions to treat in NPAN's experience. Women find that within 3 months their life is usually back on track, asymptomatic using between 20-30mg thereafter from day 12-26.

You should use your cream according to symptom relief, particularly to treat anxiety and stress. Progesterone cream has a calmative effect on the body, reducing stress (which can sometimes negate progesterone's effect on the body).

Therefore, it's a good idea to carry your cream around in your handbag so you can immediately control extreme and sometimes nasty mood swings and impeding headaches. Women report the most effective way to do this is to apply cream (dabs) to the temples and behind the neck. The effect of the application usually kicks in within the hour. Repeat as necessary throughout the day, consequently reducing stress, anxiety and headaches and associated symptoms.

Some months may be worse than others depending on whether you have ovulated and your stress levels. So dosage can vary month to month, a base physiological dose being 16-20mg, equivalent to output of a woman ovulating.

Diet and nutrition, the use of phytoestrogenic herbs and plants extracts such as wild yam can often have a huge impact on the treatment of PMS, as does weight reduction and a good exercise program (which increases the level of endorphins in the brain and helps us to feel good).

What aggravates PMS, and why are some months worse?

Some of the triggers of PMS include anovulatory cycles where the ovaries don't ovulate every month, stress, shock, relationship problems, financial problems, or fear of pregnancy, hormonal triggers associated with ageing, hormone imbalances following sterilisation such as tubal ligation, coming off the Pill or being on the Pill **(oral contraception is a synthetic hormone that stops the production of progesterone from the ovaries,** reducing the production of progesterone and inhibiting progesterone's availability to the rest of the body), poor diet high in sugars and refined foods, and diets filled with stimulants such as caffeine, heavy smoking, alcohol, substance abuse, long term medication, all of which overwork the liver and, in turn, can interfere with the breakdown, metabolism, and excretion of hormones creating further imbalance.

Other issues to consider are excess weight gain which increases estrogen dominance, poor gastrointestinal function such as inefficient elimination, constipation, infections, exposure & ingestion of environmental toxins, poor immunity with chronic infections such as Sinusitis, Candida/Thrush, etc.

Sluggish bowel and leaky gut syndrome and other bowel problems can create re-absorption of toxins leading to xenoestrogenic effect and impact on the body thereby increasing estrogen dominance symptoms. Other issues causing increased estrogen is the high consumption of chicken, and high intake of dairy products can also upset hormones.

Will progesterone help my heavy menstrual bleeding, my PMS, breast swelling and menstrual cramps?

Most women realise excellent results when using progesterone to treat PMS, breast engorgement and/or heavy menstrual bleeding. This is possible because progesterone opposes these estrogen dominant symptoms.

In the first two weeks following your last period, estrogen surges through your body. It's job being to ripen the egg and mature it ready for ovulation and prepare the bloody rich uterine lining ready for pregnancy. If this is not balanced by a corresponding surge of progesterone, that is by way of ovulation, in the last two weeks leading up to your next period, then a number of side effects develop. Breast tenderness is one condition caused by estrogen dominance. The other is thickening of the uterine lining leading to heavy bleeding and/or clotting.

Other factors such as Anaemia and Fibroids can be the cause of heavy bleeding and clotting, brought on by estrogen dominance so please get a check-up if your periods are excessive, full of clots and associated lower swelling pelvic discomfort and maybe a baring down feeling.

Introducing progesterone can actually restore hormone balance and performance. Other factors such as vitamin supplements, high antioxidants, essential fatty acids, exercise, and attention to diet can relieve fluid retention and menstrual cramping. *After four cycles, a majority of women report periods have returned to normal flow, consistency, duration, and pain-free if a PMS related problem.*

If you suffer from Endometriosis and this is the cause of premenstrual pain, progesterone will certainly help alleviate these debilitating menstrual cycles over a course of months. Bleeding problems are covered extensively in Book 2.

Can I use progesterone to control my PMS mood swings?

Absolutely! As with your migraines, you can use progesterone on regular doses throughout the day before PMS sets in, and right through until the time of menses, increasing your dose as the cycle goes on (doses vary: mild-moderate starting at 16-20mg increasing to 30-40mg; very severe between 6%-10% (100 mg maximum) dosage seems to be what is required according to the women in this category) to control the agitation, moodiness, headaches, etc.

You will find after a few months of doing this that PMS will subside and you will be back on physiological doses from day 12 to 26 (usually 20-32mg).

As your stress levels diminish, the need for high doses of progesterone for the production of high cortisol levels (brought on by stress) is no longer required. Your body is back in balance. Charting will assist you in recognising, over a period of time, when you will need to increase your physiological doses to accommodate your stress levels.

Note, variations may be required every month. Based on observation, many women with PMS tend to ovulate on an average once every three months, explaining the fluctuation in their symptoms.

Why don't progestogens work for the treatment of PMS?

Progesterone opposes estrogen dominance naturally where as progestogens (synthetic) do not. Here's the reason why.

Sadly, too few doctors understand the distinct differences between a synthetic progestogen and natural progesterone. A natural molecule such as natural progesterone has a chemical structure identical to the progesterone produced by the ovaries.

The various synthetic progestogens (such as the pill) many doctors are prescribing these days to treat PMS are often mistaken as progesterone derivatives. These patented, not-natural-to-the-body hormones carry significant **side effects** i.e., moodiness, depression, increased appetite, fluid retention, weight gain, acne, greasy skin and even increased cholesterol. These exacerbate the problems of PMS even further.

Because our body uses progesterone to make other steroid hormone such as testosterone and the three different types of estrogen, progesterone cream can have an enormous impact on your overall health.

Treating PMS is but one example. Synthetic progestogens, however, are what is termed a 'dead-end' hormone. Unlike progesterone, your body cannot use a progestogen to manufacture any other steroid hormones that your body might need (this is why progesterone is a hormone balancer and modulator).

Only natural progesterone can turn 'on' the progesterone receptor, as a key can unlock the door. A synthetic progestogens, therefore, will not have the same beneficial effect as does natural progesterone. The key does not quite fit. Any change to a molecular structure (as with progestogens) will alter the message.

At this time, the medical fraternity do not necessarily recognise that PMS is related to progesterone deficiency as brought about by anovulatory cycles or insufficient progesterone output at ovulation (diagram in this section (page 200) demonstrates PMS in relation to lack of ovulation).

Many women report how surprised they are at the irregularity of their ovulation until they become tuned into this factor. They assumed regular periods indicated ovulation, which may not necessarily be the case! They also report in many instances the return and regulation of ovulation thus the ability to reduce their doses to 16-25mg daily from day 12-26.

Does progestogen therapy do the same as progesterone therapy? I am taking a progestogen to control Premenstrual Symptoms such as irritability and depression. Is it the same thing?

Again, it gets back to the lack of understanding of the distinction and difference between synthetic and natural hormones (see previous answer).

Depression and Premenstrual Syndrome (PMS) can be caused or aggravated by synthetic progestogens such as is found in Provera. If it is not helping you and you are experiencing side effects, it is suggested you switch to natural progesterone because it is less likely to cause mood disorders like its synthetic 'cousin' progestogen (progestins).

You can be forgiven for mistaking progestogen for progesterone and vice versa. But there really is a big difference … and your body knows it. So if you are experiencing side effects taking oral progestogen tablets, why not try topical progesterone cream that you rub onto your skin. See if it doesn't alleviate your mood swings and PMS.

If you're still feeling irritable, glum, and depressed after 4 months on progesterone and your moods haven't elevated and enhanced with a sense of wellbeing you need to explore the possibility that your depression may have other origins requiring further investigation. Chances are it is more chemical depression and not hormonal.

Interestingly, some women have adopted other strategies such as magnesium, St Johns Wort, B complex and naturopathic lithium which has proved very successful in conjunction with natural progesterone, eliminating the need to resort to anti-depressant medication. Whilst other women, some short term, have needed to go on anti-depressants in the interim to support them along with their progesterone, finding later can wean off their antidepressants. Testosterone transdermal creams are proving to have great benefits in treating depression from observation and report back. But err on the side of caution with the usage of this. You need to know your testosterone reading SHGB and FAI (Free Androgen Index) and your body type. The apple shape (Android body type) carries upper body weight and stores high levels of testosterone in body fat. Testosterone is not suggested for women with PCOS.

Is my combination patch 'natural'? My doctor has prescribed it to treat PMS.

There is an estrogen and progestogen combination patch now on the market. This does not contain natural progesterone, however, it does contain natural estrogen. If you are suffering side effects from synthetic hormone replacement you may wish to investigate alternative forms of natural hormone replacement therapy. I suggest you ask your doctor to order a saliva assay / blood work to determine your hormone profile when introducing combination hormone therapy to treat PMS. Given that there is suggestion that PMS is perhaps an estrogen dominance disorder, you may not require additional estrogen in your body. Also estrogen retains fluid and may contribute to your headaches, fluid retention and other symptoms (eg weight gain).

*Note, it is the way these hormones are delivered that is **patented** here.* Certainly, the patch does contain 'natural' estrogen however it does not contain 'natural' progesterone as women are being led to believe. It contains synthetic progestogins.

There is NO patch to date that contains natural progesterone, possibly due in part because research has shown that natural progesterone is most effectively absorbed and utilised by the human body when applied as a cream. (Research tests blood serum!).

Drug companies marketing these patches indicate to women that their products are derived from natural substances such as plants and modified to copy the estrogen produced by the female human ovary.

Technically this is correct, but their constant reference to 'natural' is a play on words and *implies progestogins and progesterone are interchangeable.* One would have to understand the distinction in order to pick this up. At a time when women are becoming aware of progesterone, perhaps it's no accident drug companies are interchanging words to catch your attention and confuses our Doctors. *The term Progestogenic benefits is often used by drug companies* so little wonder confusion reigns.

Polycystic Ovary Syndrome (PCOS)
What is Polycystic Ovary Syndrome?

Polycystic Ovary Syndrome (PCOS), also called **Stein-Leventhal Syndrome**, refers to multiple small Cysts on the ovaries (polycystic ovaries) and a host of other problems that go along with them, including lack of ovulation, menstrual abnormalities, excessive facial hair, male pattern baldness, acne, and sometimes obesity (upper weight very predominant).

Some women may also have varying degrees of insulin resistance (increased incidence of Type II diabetes), low bone density, and high triglycerides.

Symptoms include:

- Menstrual periods - abnormal, irregular or scanty
- Absence of period - usually but not always, after having one or more menstrual periods during puberty - then it stops
- Obesity - beginning tummy, hips, upper body
- Infertility
- Increased body hair growth, unusual growth and distribution of body hair
- Decreased breast size
- Aggravation of acne
- A possibility of Syndrome X (Refer Dr. Sandra Cabot website and books.)

How do I know if I have PCOS?

It is where there are multiple Cysts (more than 10 small follicles per ovary, lined around the edge of the ovary), whereas in a normal ovary they are distributed more evenly throughout the ovary. It is a condition of hormonal imbalance and it is characterised by excessive amounts of male hormones (androgens) and irregular menstruation.

Women are often predisposed to it, and it is strongly linked to inherited factors that may be triggered by stress and weight gain. Polycystic ovaries can be detected by an ultrasound (vaginal ultrasound far more effective) of the pelvis, and blood results showing high levels of testosterone.

What causes PCOS, and how is progesterone used in the treatment of this disease?

PCOS occurs when a woman fails to ovulate, which results in a disruption in the normal, cyclic inter-relationship among her hormones, her brain and her ovaries.

If ovulation is unsuccessful, and a lack of progesterone is detected by the hypothalamus, the ovary is stimulated to make more estrogen and androgens (male hormones), which stimulates more follicles towards ovulation. PCOS occurs when these additional follicles are unable to produce a mature ovum to ovulate to make progesterone. These eggs won't 'pop' and progesterone isn't made. The menstrual cycle is then dominated by estrogen and androgen (testosterone) minus the production of progesterone.

High levels of testosterone not only causes male-like features, but can cause an interference with the pancreas which interferes with insulin production (consequential insulin resistance). This in turn will interfere with blood glucose metabolism, accounting for the incidence of excess weight gain, particularly upper body weight and insulin resistance thereby creating a vicious cycle. The more weight gain the more exacerbated the problem becomes.

Reducing weight helps control this problem, and enhance hormone balancing. Progesterone also assists in modulation and balancing and feminising the more male dominant male characteristics.

There are suggested links between exposure to environmental pollutants that mimic estrogen and the developing baby's tissue. Laboratory experiments, wildlife studies, and the human DES experience link hormone disruption with a variety of male and female reproductive problems that appear to be on the rise in the general human population - problems ranging from Endometriosis, testicular cancer, Infertility, and in there somewhere is PCOS.

It is argued that if a female embryo's ovarian follicles are compromised through exposure to these chemicals, this damage will not be apparent until after puberty.

Other factors that can contribute to PCOS:

- Stress - high cortisol levels, long term
- Lack of exercise - overweight
- Poor nutrition - too much sugar and highly refined carbohydrates
- Birth Control Pill - shuts down normal ovary function
- Prescription drugs - that may impair the functioning of the limbic brain
- Severe dieting at an early age inn the developing years (anorexia and severe crash diets) interferes with the developing pituitary gland and the bio feedback mechanism.
- High exposure to xenoestrogens and chemicals (recreational drugs and some medications).

NPAN has seen many young women with PCOS and there seems to be a correlation with a history of substance abuse and/or high exposure to environmental chemicals. This disease is, in a majority of cases reported to NPAN, appears to be triggered in these younger girls by high levels of stress, shock, family distress (parents divorcing or separating) and/or scholastic pressures.

Women with PCOS make up a large portion of the cases seen here at NPAN. And it is very pleasing to report, natural progesterone appears to be proving to be a major player in the successful treatment of PCOS. Progesterone used in PCOS is a controversial subject and is not keenly adopted as mainstream management and is even often disagreed with by Naturopaths as a form of consideration in treatment. Interestingly many PCOS groups through word of mouth of their members success stories are now approaching me or their Doctors to adopt the usage of progesterone in their treatment. The reason behind this solution - if you're body isn't producing enough progesterone, then progesterone supplementation is going to help maintain the normal synchronous pattern each month and women with PCOS do not ovulate regularly to produce their own progesterone.

What are the signs and tests that will confirm I have PCOS?

Tests:

>vaginal ultrasound
>
>pelvic examination
>
>ovarian biopsy
>
>blood profiles

Results of tests will show:

>increased ratio LH to FSH
>
>elevated androgen levels - testosterone
>
>urine 17-ketosteriods may be elevated
>
>relatively high estrogen levels
>
>negative serum HCG - pregnancy test

This disease may also alter the results of the following tests:

>estriol - urine
>
>estriol - serum

What is the guidelines dosage?

In early stages of PCOS where symptoms are not severe, recommended starting dose would be 32mg from day 12-26, reducing as your body responds favourably, and working towards a minimum dose where you are asymptomatic. For younger women with PCOS and no periods, it's important that they continue a regime of 12-26 days to mimic what the body would be trying to do naturally. This ensures balance.

In the more advanced PCOS cases that are observed by NPAN, the average dose most women seem to be asymptomatic at is around 54mg of progesterone cream daily from day 12-26 of your cycle (adjust accordingly) for at least the first 7 months if there is a regular cycle.

In the initial few months, however, a lot of women take 64mg-100mg of progesterone cream from day 5-26 to address many accompanying symptoms extreme progesterone deficiency, and often to address pain (can be due to the presence of Endometriosis). Ideally, after your body has settled down, you would try to wean back to a lesser dose or to extend breaks to fall into line with a day 12-26 cycle.

It's important that you have regular ultrasounds to assess the condition of your ovaries, and an indicator of treatment progression. This will also determine your response to progesterone and incorporating treatments (nutrition weight loss).

Note, if you are using a regime day 5-26 in the first 4-7 months until symptoms settle, please be aware you are using a program suggested to enhance fertility. One pregnancy has occurred where a lady stopped using cream for a couple of months because she thought she no longer needed it, had unprotected sex assuming her PCOS condition had lessened her chances of fertility, and fell pregnant. This lady is now on physiological doses (32mg) from day 12-26 and is asymptomatic.

How do I know when to reduce my dose?

The way you can tell if you're on the winning side of progesterone therapy and may reduce your dosage is by the fact that you haven't continued to gain weight, your lower abdomen is no longer swollen or tender, your sugar cravings are under control, your facial and body hair has reduced significantly, and your periods have regulated.

If your symptoms appear to be getting worse, you need to check out your testosterone levels, glucose intolerance, and ultrasound results, all of which may indicate that progesterone therapy is not enough, or you need to increase your dose. Do this only under your doctor's supervision.

NPAN suggests you refer to Dr Sandra Cabot's publication 'The Body Shaping Diet' and follow the android eating plan and feminising foods to compliment your body type and hormone metabolism. There are also some very helpful natural supplements on the market to help reduce and stabilise high blood sugar levels and insulin resistance in the treatment of PCOS. Women have found Dr Sandra Cabot's "Glucemic Balance" Formulation in tablet form very beneficial in assisting to stabilise sugar levels, sugar cravings and control insulin resistance along with dietary changes and a weight loss program high in first class protein and low glycaemic index foods with this approach many PCOS cases have avoided needing to resort to the popular prescribed medications used to help weight loss and reduce excessive hair growth due to high levels of testosterone.

Addressing weight problems is very important in the treatment of this disease. Reducing weight is imperative to a favourable outcome with or without progesterone therapy. Continued weight gain leads to continued storage of upper body fat which, in turn, generates higher levels of male hormones, and further hormone disruption and insulin resistance results. This cycle becomes vicious, and the disease worsens. Dr. Sandra Cabot's new book ("Can't Lose Weight? You could have Syndrome X the chemical imbalance that makes you store fat") addresses insulin resistance and the chemical imbalances that make you fat. Also see 'Weight Issues' Chapter 14 and Chapter 17 on phytoestrogens and the benefits of estrogenic foods. Refer to my Book 2 More Secrets Revealed.

What may I expect to experience while using progesterone if I have PCOS?

Women have reported, several months into progesterone therapy, *episodes of ovary popping* which can result in severe pain. Patterns occur around 4 and 7 months. And can, for some, be a very frightening experience, especially when they do not understand what is happening in their body after months of stability and a sense of wellbeing.

This period of discomfort generally lasts for a couple of days. It may bring on unusual bleeding (often trauma induced following a egg being released from the ovary) and it may even be very unusual in colour, reported by some women as being watery and pale (serum-like). These episodes of ovary activity may set off fortnightly periods for a while, until the body resettles again.

It is important that you do not mistake this bleed as your true period thus breaking from cream, as this could further disrupt your cycle. Just continue on your established cycle, and take your cyclic break when it falls due to true expected menses time.

Synchronisation will be re-established despite this follicular disruption. I try and explain to women that, based on the many reports provided to NPAN, this is quite a common occurrence. But just to be on the safe side, and for your own peace of mind, see your doctor, ask him to order another ultrasound and/or hormone profile.

NPAN interprets these displays of activity as progesterone's positive action in the body.

I'd like to include here an account of one woman named Fiona who had severe PCOS and who had been trying to conceive for two years. She found that **this episode of pain and popping heralded a renewed fertility**. And from this point on became vigilant with her blood profiles and saliva assays to check FSH and progesterone levels.

Within seven months Fiona went on to conceive and is now the mother of a very healthy baby boy. Her doctor wanted Fiona to cease progesterone to provide an accurate FSH reading (without the influence of progesterone) but Fiona, being well read, refused. Fiona went on to become pregnant the following month, and had she stopped progesterone, perhaps this drop may have compromised her chances of fertility.

I bring this story to your attention so that you may become aware of the need for contraception if you have been led to believe you are infertile (avoid synthetic hormones as it will undo all the good work). I hope it sheds a ray of light and hope to women attempting to conceive and may be disillusioned at this point in time. Since the first publication many other so-called infertile women with PCOS have had babies. See our latest pregnancy in Kate's story 'My Miracle' in Book 2.

Please note, until you achieve physiological doses (up to 4% for some women) on a 12-26 day program that is 14 days on cream, mimicking nature, please take extra precaution with contraception as ovulation is very unpredictable. A pattern usually emerges, and after 7 months women wean back, if on high doses, working towards a more natural cycle. Refer to question 'How do I know when to reduce my dose'. Resting the ovaries on high doses then dramatically reducing (or stopping for a month) once symptoms have been abated can surge the ovaries to ovulate. Usual time round about 6-7 months before returning to 2 weeks on 2 weeks off. Please visit Fertility section in Book 2 'Natural Progesterone More Secrets Revealed' and Kate's testimonial.

What else can I do to improve PCOS symptoms?

- Pay particular attention to diet and nutrition
- Avoid all refined carbohydrates and sugars
- Get plenty of balanced exercise and anti-stress activity (don't overexercise)
- Drink lots of filtered water,
- Reduce weight and maintain correct weight
- Avoid diary products (particularly if trying for pregnancy as they may glue or sticky up the fallopian tubes as it has mucous like effect on the body)
- Reduce estrogen dominance Book 2 'Natural Progesterone More Secrets Revealed' delves into this in greater detail
- Learn to manage your stress levels, and rest up
- Use a combination formula designed to address the Android Body Type can assist stabilisation. (Included in my next book).
- Incorporate appropriate nutritional supplementation and estrogenic foods
- Adopt liver cleansing program to assist hormone balancing and weight reduction (and pregnancy).
- Stabilise blood sugar level instabilities.

Migraines / Headaches

I have always suffered Migraine headaches, nausea and vomiting during the time of my period. Will progesterone help this?

I see many successful outcomes using natural progesterone.

Migraines are very debilitating. And this ailment can plague women over a lifetime. They are rarely pain-free much less able to clear the fogginess in their head. Estrogen dominance has a great bearing on this condition.

While headaches and migraines are multi-factorial, when hormonally induced, progesterone therapy has rendered remarkable results. Hormone balancing via progesterone therapy will eventually resolve estrogen dominance induced headaches and migraines, however, it will take time, especially if you have suffered with chronic headaches for years.

One of the causes of headaches can be the result of too much estrogen in your body. Or there may be other contributing factors such as liver dysfunction, chemical sensitivities, toxins, food allergies, stress induced or perhaps something more sinister.

Given that you have indicated your headaches, nausea and vomiting are cyclic, there's a very high probability that they are hormonal. Following a monthly pattern suggests estrogen dominance.

*Too much estrogen in the body causes **intracellular edema/oedema*** (creating pressure from the internal swelling of the cells). When this occurs, it allows the sodium (salt) in the body to permeate (pass through) the cell membrane, bringing water through. Retaining body fluid on the wrong side of the cells creates a condition termed intracellular edema and fluid retention which often causes headaches. In other words the vessels swell causing pressure and discomfort due to osmosis.

Chickens, for example, are fed high levels of estrogen-laced grain to plump up their cells, accelerate growth rate, thereby increasing body weight which, in turn, increases sale value.

A lot of women fail to realise that even though they may have a lot of fluid retention such as puffy feet and hands, particularly around this time of the month, they can *actually be dehydrated* because the body fluid is on the wrong side of the cell. So it's important, if you're a headache sufferer, to drink ample pure water, to flush out the excess estrogens and toxins and to re-hydrate your body. You may not be thirsty even though you are dehydrated.

Contrary to what you might think, this will NOT increase your fluid retention. In fact, it will help you eliminate the excess estrogens and balance your fluids. *The more hydration is restored the more natural thirst returns!*

The usage of chemicals, stimulants or codeine based drugs can actually make headaches worse because of withdrawal symptoms which they can create headaches including migraines. I personally was a codeine addict and was unaware of this and it took me a long time to discover that the withdrawal from this substance was actually creating more pain in my body. I now use Magnesium in its place. Many people are addicted to such things as coffee and don't even realise it. To test this out try seeing if you can go without a cup of coffee for a few days without getting a headache or the shakes.

I see many women resort to diuretics (fluid tablets) to correct fluid retention but it can create an electrolyte imbalance because they are urinating lots of valuable minerals. If you choose to go off diuretics it must be done under your doctor's supervision.

A safer way of correcting sodium retention is with the use of natural progesterone. Over a period of time, progesterone stops the permeability of sodium through the cells which helps balance the fluid within the blood. Reduced fluid retention will result, relieving headaches and blood pressure if it is hormonally influenced.

If you are already applying progesterone cream and continue to suffer headaches and/or fluid retention, look at other possible causes, maybe speak with your doctor, get saliva levels done along with possibly a kidney test and a blood pressure reading.

HRT and the Pill are high players here and often not linked to headaches. Some women find by stopping the oral contraceptive pill is enough to eliminate headaches and migraines. **Of course you cannot be on the pill and progesterone at the same time.**

Will taking estrogen with progesterone affect my headaches?

Yes, it can. Please refer to comments above on intracellular edema and fluid retention.

This is why it is important if you are taking a combination of estrogen and progesterone replacement, I suggest you assess your estrogen dosage.

Also note *that you must break from estrogen at the same time you break from progesterone cream, otherwise you will fail to break the estrogen dominance cycle, and headaches and migraines will persist.*

If you are using vaginal estrogen pessaries or creams, make sure you know why you are using them because there are various types of estrogen and dosage prescribed on the market. A popular form of estrogen via this route is estradiol rather than oral estrogen.

Estradiol dosage could negate or override your progesterone thus creating a estrogen dominance environment. If this is the case, you won't feel many benefits of using topical progesterone at physiological doses of 20-32mg.

If headaches fall into this category, progesterone effectiveness will be compromised in headache management. Higher doses will be required using progesterone and strong estrogens (Estradiol and Estrone) together. Switching to a low dose Triest transdermal cream which combines all three natural estrogens in proportional ratio aligned with the bodies natural estrogen ratio is often more suitable or using a gel (Sandrena - Estradiol) where you can control administration as required, perhaps not every day. Separating estrogen from progesterone has proven useful for women attempting to control balance (especially if they need some estrogen top ups). Which may be the case with women weaning off estrogen. For other women the weakest estrogen Estriol vaginal cream ("Ovestin" 1mg) is all they may need. Using this form of estrogen and dosage of 1mg does not normally tilt the progesterone ratio and women will not need to increase their progesterone doses.

I suffer vaginal atrophy and dryness, and use estriol cream. Will this create hormonal headaches?

There are some women who are super sensitive even to the mildest for of Estriol administration however in most cases the answer is no.

Estriol is a very mild and safe form of estrogen. And the creams tend to be at lower doses such that they do not compromise progesterone therapy. It's an ideal approach to maintaining healthy vaginal mucosa (mucous membrane), vaginal integrity without causing increased side effects of estrogen dominance such as headaches.

However, about 2% of women have reported that they are so sensitive to any form of estrogen that even the slightest overdose will bring on an instant Migraine or breast swelling (engorgement).

I am not usually a headache or Migraine sufferer and I fall into this category but acknowledge the need for vaginal maintenance. This is why I now mix "Ovestin" (estriol) with progesterone to avoid the onset of severe headaches/migraines which I experienced in the past.

It took me a long time to recognise my sensitivity to estrogen, that can vary month to month, or how often I use "Ovestin". I have found over the last few years it is better for me to do minute doses daily to achieve the recommended dose of 1-3 times a week dose requirement of vaginal estriol. The way to gauge your dose administration is by the health state of the vaginal walls, correct lubrication, painless intercourse (i.e. Not gritty and paper thin) and of course no bladder problems. When my bladder along with other women's reports feels sensitive this is an indication of a need for more Estriol. Bladder sensitivity can be displayed in a slight twinge, loss of tone, not being able to empty completely and Stress Incontinence. All these (also and/or vaginal dryness), are markers to increase use or frequency of Estriol vaginal cream. Refer to pages 244, 248.

I am getting very bad headaches/migraines on progesterone cream. I thought progesterone was meant to stop all this.

Eventually it will, and headaches should lessen month by month. Some women have taken 7-12 months (a few up to 18 months) of persistent effort and adjustment on progesterone creams to see fabulous results emerge. It has been for some, a time of trial and error and debilitation. These women diligently followed nutritional guidelines and methodical application of progesterone cream to see their efforts pay off.

When you commence progesterone supplementation, in the first 8 weeks in particular when estrogen receptors are being woken up in the body as a result of the re-introduction of progesterone, headaches can actually be exacerbated. This is why it is suggested that you double your dose of progesterone cream (up to 10% 100mg - some go as high as 200mg) and introduce phytoestrogens and magnesium to help counteract the side effects of estrogen wake up. And get in early, apply cream before you feel a headache coming on. Learn your headache onset signs. Increase gradually, hourly (it helps to put on temples) to the level where you can prevent the headache emerging.

Additionally, between the 8 week to 4 month time frame while the body is adjusting to renewed progesterone levels and utilising progesterone to oppose estrogen dominance, that women **try to avoid codeine-based analgesics.** I have observed that codeine can often set up a pathway of increased pain due to withdrawal symptoms, while overloading the liver. Long term analgesic use can accumulate in the body, and may take quite some time to be removed it may take time to wean yourself off these also don't go cold turkey if you have been using analgesia over many years to treat headaches.

Of equal importance is the need to detoxify via a liver cleansing diet. And avoid trigger foods and substances that may set off allergies. For once the liver is no longer overburdened, progesterone will work more effectively. All our hormones are broken down by the liver and if the liver is fatty, has accumulated toxins through drug ingestion for pain management, it means progesterone will further burden the liver.

A lot of women are not aware of this. In fact, if a woman reports nausea when starting progesterone it is often reflective of her poor liver functioning status, and the need to assist it by way of a detoxification program.

Journal charting can assist women in identifying their triggers and when they occur, note how long they may last, degree of intensity, associated stresses, whether it be internal, hormonal, chemical, medications, food or toxic. Patterns will emerge over the 7 month period.

Evidence NPAN has gathered to date suggests that women who follow a strategic health plan that incorporates regular massage, where possible meditation, detoxing the body, and substituting pain killers with high levels of magnesium, St Johns Wort, and other natural anti-stressors and calmers in the form of natural herbs, the end result is far more rewarding and longer lasting than the more traditional drug-induced 'instant pain relief' approach.

Use a premium phytoestrogen to protect estrogen receptors from the more toxic estrogens (xenoestrogens) and more potent estrogens manufactured by the body, thus toning down the impact of estrogen dominance, calming and blocking these receptors with plant estrogens. *Essential fatty acids (Omega 3,6 & 9) are also essential for brain integrity and protection and to produce anti inflammatory chemicals.* Ensure high fibre to assist regular bowel elimination of the potential aggravating, damaging and circulating toxins and poisons.

Progesterone will work if you hang in there, however, it may be a long haul, and initially it may not appear to be giving you results. It's a case of persistence and patience, and following strategies that will be long lasting.

Progesterone is a journey ... not a quick fix. Headache management is complex, and needs to be approached holistically.

How can I use natural progesterone to control my headaches/migraines?

Your approach to cyclic headaches and migraines is to tackle estrogen dominance head-on. And the best way to avoid monthly migraines is to recognise when they start (in your cycle)and start applying cream a couple of days prior. So that you're treating the (hormonal) condition that would bring on the headache. And as the cycle progresses you can increase your dose accordingly.

Work in the vicinity of 50-100mg if you have to. Some women have gone as far as 200 and higher for a few days to control the onset of migraines. It has been found that if women do hourly doses - dabbed onto their temples and behind the neck when they feel most susceptible and stressed - the higher levels may not be necessary, because they have managed to control and assess their symptoms on a 1-2 hourly regime. It's amazing how, when you become calmer, the curtailing of stress may be all that's required to reduce the triggers of the onset of a Migraine. Also bump up your intake of magnesium supplements which is a muscle relaxant, invaluable in the treatment of muscle spasms, cramps, nervous tension, and pain management.

Progesterone exerts a vasodilator (relaxing) effect on the blood vessels further assisting anti-spasmodic action that can set off headaches. It also helps control the sodium balance on the right side of the cell membrane preventing osmosis (fluid being pulled into the cells) causing intracellular edema. It is this extra fluid that creates the pressure and can cause the headaches. In other words the fluid is on the wrong side of the cells.

Drinking heaps of pure water also prevents toxic build up, flushes out body wastes and toxins, and maintains fluid balance preventing dehydration.

Suggestions - Intravaginal application and warnings in Migraine management

If you can't recognise the onset of a headache/Migraine or it strikes unannounced, try adopting an intravaginal dosage starting at 20mg (which would effectively double your dose to that equivalent of 40mg topically). Wait a couple of hours and reapply if symptoms are not abating (with caution dosage of another 10mg). Repeat until headache subsides. This can markedly reduce the impact of your headache, occasionally thwarting the onset of a Migraine. I have resorted to this route successfully. ***This is not** a standard procedure for Migraine treatment with the use of transdermal progesterone cream. IN FACT IF YOU HAVE NOT USED this route before and you administer a high dose (even a physiological dose of 10-20mg) you can actually create a headache, fogginess and even a Migraine along with an onset of a period.* This is because it is targeting new receptors and bringing the body into a state of Estrogen Dominance Wake Up Crisis (as in the beginning which some of you may have experiences).

Even if your body is used to the topical application route i.e. Transdermal on skin and you have been asymptomatic and your body has been settled the ***intravaginal administration route can bring on the estrogen dominance crisis.*** This is why I warn women as my first attempt induced a Migraine which took a couple of days to settle. I pulled back and slowly/minutely introduced progesterone vaginally 1-2 times a week of 5mg which equals 10mg transdermal, gradually and more frequently increasing until my body adjusted and accommodated the topical cream intra vaginally by this administration route. After 3 years I can now tolerate between 32mg-100mg intra vaginally alternating this administration route with transdermal application. Just to remind you 16mg transdermal (applied on the skin) equals 32mg vaginally, 50mg transdermal equals 100mg vaginally. You can appreciate why you need to start off with minute doses. Because of this powerful absorption route of an equivalent increased dosage.

Be aware that the vaginal route has a high impact (equal to double the topical equivalent)on your body through direct absorption, so go easy on how much you apply. *I suggest to women that they experiment with this unique approach before actually relying on it to treat the onset of a Migraine.*

Note: If a full-on Migraine has already begun, progesterone will not be able to stop it or reverse it. You may need to resort to medical treatment or see your doctor. Progesterone will not help prevent nausea and vomiting if your Migraine has progressed. Progesterone however will assist in keeping you calm along with the use of Magnesium.

For introduction of the intravaginal application method once you have mastered this route of administration.

Summary:

A good starting point:

Suggested guideline for introduction to vaginal dosage is 10mg (1%) once a week, to allow your body time to adjust to this method, and for you to assess your sensitivity and response to intravaginal progesterone application. The first few applications can bring on estrogen dominance wakeup, and this is the last thing you need when you are battling a headache. In fact, it could possibly make the headache worse. So introduce very gradually and with caution.

Once you have adopted this route:

Suggested guide to alternate transdermal and intravaginal dosage according to your needs.

Women who have mastered this method find it a reliable emergency deliverance system with excellent outcome. These women have been on progesterone for many years and know their bodies.

PLEASE NOTE, NPAN WOMEN AND MYSELF HAVE ONLY TRIALLED ONE PARTICULAR MANUFACTURED PROGESTERONE CREAM IN THE INTRAVAGINAL METHOD (PRO-FEME). WE CANNOT VOUCH FOR OTHER CREAMS, NOR ARE WE IN A POSITION TO RECOMMEND THEIR USAGE AND LEVEL OF SAFETY IF USED IN THIS MANNER. PLEASE READ SECTION ON CREAMS USED VAGINALLY. CRINONE GEL BEING NOT AVAILABLE IN AUSTRALIA MEANS WE HAVE NO EXPERIENCE IN ITS USE FOR HORMONE BALANCING.

THE MANUFACTURERS OF PRO-FEME DID NOT DESIGN THE CREAM FOR VAGINAL USE BUT IT CONTAINS NO KNOWN INGREDIENTS THAT ARE LIKELY TO BE HARMFUL. WE CANNOT VOUCH FOR ANY OTHER CREAMS AND THEIR CONTENTS AS WE HAVEN'T USED THEM.

See reference section for references on vaginal delivery and progesterone. My second book also mentions more vaginal usage. See Book 2 'Natural Progesterone More Secrets Revealed'.

I have been free of headaches for over twelve months on progesterone, but now they are suddenly returning again. Why would this be?

Reports of headaches and migraines re-emerging after a headache-free period are not uncommon. **This I term Estrogen Dominance Wake Up Crisis** which I deal with very extensively in my second book covering causes and management.

There are many reasons why this may occur. Ruling out conditions that are currently under the watchful eye of a qualified healthcare professional, I pose the questions, "What has been going on in your life?" "Are you still taking your phytoestrogens?" "Have you been under any extra stress lately?" or "Have you been exposed to unusual toxins?" (for instance repainted your house). Other toxins being new carpeting, new office equipment and recent renovations.

And usually women can recall, perhaps one to two months prior, an incidence of unmanaged stress, a shock, an infection, illness, or the introduction of some other form of medication, or lifestyle change such as a new job or new environment, travelling, changing climate.

There are many aspects that can cause an imbalance in our hormonal constitution. Stress for example. Normal physiological doses can maintain hormonal health beautifully until the body has to call on its reserves of progesterone to perform other roles in the body such as handle stress or create cortisol to handle infections. In which case your dose needs to be increased for a short period of time to accommodate the body's need for higher levels of progesterone. You may also need to increase dosage for a month just to resaturate your now diminished reserves, to restore them back to equilibrium if it is a progesterone deficiency problem. Remember stress always robs your progesterone to make the survival hormones.

This quick check solution is often as simple as doubling the dose for that month and then reducing gradually back to the physiological dose. It does not take long to quickly get the reserves up and to refuel the body with progesterone if the body is normally in balance. You will notice a remarkable difference and improvement if this is what your body needs.

Additionally, if there are stress factors that are ongoing, it may pay to slightly increase dosage (by 1-2%)over that period of time as a buffer. And to also look at improved nutritional and vitamin supplementation that will support the body. Perhaps a super multivitamin B complex magnesium complete, and other calmative herbs. Perhaps more sleep or a holiday.

Charting can actually help you identify where the triggers are and what your body is actually telling you. Is the physical born of the metaphysical? Certainly headache, a heavier period, sore breasts, sleep disturbances, agitation or whatever are all early warning signs of estrogen dominance needing to be heeded to.

At NPAN I have observed that women who are 'headache people' tend to remain 'headache people'. It doesn't take much for them to become imbalanced and their headaches act as a barometer that they are in overload and need to rebalance and revisit basic principles.

Pose these questions to yourself, "What has been happening in my life?", "Have I been under extra stress?", "Have I been exposed to any chemicals (renovated your home/office)?","Have I eaten incorrectly (junk food)?","Am I allergic to something?","Do I feel unwell, perhaps there is an illness in my body that needs to be addressed?", "Do I need to lose a little weight / have I gained weight?","Am I becoming estrogen dominant again?", or "Do I need to detox my liver or change my eating plan?". "Do I need to reduce my stress and lifestyle or change my job?", "Am I taking phytoestrogens?", "Am I using adequate amounts of Magnesium?","Am I drinking adequate water?","Am I exposed to toxins?", "Where am I in the stages of my progesterone journey?", "Am I estrogen dominant?".

I cannot emphasis enough the importance of phytoestrogens and the relationship between these and progesterone. Far too often women abandon this principle and the vital components of phytoestrogens which have a huge influence in the interplay of progesterone's performance. They also assist the body to tone down estrogen dominance.

I'm having Migraines after my period, not before. What does this mean?

If the Migraine occurs after the period, this indicates you are still estrogen dominant and that you have yet to realise the full benefits of progesterone therapy. I suggest you take shorter breaks rather than start day 12. Instead start day 5 for a few months and assess your periods, then extend your breaks as your headaches lessen.

Charting will help you identify triggers, recognise when migraines and headaches are likely to occur so cream dosage can be increased prior to the onset. Women have found that if they increase their progesterone dosage prior to their periods, particularly if this is when their migraines occur, pain can be managed without the need for pharmaceutical pain killers.

There is one particular case that comes to mind. Susan reported debilitating migraines 3 days after her period started. She was a 28 day cycle. Using personal charts to aid me and I discovered that in actual fact she continued to be progesterone deficient despite applying cream from day 12 to 26 over 4 months. Susan wasn't seeing any results.

It was obvious that her body had not replenished or sustained its stores of progesterone. Of note was her history of heavy analgesic and substance use, her considerable intake of alcohol and nicotine. I found the way around this particular case was for Susan to take very short breaks from cream each month. Stop using progesterone cream for only 5 days instead of 11.

Susan followed my suggestion, taking 32mg at the beginning of the month increasing dosage to 64mg just prior to her period. After a few months she began to see results, and Susan was then in a position to wean back accordingly.

It was also suggested Susan go on a liver work program to allow her liver to function more adequately thus allowing her body to utilise progesterone more effectively. After a liver detox and weight loss program, increased phytoestrogens and eating the right foods, Susan was able to resume day 12-26 within a 4 month period.

This was brought about as a result of reducing her estrogen dominance naturally, thereby reducing the need to administer high levels of progesterone dose to oppose (which can render progesterone ineffective if used long term without addressing the underlying problems).

I've been on progesterone for 4-7 months and have not experienced any relief from headaches.

If progesterone therapy is not having any positive bearing on your hormonal health in the first few months, especially around 3-4 months when progesterone reserves should be topped up and levelling out, and if you still find yourself battling intense cyclic headaches, there's every indication cell receptors are not very responsive.

Often you need to work on the liver (detox) to facilitate higher levels of activity and greater assimilation of progesterone. Also note that magnesium can have a tremendous effect on assimilation in these cases, particularly in assisting progesterone conversion, and the messages received by progesterone receptors.

My observation, progesterone has little impact on women who have suffered long term chronic conditions such as Chronic Fatigue Syndrome (CFS) and Adrenal Exhaustion, or may have had glandular fever during their lifetime. These are health conditions, for example, where progesterone and complementary nutritional supplementation appear to have such little impact at cellular and receptor level.

The body appears to have shut down. Progression is usually slow and steady, so even headache episodes may take considerable time to abate. A retrospective look over a twelve month progesterone therapy and some progress can be acknowledged.

These women need nurturing because it's a long, hard haul back to good health and can be frustrating bringing about despondency.

Again, it is an individual thing that needs to be monitored and all aspects of your health and health history taken into account. You can never assume your symptoms are hormonally related. I vehemently stress that all health issues or concerns you might have, be investigated by a qualified healthcare professional.

Fibromyalgia/Chronic Fatigue Syndrome
What is Fibromyalgia / Chronic Fatigue Syndrome?
Fibromyalgia

Fibromyalgia means pain in the muscles, ligaments and tendons - the fibrous tissues in the body. FMS used to be called **"fibrositis"**, implying that there was inflammation in the muscles, but research later proved that inflammation did not exist.

Sufferers of FMS will invariably suffer from Chronic Fatigue Syndrome (CFS) and often bouts of Depression as a consequence of their exhaustion battling with this disease, but CFS sufferers are not necessarily victims of the pain associated with FMS.

Most patients with Fibromyalgia say that they ache all over. Their muscles may feel like they have been pulled or overworked. Sometimes the muscles twitch and at other times they burn.   Pain is often migrational.

Women tell me that it's extremely difficult to distinguish between what is a benign isolated incident of pain versus something more sinister. Should she be concerned about that pain in her chest, or dismiss it as just another chapter in the progression of this disease? A very hard call for discernment.

Fibromyalgia is defined by pain. There are really no visible manifestations of this disease. For that reason, victims of Fibromyalgia are often viewed as hypochondriacs, malingerers, poor souls seeking attention through illness and for some they have lived chronically like this, have lost a sense of achieving a healthy status becoming entrenched in their pain and disease. A hard circuit to challenge let alone break. I have witnessed some women become consumed by the disease in their search for answers to a point of losing themselves and becoming their disease. Their cries for help eventually fall on deaf ears and empathy is no longer forthcoming. Because these people look so well on the outside people do not understand their frustration and insistence on being affirmed.

For example, when we're in pain, perhaps we've hurt our ankle, we expect a degree of understanding that, yes, ankle sprains hurt. A toothache hurts. Sinus congestion is painful. To some degree, people generally appear capable of empathising openly with another's suffering when there is evidence of injury or disease and can relate.

But given that Fibromyalgia patients present as perfectly normal, otherwise healthy individuals who appear to be simply recovering from a bad dose of the flu, this life-altering disease is dismissed by family, friends and work colleagues as either a passing condition or entirely psychosomatic. The circle is vicious.

So, one must not only contend with the debilitating symptoms of Fibromyalgia, day in day out, maybe for the rest of her life, but she must also brace herself for the ignorant backlash she will invariably receive from those who should, during her time of need, be extending emotional and physical support. She must also challenge not becoming her own worst enemy and a victim of this disease (of unknown cause). It takes courage to change programs, belief systems and negative self talk. It takes awareness and effort to stop subconsciously feeding our mind with reinforcing negative thoughts such as "I am ill", "I am like this because", "I cannot do this because" and "I cannot go there because". It is a fact deprivation lowers immunity. So I encourage women to find the antidote and not feel so deprived by focusing on a more positive outcome even though there are no answers to this disease. Progesterone is the first step to helping a women return back to herself.

Traditional treatments are geared toward improving the quality of sleep, as well as reducing pain, because deep level (stage 4) *sleep is so crucial for many body functions, such as tissue repair, antibody production, adrenal regeneration and perhaps even the regulation of various neurotransmitters, hormones and immune system chemicals.*

The sleep disorders that frequently occur in Fibromyalgia and Chronic Fatigue patients are thought to be a major contributing factor to the symptoms of this condition. Medicines that boost your body's level of serotonin and norepinephrine - neurotransmitters that modulate sleep, pain and immune system function - are commonly prescribed. Olive Leaf Extract has had positive effects on some sufferers. More and more women are responding to long term use of progesterone, Olive Leaf liquid, B complex liquid and essential fatty acids and a nutrient rich diet full of natural antibiotics. Exercise is vital as is sunlight as these increase the production of happy chemicals (endorphins).

Chronic Fatigue Syndrome

Chronic fatigue syndrome, or CFS for short, is a poorly understood condition or collection of conditions that cause a variety of symptoms such as substantial fatigue, muscle pain, sore throat, emotional instability, and difficulty concentrating. These symptoms persist for six months or more and are not explained by any other known medical condition.

One distinctive difference between CFS and FMS is their sleep patterns. CFS sleep for more than what is considered normal and yet do not wake up feeling fresh and rested, while FMS patients cannot establish a restorative sleep pattern because of the constant presence of pain. They are deprived of sleep.

Experts are in disagreement as to the cause or causes of CFS, but a popular theory today is that it is an auto-immune disorder. This means that the immune system has somehow been directed to attack the body itself. Many CFS experts have changed the name of this disorder to *Chronic Fatigue and Immune Dysfunction Syndrome (CFIDS)* to reflect the role of the immune system. Observation on my part witnesses both disorders as years of progesterone deficiency along with majority of women who have a history of glandular fever.

You might like to visit the "Co-Cure" website (http://www.co-cure.org) for more on Fibromyalgia & Chronic Fatigue Syndrome. The name stands for "Cooperate and Communicate for a Cure."

Also visit product information on testosterone usage (now being recognized in helping CFS) http:/www.lawleypharm.com.au.

What causes FMS?

The exact cause of Fibromyalgia Syndrome is unknown. Many different factors, alone or in combination may trigger this disorder. In recent years, studies have shown that in FMS, the muscle is especially vulnerable to decreased circulation and minor injury.

Research has also looked at the role of certain hormones or body chemicals that may alter pain, sleep, and mood. Factors that possibly aggravate FMS are changes in weather, cold or drafty environments, hormonal fluctuations (premenstrual and menopausal states), stress, depression, anxiety and over-exertion can all contribute to symptom flare-ups.

FMS is more common than most people think. And once diagnosed, there appears to be very little physicians can do in the way of treatment beyond drugs and coping skills to manage pain. Invariably, the onus is placed back on the individual to deal with this condition as best she or he can.

Support groups that offer information and pain management seminars are invaluable. But basically Fibromyalgia represents a lonely, agonising road of silent suffering that continues on for years, for some a lifetime.

NPAN does not have the statistics for Australia at this time, but we do know that over 6 million Americans, 90% of them women in the prime of their life, suffer from FMS and sometimes struggle for years before being correctly diagnosed.

Symptoms usually appear between 20-55 years of age, but children are also diagnosed with Fibromyalgia syndrome. Pain and severe fatigue may keep FMS sufferers from their chosen profession and unable to perform common daily tasks.

It would have to be questioned how much of our xenoestrogen environment and exposure has an interplay on the endocrine and immunity system resulting in massive health disruption and havoc to our well-being.

What are the signs and symptoms of FMS?

- FMS produces chronic body-wide pain that has a 'burning' sensation, which migrates and can be felt from head to toe.
- Sleep disturbance and non-restorative sleep
- Persistent fatigue, lethargy
- Headaches
- Cognitive or memory impairment
- Morning stiffness
- Pain that migrates from day to day
- Symptoms shown to be chronic, but may wax and wane

My observations of FMS and CFS sufferers who may also have:
- Depression, suicidal thoughts, self absorbed, withdrawn, insulated
- Endocrine disruption, hormonal imbalance, sluggish thyroid function
- Lowered immunity and a tendency to contract colds and viruses
- Poor nutritional assimilation and/or response, poor cell response
- Lack of essential fatty acids and nutrients particularly minerals
- Origin of virus for instance Glandular Fever
- Early Tubal Ligation
- Chronic stress and Adrenal Exhaustion, may have very low DHEA
- Possible connection to sexual abuse related issues

Recent scientific research studies have shown central nervous system involvement in FMS.

Dealing with this chronic pain, day in day out, and exhaustion year after year, wears the individual down.

Can natural progesterone help ease, if not cure, Fibromyalgia?

A number of our women battling chronic Fibromyalgia have reported significant pain relief and long term improvement of symptoms using natural progesterone cream. There seems to be no doubt in these women's minds that progesterone has a positive impact on sleep and mood modulation.

Julie, for example, is one of so many women who are reporting promising results when natural progesterone is incorporated in the treatment of Fibromyalgia. Combined, with nutritional supplementation.

Julie's case mirrors many others NPAN has observed and monitored. She was first diagnosed with Fibromyalgia, around the time she began experiencing the early warning signs of hormone imbalance.

In her search for answers, Julie visited a leading Rheumatologist and a Doctor specialising and researching in the field of Fibromyalgia. However, beyond lifestyle modifications, rest and attention to diet, nothing much was gleaned from the appointment that she didn't already know. She was told to go home, get on with her life and learn strategies to cope with this debilitating condition.

Then, about seven years ago, Julie became informed about natural progesterone cream (some testosterone which has been incorporated in the last 12 months with positivity). Now she's drug free. Julie controls her symptoms with progesterone cream and magnesium supplements. However, she points out there's a fine line between stress, diet, nutrition, lifestyle, hormone balancing and Fibromyalgia.

She maintains progesterone helps her to remain calm and level headed. That her coping skills are markedly improved, and that her sleep, most days, is deep and restful. Julie however still battles with poor Gastro Intestinal Absorption and assimulation of nutrients.

That's not to discount the many years that Julie struggled trying to achieve hormone balancing with topical application to the point of overdosing. She was never able to arrive at a correct dosage that would overcome estrogen dominance. While her saliva levels showed exceptionally high absorption there was little evidence, judging by her symptoms, that her body was utilising it effectively.

Julie abstained from progesterone for several months to clear the excess progesterone from her system which was confirmed with ongoing saliva assays.

Julie went back and tried again, using physiological doses of a less potent cream (4%). It was suggested she try intravaginal application at 2%. The results were remarkable.

Julie entered immediate estrogen dominance wake-up (where it was not evident topically) suggesting that her receptors were responding to this form of application.

She has continued to alternate between vaginal and topical applications so that her receptors respond optimally. And feels, after using progesterone cream for seven years, that her cells are once again waking up and giving her a renewed, more positive response to progesterone therapy. Testosterone (natural) transdermal is supporting Julie with more energy and helping to control her low grade depression.

In Julie's case, stress and anxiety are her biggest triggers of Fibromyalgia. So when she feels her symptoms creeping back in, she applies a intravaginal dosage equivalent to 20-30mg or up to 64mg topically to compete with the cortisol output (as there will be competition for the same receptors), and she includes high potency magnesium supplement rather than reaching for an analgesic.

According to Julie, pain does not interfere with her daily life when her hormones are balanced, she's eating, much better now juicing and taking nutritional supplements, getting regular exercise, resting when her body tells her to and, above all, having a good belly laugh every chance she gets. In other words, she tries not to take life too seriously and become her ailment. She has more control.

Of course, the solution is not always that simple for every woman. It's awfully difficult to treat a condition with unknown origins. And yet, the introduction of progesterone - our mother hormone - appears to have a favourable impact in the treatment of Fibromyalgia. That much is clear.

Chronic Fatigue Syndrome (CFS), often referred to as an Auto-immune Disease, is widely researched but little is known of it's origins. Like FMS, CFS is hard to treat with progesterone alone. Nonetheless, intravaginal application seems to target cells and receptors more directly, bringing about beneficial responses of this *multi-factorial hormone, one being the rebuilding of the auto-immune system.*

In the case of FMS and CFS, I suspect that topical application is hindered either due to poor skin absorption, sluggish cell receptability, poor blood circulation, impeding conversion between the cells, or its capacity to collect progesterone from the fat tissue and deliver it to the receptor sites. And even if it does get to the receptors, there may be an inability for the receptors to respond (wake up). Observation is that intravaginal application appears to bypass the opportunity for progesterone to be stored in fat before it gets used. But this is only a theory of mine. Refer to chapter 11

Fertility/Infertility/Contraception/Postnatal Depression
Can I use progesterone for contraception?

Theoretically, a surge of progesterone in the body would 'trick' the biofeedback mechanism between the hypothalamus, the pituitary gland, and the ovaries that ovulation has occurred, thus inhibiting ovulation.

In simple terms, progesterone gives the body the message that one of the ovaries has already ovulated so therefore the other ovary doesn't need to. And without an egg being released from either ovary, conception cannot take place.

But this is in theory only. It is not known what safe level of topically applied progesterone would be required to inhibit ovulation (contraception).

Until more conclusive evidence is available, NPAN advises women NOT to rely on progesterone supplementation as a form of contraception. I believe, in the future, natural progesterone will be developed as a natural form of contraception just as it is now being administered in fertility clinics to help sustain pregnancy.

Please note, you cannot use the Contraceptive Pill and natural progesterone concurrently and get good benefits, since both will compete for the same receptor sites. And progestogens used for fertility control ie. oral contraceptive pill (OCP) are NOT progesterone. They have two very different molecular configurations. The pill is a meagre dose of the altered progesterone molecule to progestogens, designed to stop fertility. The pill would not sustain pregnancy and possibly harm the foetus or bring about a miscarriage if continued to be used throughout the pregnancy.

Progestogens (in The Pill) is designed to stop fertility whereas natural progesterone made by the body enhances and maintains conception. *Progesterone is for PROGESTATION*, this is where the name progesterone comes from. Having made the distinction, you can see why the two are not compatible when used together. Refer to page 346.

The Morning After Pill

Some of the women in the group on Natural Progesterone cream have resorted to using the The Morning After Pill for the purpose of abortion. It has been observed that women experience a huge backwards step as a result of the high levels of progestogens introduced into the body, short term. The effects have varied with each woman. We cannot determine how long it takes for the progestogens to move off the receptor sites to allow progesterone access once again. (Observation is days to months for availability for these receptor sites). Refer to page 346.

Women have asked me if they should stop progesterone when using The Morning After Pill, and I suggest they continue on with progesterone supplementation as usual, otherwise it could cause a greater disruption to their cycles. I also suggest the Liver Detox Formulation and MSM to assist in the removal of these powerful progestins.

What's a SAFE, easy to use alternative if I don't want to use The Pill?

During a woman's menstrual cycle, there are only about 3 days (72 hours) when her egg is available for fertilisation. **Sperm can survive up to 72 hours (3 days) in the vagina and uterus**, so if sexual intercourse occurs up to 3 days before a woman is fertile, she can still potentially become pregnant.

Thus, there are about 6 days per month (3 days prior to fertility, and 3 days of fertility) that a woman can conceive and it is not always at day 12-14. Some women ovulate as early as 5 days (from their bleed). It is important to know your own body's ovulation pattern and rhythm.

There are devices on the market now that detect fertility through saliva method. This fertility detector device is a hand-held mini-microscope about the size and shape of a lipstick holder.

It is scientifically well established that hormones filter into saliva and that during fertility a 'ferning' pattern can be seen in saliva under a microscope. Just prior to or during fertile days the sample will typically resemble "ferns" while during non-fertile days, only random and shapeless 'dots' will be visible.

Cycle awareness can be especially helpful for women who tend to have anovulatory cycles (no ovulation occurs, Infertility results, no progesterone is made by the ovary). If you know that you haven't ovulated in any given cycle, and thus your ovary won't be producing progesterone, you can then supplement with progesterone that month and avoid estrogen dominance symptoms such as PMS.

These kits come with a life-time guarantee, and can be used over and over again unlike the conventional urine tests to determine fertility that tend to be expensive, messy, and can only be used once. They are like a lipstick compact and can be carried in your handbag.

You may wish to refer to the question on the next page "If I'm not ovulating and not producing progesterone every month, how come I'm getting a period? Section on Saliva Assays.

Advantages of Fertility Detector:

- You're trying to become pregnant
- You're trying to avoid pregnancy
- You want to determine whether you're ovulating
- You want to enhance your awareness of your menstrual cycle
- Convenient to carry around applicator in handbag and not dependent on temperature method

Can I use progesterone for Infertility?

Progesterone is widely used in conjunction with Infertility, already extensively used in fertility programs. In Australia, vaginal pessaries are used, and in the USA Crinone Gel (8%) has been developed for such a purpose it is now in a 4% strength and studies have shown benefits at this 4% strength (40mg).

When used topically, benefits are quite significant in helping to regulate periods and bringing the body back into synchronisation, and in some cases, triggering ovulation.

Often the introduction of progesterone back into the body can 'crank up' the ovaries, particularly where there has been a   considerable shortfall of this hormone in the body. Consequently fertility may follow. *However, if your follicles are depleted, progesterone cannot restore fertility* (ie not enough eggs left). Appropriate tests can establish your state of fertility.

Women often come to me after all other avenues have failed. So I have needed to keep a very open mind about the power and possibility of transdermal progesterone cream in regards to fertility.   Many pregnancies have been achieved so progesterone cannot be dismissed or these pregnancies considered co-incidental. It is such an exciting prospect but I emphasis success appears to come when a holistic approach is adopted thus suggesting fertility is multifactorial process.

There are many reasons for Infertility not just a progesterone deficiency.

IMPORTANT MESSAGE: *If you have been using progesterone in order to get pregnant and you are successful, **DO NOT** withdraw the progesterone cream suddenly.* Regular dosage can be maintained and gradually increased to 80mg right through until the last trimester.

At this stage the placenta is well and truly producing adequate levels of progesterone to maintain the pregnancy. The baby's placenta takes over the production of progesterone at the beginning of the second trimester, and this is when a miscarriage is likely to occur if this production is not adequate.

Women with a history of miscarriage or premature delivery choose, for their own peace of mind, to continue using progesterone through to the week prior to expected delivery. The placenta is producing such huge amounts of progesterone (300-400mg per day in the last trimester), that any extra progesterone over and above will not harm the baby (see research by Katharina Dalton, MD (UK)).

THE LATE DR. LEE WARNED THAT IF YOU ARE GOING TO STOP YOUR PROGESTERONE, WEAN OFF YOUR DOSE EVER SO GRADUALLY BECAUSE ANY SUDDEN DROP CAN TRIGGER A MISCARRIAGE.

If I'm not ovulating and not producing progesterone every month, how come I'm getting a period?

Sadly, many women think regular periods equate to regular ovulation. Getting a period does not depend on ovulation, and therefore the presence of progesterone. It is the presence of estrogen in the body that prepares the uterus each month for the possible fertilisation of an egg. This results in the uterine lining building up with a thickened, bloody lining of the uterus in preparation for the fertilised egg to embed itself in to. It's the failure of conception that brings about the shedding of the uterine lining which is known as the menses (menstruation). It's the fluctuation of the hormone estrogen that brings on this activity.

Therefore, a woman with normal or elevated estrogen levels in her body will have a period (perhaps at times irregularly). So if you are menstruating you have adequate levels of estrogen, contrary to popular medical belief.

Women assume that their regular period indicates they are ovulating. And this is not the case as demonstrated above. A period can occur regularly in the absence or presence of ovulation. It is only when ovulation has occurred and conception takes place that the shedding of the uterine lining is prevented, remaining intact (no presence of a period due to confirmation of pregnancy).

And progesterone is the hormone that is maintaining the integrity of the uterine lining to promote gestation (pro-gestation, that is supporting the pregnancy).

If conception doesn't take place but ovulation has occurred that month, both hormones drop off signaling the onset of menstruation. And then the cycle starts again. First estrogen to ripen and mature another egg and prepare the uterine lining, then progesterone from around day 12 when ovulation has occurred to promote fertilisation and maintenance of pregnancy.

Progesterone can only be manufactured as a result of the egg being released from the ovary. *So if you're not ovulating, you're not producing progesterone from your ovary each month. Progesterone is manufactured in the corpus luteum after ovulation.* (Small amounts of progesterone are made in other specific glands such as the adrenals).

It's quite common for women to not ovulate every month. This gives rise to estrogen dominance. It also explains why some months you may feel more PMS, and have a heavier shedding (perhaps with clots), indicating a build up due to estrogen influence with no opposing progesterone.

When a woman is physiologically balanced with estrogen and progesterone, *ceasing progesterone supplementation can bring on a period within 24 to 36 hours.* This is why women are advised to continue taking their progesterone if they suspect they are pregnant because stopping cream can actually bring about a miscarriage. See information on Saliva Kits previous 2 pages.

Can I use progesterone for Postnatal Depression?

One of the factors of Postnatal Depression is the sudden drop of progesterone once the baby is born. When you consider that a women in her last trimester of her pregnancy is producing up to 400mg of progesterone via the baby's placenta, after the baby is born and the placenta is expelled, the progesterone factory is literally turned off. This drop in progesterone is necessary to stimulate another hormone (prolactin) to bring on lactation (breast milk).

Most women will be familiar with the term **'baby blues'**. With the sudden withdrawal of progesterone, depression can be triggered, known as Postnatal Depression. This can vary for every woman in the time of onset, severity, and duration. And for other women, it can be insidious, undiagnosed and left untreated for many years after the baby is born.

But it's now recognised that women generally do go through a brief period of depression following the birth of their child which they usually get over in no time. Now, with the discovery of progesterone supplementation, it has been such a breakthrough in defeating Postnatal Depression and the avoidance of antidepressants in many.

For mild to moderate depression, natural progesterone has proven quite adequate in small doses (15-20mg) for approximately 4 months uninterrupted. I suggest you start at lower doses and assess to see if your depression is lifting, and only increase if you feel you are not responding at that dosage. Give yourself a week to feel the benefits.

Unlike women who have to wait 6-8 weeks to reach saturation level in the body to feel the benefits of progesterone, new mothers don't need to go through this process because their body, being familiar with this hormone, will respond very quickly with the reintroduction of natural progesterone.

Moderate to severe depression may require higher doses (32-64mg), then wean back gradually. It is advised you make your GP aware of the fact you have chosen to trial natural progesterone and seek his support, rather than resort, at this point, to traditional anti-depressant drugs that might expose you and the baby to these substances. (See the section on 'Can I take progesterone while I'm on my anti-depressant drugs?')

My observation has been that progesterone has provided women with a 'happy' and safe solution for mum and her baby, and has not interfered with her milk production.

Some women have even commented that they've been able to relax, cope better and enjoy the experience of motherhood and breast feeding for the first time, where their previous accounts battling depression and their refusal to resort to medication, or the side effects of the medication they were encouraged to take may have left them feeling quite cheated of the whole mothering experience.

Women share and express their feelings of shame, guilt and failure associated with Postnatal Depression, particularly when it has not been explained to them that Postnatal Depression is the result of a hormone imbalance over which they have no control over. My well read followers are reporting frequently their satisfaction and relief of having had Postnatal Depression, some for the first time 3 or 4 children later, not experiencing this again. I have had one lady who is up to her 9th baby and with every pregnancy her Postnatal Depression worsened, she is in full bliss with this baby because for the first time she is depression free because of her use of progesterone. (All pregnancies had been planned despite her horrific experiences with Postnatal Depression).

There are cases where Postnatal Depression is very severe and requires you to be under the care of a specialist. If you wish to incorporate natural progesterone using high doses, you will need to find a doctor who will support this therapy. Another world known pioneer in progesterone usage is Katharina Dalton, MD (UK) who is famous for her work and research in the treatment of Postnatal Depression (and PMS) using very high levels of progesterone (100-300mg) daily. Here in Australia, there are doctors who will adopt the troches/lozenges and pessaries at high levels, but this falls outside my arena of experience and as I do not have sufficient correlated observational data.

Note, please take precaution during lactation that you do not become pregnant. Breast feeding in conjunction with natural progesterone is not a substitute for contraception. Some women are, by nature, very fertile and have conceived while breast feeding (not on progesterone).

Menopause
What are the symptoms of menopause, and what causes them?

Menopause means the end of menstruation, and the end of your reproductive years (for some a joy, others a strange kind of sadness).

Menopausal symptoms are triggered by the drop of estrogen, and varying in intensity. These are the most common:

- Absence of periods
- Hot Flushes / flashes, night sweats

- Aches and pains - joint, neck, backache, restless legs, stiffness
- Dizziness, vertigo, Tinnitus
- Headaches, head congestion-sinusitis
- Vaginal dryness or itching, painful intercourse and loss of libido
- Bladder problems - Stress Incontinence, other irritations, prone to infections
- Dry and ageing skin - loss of elasticity, weight gain (flabby stomach)
- Crawling or itching sensations under skin, scalp itchiness/tightness
- Poor sleep patterns - commonly waking 12pm, 2am and 4am
- Foggy thinking, loss of concentration, inability to recall
- Emotional changes - anxiety, irritability, depression, loss of self-esteem, lacking confidence, panic attacks, palpitations, crying, social phobia and many more
- Physical exhaustion, mental fatigue, obsessional worrying/thoughts

Compare these symptoms to those listed on Estrogen Dominance checklist and you would be understandably confused. Even though you may be low in your production of estrogen (because of ovarian failure) causing your periods to stop, you may yet be estrogen dominant as your progesterone levels drop to zero at menopause.

The sudden drop and surges of estrogen bring on these hot flushes and other symptoms, that vary in severity and duration for every woman. Women who are not menopausal can experience these same symptoms when there is a huge ratio imbalance between these two hormones (as early as their mid-thirties). I have seen young women from 18-20 years with extreme severe symptoms seen mostly in peri menopausal and menopausal years as a result of this ratio imbalance.

Hot Flushes (Flashes)
How can I stop Hot Flushes?

Women have found that they can usually gain control over the intensity and frequency of Hot Flushes after 3-4 months on progesterone. Initially in the first 2 months high doses are recommended to overcome the "estrogen dominance crisis" wake up time and to re-saturate the body with a long overdue lacking hormone. Bringing this hormone back tends to help settle down the body and modulate the effect on the estrogen fluctuations, thereby reducing Hot Flushes. It is thought that it is *when estrogen levels drop quickly the brain releases a signal to tell the body it is overheating. It is this signal that prompts the stimulation of adrenaline like substances that result in what most women experience as a sudden intense heat, Hot Flushes, sweating and often a rapid heart beat.* The body is also experiencing panic mode, attempting to wake up the ovaries to mature (now gone) eggs. The follicular phase and the sleeping non responsive ovaries creates a high Follicle Stimulating Hormone reading. This FSH determines a huge reflection of menopause. Refer page 235.

Most flushes can last from a few minutes to an hour. They can be generalised or localised to one specific area. Some women say they know when they are going to have a hot flush, as they may get cold or shiver prior or may sense a heat surge or experience sensation from their lower legs or feet which moves up over the body. Others may just flush around the neck and face. **Night sweat**s usually are described as overwhelming body heat and perspiration, resulting in saturated nightwear and sheets. It usually interferes with the sleep patterns, which may cause serious fatigue and depression. This is the most common complaint as they can be debilitating interfering with work, quality of lifestyle, not to mention the embarrassment women feel with Hot Flushes. Comments are constantly passed "I feel like a neon light", "People laugh at me" or "Make derogative comments", "I feel I'm suffocating", "I just want to strip off", "I cannot attend social functions", "I cannot concentrate because of these annoying Hot Flushes", "My husband can't stand sleeping with me" or vice versa "I'm just sheer exhausted and can't function", "I'm sick of changing the soaked bed linen half way through the night" or "Carrying my deodorant and a change of clothes around with me". The list of lines are endless and I'm sure if you are one poor suffering soul you could add another 10 of your own. Not much fun is it!

Many factors can set off and worsen Hot Flushes. So there is a lot you can do to help reduce and control these unpleasant, exhausting and often debilitating experiences not to mention the inconvenience, embarrassment and annoyance of their unannounced arrivals! Women come to NPAN on this factor alone, very distressed over Hot Flushes and the disruption to their lives. Life can be very miserable at this time for the severe sufferer of Hot Flushes and night sweats, experiencing up to 30 a day which can go on for years.

Suggestions offered to women are:

Use progesterone as recommended. Don't be frightened to apply during the night after Hot Flushes, sweats in the initial stages. I did for 7 months until I gained control.

Use a premium phytoestrogenic menopausal formulation

This will assist the body by providing estrogenic benefits without the high level of side effects of stronger estrogens. Progesterone also works brilliantly in the presence of a good phytoestrogen. Look for formulations that include high levels of isoflavones, these have been shown in studies to play an important role in maintaining health during and after menopause, particularly in relieving Hot Flushes and night sweats. Myself and hundreds of women I have consulted have been using ' Femme Phase' powder for years with great success, but there are many premium products out there. A good formulation will include a variety of supporting factors. I use Femme Phase because it covers and multiple number of phytoestrogens B's, Calcium, Zinc and Copper to name a few important components.

Avoid triggers that set off Hot Flushes such as:

- Alcohol
- Caffeine
- Hot-spicy food
- Stress
- Over-heated stuffy rooms
- Sweet "fizzy' drinks

- Rich foods, those high in sugar or fat
- Sun baking, hot baths, saunas, solarium
- Exhaust fumes from motor vehicles, petrol vapours
- Chemical sprays including household cleaning agents
- Paint fumes, solvents, hair dyes, check your cosmetics ingredients
- Other toxic fumes, pollutants and radiation
- Unventilated rooms, heat trapping clothing

Situations that may trigger Hot Flushes are flying and a change of time zone. It is in my case, even occasionally still now 8 years surgically induced menopause, interestingly, I am otherwise hot flush free. I have linked my problem to high altitudes and airport plane fumes. Also there is a skin tannery in Melbourne that never fails to set me off even blind folded and with the windows up. I control these symptoms by using an extra dose of progesterone 12 hours before flying and after arriving at my destination. I have also found that it helps to increase the dose of phytoestrogens at the same time.

CERTAIN MEDICATIONS CAN INCREASE HOT FLUSHES, for example, starting a course of *anti-depressants* or some *anti hypertensive drugs*. (Addressed in Book 2).

Tamoxifen is a special case, this drug often causes Hot Flushes on starting therapy. This will often settle down with a continuous course of progesterone.

Other treatments and suggestions to follow until the progesterone starts to bring Hot Flushes under control are:

Keep your fluids up, drink cold water or suck ice cubes. Carrying a water spray or moist towel can be useful. In the early days I found applying progesterone cream to the temples when under stress helped. Dress appropriately to accommodate hot or cold fluctuations, in other words, layer dress so you can quickly remove clothes if necessary. Choose materials that breathe and do not trap heat in, such as nylon. Cotton and wool are useful choices. Use night attire that soaks up moisture and swap synthetic sheets and bedclothes for natural cotton. Sleep on a towel in a cool, controlled, calm and quiet environment. Use aromatherapy if this creates a calming effect for you. Avoid hot baths too close to retiring for the night. Take a magnesium complex supplement and progesterone 20 minutes before bed and empty your bladder and avoid the temptation of a late night caffeine drink. Try adopting herbal teas such as chamomile before bed.

Avoid moisturisers that are greasy as they trap heat in, use moisturisers that contain natural oils with vitamin E. The skin is a cooling agent for the body, and sweat is one way the body releases heat and controls body temperature. A large skin area allows evaporation and cooling. If the body is constantly over-heating, this may reflect a dysfunctional liver, so a liver detoxification program may be useful. It is amazing the impact this will have in conjunction with the adoption of the above suggestions. A fan over your body can do wonders. It is easier to keep warm than to cool off quickly.

If after 7 months of progesterone therapy and adoption of these suggestions, Hot Flushes continue, you may need to introduce a small amount of natural estrogen or re introduce small amounts of estrogen. Especially if you have been on estrogen or are weaning off, as the body cannot cope with the drop of such pre conditioned estrogen status administered (to prevent estrogen drops thus putting the body in a false pre menopausal state), without a gentle reduction the shocked body has not had time to adjust and other areas have not learnt to accommodate adequately to take over estrogen manufacturing Before doing so please read section on estrogens.

NOTE: If you have been on HRT long term and have switched to natural progesterone, it is unwise to go off estrogen cold turkey. Whilst you have to stop progestins, it is wiser to wean off estrogen and adjust dose variations accordingly.

What is the alternative treatment to menopausal symptoms other than conventional estrogen replacement therapy or HRT?

Progesterone supplementation can reduce the ratio variations, restoring hormone balance, resolving most of these symptoms without the need to supplement with estrogen. Please refer to the chapter on 'Phytoestrogens' which play a major role in providing estrogenic benefits in the body without the need for supplementation in the form of estrogen therapy so readily prescribed.

Women, reluctant to taken HRT due to a history of blood clotting or adverse reactions to HRT in the past, or a history of Breast Cancer, prefer to try progesterone and phytoestrogenic therapy in conjunction with mineral and vitamin supplementation, and a good diet plan. They have found this approach to be most effective in the control of menopausal symptoms with greater peace of mind minus any nasty side effects such as weight gain.

The only form of estrogen that they may require is a form of vaginal estrogen cream to maintain healthy vaginal tissue and protect against atrophy and dryness. Interestingly, a lot of women don't even require this, progesterone therapy being sufficient to keep women healthy and well lubricated. If your vagina is dry it is a good indication Estriol (Ovestin, containing the safer estrogen) is necessary and why risk estrogen supplementation or of higher levels and of a stronger and perhaps cancer promoting, form (Estriodol/Estrone). If this is all you need it for. NOTE: Estriol levels actually are elevated in pregnancy which make one believe they have a protective factor or oppose the stronger estrogens - perhaps protecting the baby and body.

Regular blood work and saliva assays should be ordered to ensure adequate hormone levels.

Please also refer to the section on 'Hormone Replacement Therapy (HRT) and/or Natural Hormone Replacement Therapy (NHRT)' chapters 16 & 17.

What's the reason behind prescribing estrogen replacement therapy at menopause?

There are two reasons. Firstly, to stop all the symptoms that occur as a result of the sudden drop of estrogen that is designed by nature to stop your periods. Sadly many doctors do not understand that progesterone will in fact address most if not all these symptoms without the danger of introducing high levels of estrogen back into the body. Unopposed estrogen increases the risk of uterine cancer and Breast Cancer. That is why it is medical practice to incorporate synthetic progestogens with estrogen replacement therapy (termed HRT) to protect women with an intact uterus, from uterine cancer.

Secondly, estrogen replacement therapy is routinely prescribed "to protect a menopausal woman from Cardiovascular Disease and maintain bone density to prevent Osteoporosis". Please refer to latest medical references and findings suggesting they have been wrong.

My understanding has been you have to be on estrogen more than 5 years to derive any real benefits of estrogen in the delaying of bone resorption and further bone deterioration. And yet drug companies warn that long-term use of estrogen carries significant health risk, particularly the risks of cancer (increases after 5 years).

Women contemplating hormone replacement find themselves between a rock and a hard place, and little wonder they are resorting to natural progesterone. Progesterone is a safe but as yet unproven alternative in the prevention and treatment of these two conditions viewed as complications of menopause (now appearing to become medicalised).

It's certainly a more attractive option for those women who have a history of cancer, blood clotting, Fibroids, or any other estrogen-driven conditions.

So, what about those women who have a family history of Heart Disease and Osteoporosis, or have these conditions themselves? Doctors scoff at their decision to take progesterone. Certainly, it is a difficult call. I urge you to jump to the 'Medical References' (page 420), and read carefully to help you form a balanced opinion. I encourage you to take these references to your Doctor. You can print them off from my website www.npan.com.au. I designed it this way for this purpose, to help you with your approach to your Doctor.

You may also wish to read more on this subject in books such as HORMONE HERESY BY SHERRILL SELLMAN and PROGESTERONE BY KIMBERLY PATTERSON.

NOTE: In Kimberly Patterson's book she refers to my service and information as free. Yes in earlier days quite so, however, the information provided in my own books and the services provided by me are on a fee paid basis for consultancy and seminar work. Also information packs are not free as Kimberly Patterson's book implies. My business is not an 1800 free call line and it is wrongly assumed that my business runs a 24 hour service funded by the government.

Is there a test to determine menopause?

Yes, there is. It involves a blood test where pathologists measure estrogen levels, the most active form of estrogen being estradiol.

- Generally less than 200 pmol/L indicates menopause and post menopause.
- Follicle Stimulating Hormone (FSH) will be high, usually between 40 and 200 mIU/mL (levels tend to be 10-15 times higher than the normal levels of a premenopausal woman).

The reason for elevated FSH levels is the body's attempt to reactivate the flagging ovaries as you draw to the end of your reproductive years. This is nature taking its course, and will settle in time once the signals between the brain and the ovaries (biofeedback mechanism) have accepted that the ovaries have gone to sleep, and the body makes other adjustments to compensate for this, but the FSH stays high.

What causes menopause? Will progesterone interfere with this?

No, natural progesterone will not interfere with your passage through menopause (unlike synthetic progestogens used in HRT).

Briefly, menopause is the cessation of menstrual bleeding signaling that estrogen production has fallen to a very low level, preventing the build up and shedding of uterine tissue every month (menstruation). It is the mark of the end of reproduction.

The drop in levels of estrogen is due to the inability of the ovaries to manufacture the sex hormones estrogen and progesterone. A woman is never totally deficient of estrogen, although her estrogen levels drop below a point that creates monthly menstrual cycles. The late Dr John Lee says it only drops 40-60 %.

Menopause is a marker of ovarian failure, because the body can no longer ripen and mature the remaining follicles into eggs for fertilisation. This happens around about age 50-55, although women are entering menopause much earlier now. It is the follicles within the ovaries that produce the vast majority of estrogen and progesterone which is produced after the ovary has popped - (ovulation).

Progesterone therapy will not cause a woman to go back into monthly cycles if she has truly entered menopause because it is estrogen that creates the monthly cyclic bleeds not progesterone. The build up of the endometrial tissue is under the influence of estrogen, not progesterone. And it is the drop of estrogen that signals menopause and stops your period. A woman can have stopped ovulating, and be infertile many years before her periods stop.

If you have a bleed when you start progesterone and are by test confirmation menopausal, do not be alarmed. This is a common phenomenon and I believe it is due to the remaining uterine bloody tissue build up, that upon reintroducing progesterone, stimulates these uterine receptors causing a bleed (shedding). I call this housekeeping. One period is usually all that is seen. Of course if bleeding continues seek medical attention.

When will I go through menopause?

All women are unique so it stands to reason each will enter menopause according to their biological clock. However, the average age at which women enter menopause tends to be around fifty years of age. Times are changing though. Women are entering menopause earlier, some around 40 starting as early as 35 years and I believe this shift has root in the endocrine disrupters present in our environment and food chain. Other causes contributing may be a Tubal Ligation or partial Hysterectomy for example. These women enter far earlier.

My doctor says I've had premature menopause. I'm a little bit confused.

This means that you have entered menopause earlier than the normal average menopausal age, and that your periods have permanently stopped. *The term menopause means final cessation of menstruation, or the last menstrual period and the guideline to this is **one year***. (See question 'Why have I gone through menopause early?')

What is meant by perimenopause?

'Peri' menopause denotes the months or years 'round about' or nearest to menopause. To be diagnosed perimenopausal is to exhibit signs and symptoms that your reproductive years are winding down. You are having occasional anovulatory cycles. By this I mean you menstruate but perhaps you are not ovulating every month. The age is roughly between forty to fifty-five, although many women are going through perimenopausal symptoms earlier, particularly those who have had tubal ligation or some form of disruption to their hormones.

This is a time when progesterone levels are likely to drop and estrogen dominance set in.

What is meant by premenopause?

'Pre' menopause denotes the years 'before' or leading up to menopause. However, it generally spans 4-5 years and starts in the late forties. Again, it can begin any time after the age of thirty-five and is characterised by hormonal imbalance in a woman.

How long does menopause last?

Menopause signals the end of your reproductive years. We are now seeing women enter menopause at an age far younger than their mothers before them. Increasing numbers of women are having anovulatory cycles beginning in their mid thirties where they continue to menstruate but they are not ovulating (contributing to Osteoporosis).

Which bears out the fact that loss of fertility is due to the disappearance of follicles and their eggs rather than age. Of the 300,000 follicles present at puberty from which eggs can be matured, **ovulation rarely occurs when only about 1,000 eggs are left.**

Once your periods stop and you enter menopause, you become infertile. You will never have another period. You move beyond the reproductive phase of your life into another. You have completed your childbearing years, and now have the opportunity to pursue those things that will facilitate a deeper level of self-discovery.

Menopause is a time to start putting YOU first for a change! It can be the best years of your life, see my chapter on 'The Spiritual Side of Progesterone' page 70.

Will my periods return if I have entered menopause and my doctor has prescribed estrogen in the form of HRT?

Yes and no. An 'unnatural' period will return if you are put on estrogen replacement therapy and forced to take breaks (which is a routine procedure to prevent the dangerous build up of the endometrial lining).

If you are on estrogen continuously (with an intact uterus) and were not advised to have a periodic break, you would experience break through bleeding and would probably warrant a curette. I have a suspicion that estrogen therapy alone is one of the causes of so many women getting Fibroids sometimes long after therapy has stopped. Too many women have discovered this themselves. This is why progestogens are prescribed along with estrogen to prevent thickening of the uterine lining, and the regime provided with HRT is designed to bring about a chemically induced period every month.

Note, this will not render you fertile if your ovaries have ceased to function.

It goes without saying, a woman who has no uterus and is on estrogen replacement therapy alone (dosage may be continuous) cannot possibly have a bleed or build up of endometrial tissue because her uterus has been removed.

Can natural progesterone replace synthetic progestogens at menopause if I'm on HRT?

Yes, but there is a need for caution during this change-over phase.

There is considerable debate as to whether progesterone can actually prevent thickening of the endometrium. Although, based on observational experience, women do not suffer the same degree of tissue build up once they start progesterone. The medical fraternity are not convinced natural progesterone alone at physiological doses will adequately protect women from Endometrial Hyperplasia (excessive cell growth of the uterine lining). Please refer to the 'Medical References' page as it explains why the medical fraternity hold this opinion.

Women who have an excessive build up of bloody uterine tissue, even after menopause, may have a shedding once they start progesterone upon initial stimulation of cell receptors activity in this area. *But periods will not continue with regular progesterone application* **unless** *a woman is on estrogen therapy and taking breaks* (as periods have stopped, i.e.., menopause).

In short, natural progesterone cannot be relied on to prevent Endometrial Hyperplasia if you are taking estrogen replacement therapy. We don't know, at this stage, what dosage administration is required to oppose estrogen replacement therapy, specifically preventing thickening of the uterine lining. Chances are your doctor will insist you take a synthetic progestogen to complement your ERT to protect you against thickening of the uterus. Compounding pharmacists are, therefore, matching natural progesterone therapy, usually in the form of troche, at doses that are equivalent to doses of progestogens. This approach appeases the doctor.

Of interest is the introduction of 10% natural progesterone creams that have perhaps been manufactured with this purpose in mind.

However, any bleeding that occurs during this stage of your life should be investigated.

When is menopause not menopause?

Several women in their late thirties early forties who'd been told by their GPs that they had entered menopause and hadn't had a period for years, started to menstruate again on a regular cycle once commencing progesterone therapy. Clearly, these women were not in menopause and were misdiagnosed. Nutritional supplementation, good diet, exercise, and the use of progesterone has returned a healthy body.

Often these women, because they have been diagnosed premature menopause, without correct diagnostic tests, have been put onto HRT over many, many years. They report contemplating why they never felt quite right. Some of these women, once commencing progesterone supplementation and realising that they weren't menopausal at all, have become very angered that their opportunity for fertility may have been cut short simply because of a misguided diagnosis.

Three women come to mind on this issue alone. These women, now aged between 40-60, tried desperately to have babies in their prime, and went through all sorts of fertility programs and experimental drug trials, one being Tamoxifen for fertility which proved successful (15 years ago), and eventually gave up, thinking that their reproductive years were well and truly finished. They were put on HRT for what their doctors termed premature menopause.

You might like to read Klara and Margaret's testimonials, two women who were diagnosed as menopausal and have begun regular menstruation using progesterone. Margaret has battled Fibroids (and beaten the threat of a Hysterectomy) only to now be entering her menopausal years (then 55 now at 58). Interesting her Fibroids have disappeared having had years of estrogen implants. But in the last 2 years Marg's Hot Flushes started to emerge and progesterone alone was not maintaining her. Having clearance of no more Fibroids Marg has, in the past 18 months, gently introduced some Sandrena (natural estrogen gel/estrodial). She applies minimum amounts to top up (not daily) when she finds her energy flagging and Hot Flushes emerging. She also has Insulin Resistance which she is addressing along with weight reduction.

Are the ovaries beneficial or do they have any purpose after menopause?

They certainly do! I urge women who have been told they need a Hysterectomy to hang on to their ovaries regardless, unless life-threatening or a family history of ovarian cancer.

Even though a Hysterectomy will interfere with the blood supply therefore will eventually result in complete dysfunction of your ovaries, leaving them where they are will benefit your overall hormonal health providing they are healthy. You will derive some benefits although severely compromised due to blood supply interference. For this reason, there's no time factor. It will vary for each woman. On observation I have seen the lucky women get 6-7 good years mileage out of their ovaries.

Healthy ovaries continue to function well and truly beyond menopause.

Ovaries that have not been damaged through surgical interference or through chemical damage, do produce small quantities of estrogen and significant amounts of testosterone for a period of at least a few years to twelve years or so. They certainly have their place in maintaining your overall wellbeing.

Despite the fact that you have entered menopause and your ovaries don't produce ripened eggs every month, they do still continue to secrete hormones and perform other activities in the body.

It is probable that the ovaries, postmenopausal, have a capacity to produce testosterone in greater quantities than the adrenal glands. Maybe this is why women constantly report increased libido and sexual enjoyment during their postmenopausal years. Not all with high testosterone production reap the improved libido.

The downside to this masculine hormone is more hair on your face and less on your head, and perhaps unsightly pimples or acne. Shrinkage of the breasts has also been reported.

It is therefore understood that, after menopause, the ovaries have a great impact on our sex hormone testosterone more so than our stores of estrogen (but let's not forget our food sources can supply a great deal of our estrogen, and the stored estrogen in our body fat).

Where do you get estrogen from after menopause? And is it necessary to take estrogen therapy?

Estrogen can be manufactured in various ways depending on the amount of body fat we have, the health of our adrenal glands & ovaries, the food we consume, our body type (shape) and our health in general. Women with considerable body fat tend to have higher levels of estrogen than thin women. This is because there is a **hormone called androstenediol found in body fat and muscle cells that is converted into estrone** - one of the three natural estrogens produced by the body - before and after menopause. The more fat the more estrone that is made.

Gynaeoid women (pear-shaped) have a tendency to store lots of estrogen in their lower body fat (buttocks, hips, tummy & thighs). If you are this body shape and carrying excess weight (and cellulite) think twice about taking estrogen therapy at menopause. You already have adequate stores (in body fat).

Our ovaries do not produce progesterone after menopause, and often don't produce it in the years leading up to menopause because progesterone is manufactured by the ovaries upon ovulation. And as discussed in earlier chapters, many women experience anovulatory cycles (where they fail to ovulate) as early as thirty something and even teenagers now (PCOS is a classic case).

The question is often raised why do women need progesterone after menopause more than estrogen? In my opinion, it stands to reason a woman needs progesterone supplementation because her ovaries are continuing to put out some estrogen and some testosterone but no progesterone and she lives in sea of estrogen.

In times gone by this would not have posed a problem. However, given our day and age and the way we live, our hectic lifestyles, our refined sugars and high carbohydrate diets, estrogen levels, whether produced by our body fat or via exposure to xenoestrogen, never drop to zero as does progesterone which our body cannot derive from anywhere else to any large degree to balance these excess estrogens except in supplementation form. This is my logical interpretation for the ever increasing need for progesterone supplementation as we go into this century having less babies later in life.

PHYTO-PROGESTERONE (PLANT DERIVED PROGESTERONE) DOES NOT EXIST IN THE PLANT KINGDOM LIKE PHYTO-ESTROGENS, TO SCIENTIFIC OR ANY OTHER STUDIES TO DATE.

Why have I gone through menopause early?

When women go through menopause earlier than one would expect, this is known as premature menopause. And when this happens, it usually strikes women in their twenties and thirties. Women who menstruate early in life are often earmarked for early menopause.

A tubal ligation and/or Hysterectomy can cause a woman to enter menopause by at least 4+ years. Women who have their ovaries removed through surgery or damaged by say, chemotherapy, will automatically go into menopause (medically termed surgically induced menopause). This can occur at any age where these two factors exist. See question 'What is premature menopause?' I recently heard (at the tail end) on radio, about a book that had been written by a Doctor/Researcher. The title was something like "Menopause Why Me", I didn't get the author (stuck in traffic without a pen) so I have not been able to track this book down. The Doctor was stating the cases of world wide children not even going through puberty, having entered menopause. I wish I could get hold of this information. If you know of this book please jump on my website www.npan.com.au and email me the details. I would be ever so grateful.

Why is it I'm becoming more masculine since entering menopause?

A lot of women experience increased facial hair and obvious male predominant features once they have gone through menopause and continue to experience andrenous effects such as male pattern baldness and more masculine characteristics. Their body shape may change a bit. This is due to their hormonal imbalance and often comes as a result of the drop in estrogen which is more a feminising hormone. Women with PCOS also show these male-like features and androgen patterns where there is excessive testosterone levels and have little, or no progesterone.

After the woman's ovaries cease to ovulate and cease to produce a period each month, estrogen continues to be made but to a lesser degree. The ovaries continue to make androgens, the so-called male sex hormones, which promote the masculine characteristics. Breasts may also shrink and the skin and facial features may become more rugged, coarser, more angular looking, lots of annoying facial chin hairs, may start to warrant tweezers. I laugh when so many women tell me the best place to pluck these is in the rear vision mirror while waiting at the traffic lights! I wonder how many women are relating to this comment. This is easily fixed by taking more natural estrogen replacements and often I suggest phytoestrogenic formulas, lots of essential oils (omega 3-6) and phyto-sterol foods to increase the amount of feminising hormones in their body, while at the same time reducing the production of the masculine hormones in the ovaries which will, in effect, reduce the masculine features.

Progesterone also will help balance and stimulate estrogen receptor sensitivity and bring about a modulating effect. It will also improve skin hydration, softness and elasticity, stop hair loss, and for others may even slow down the 'greying' process. Acne may also improve if it's related to high testosterone levels as progesterone restores harmony.

I thought once my periods stopped and I was menopausal that all my symptoms would stop. Why haven't they?

Menopause means the cessation of the menstrual period therefore the end of the reproductive years, but it doesn't mean your symptoms will magically disappear. Rapid fluctuations of a number of the steroid hormones can create a roller coaster effect and our mothers have probably passed comments such as "I never went through all those problems!" Or "it is a state of mind, get over it!". The saga goes on.

This period of time is often called the perimenopausal time, or climacteric period, *where the symptoms of Hot Flushes, sweating, headaches, PMS, menstrual bleeding changes and irregularity, mood swings and all the symptoms of estrogen dominance can exist.*

These symptoms can vary from woman to woman, and *last for a few months, even 10-15 years* (scary concept don't you think). Following menopause, there is a period following the cessation of your period where things are still settling down and you can still experience debilitating symptoms. Just because your periods stop need not necessarily mean that symptoms subside. A lot of factors come into play, particularly estrogen dominance and the circumstances that promote it.

All these symptoms are viewed and linked to estrogen deficiency by doctors due to large drops of estrogen at menopause. Confused? Even a woman with low levels of estrogen can have estrogen dominance symptoms if she doesn't have any progesterone to balance the effects of estrogen in the body. See the question on 'What's the reason behind estrogen replacement therapy at menopause?' on page 234 and 'Hot Flushes – How can I stop Hot Flushes?' on page 231.

I'm entering menopause and my periods are erratic. What days would I apply cream?

For women entering menopause, erratic periods go with the territory. Some women report intermittent bleeding that goes on for years, others tell of how their period just stopped all of a sudden.

So progesterone isn't really going to regulate monthly bleeding when Mother Nature is signalling the end of your reproductive years. What progesterone supplementation can do, however, is make the going a little easier. If the periods are beginning to wander. Lengthening or shortening or unpredictability erratic and menopause is nearing, progesterone will not regulate these (may so temporarily). I call this the **pre menopausal dance** and it expresses itself uniquely.

It is important not to try and align your breaks with unpredictable periods but to stick with a regular monthly cyclic break and follow this pattern (even if a period may appear one month during break here).

So using a calendar month, apply cream 3 weeks out of 4, breaking from cream for 7 days (20mg is usually sufficient if asymptomatic, higher doses if not). Perhaps incorporate vitamins and phytoestrogen supplements, and address your stress levels. Choose your monthly (28 day) break to align with where your bleeding used to occur! i.e. stick with your original normal bleeding cycle following the bio rhythm you had.

If you have numerous estrogen dominance symptoms then you will need to work on higher doses to bring symptoms under control. 32mg appears to be a comfortable dose for most (after initial high doses, if required).

A lot of women benefit immensely by incorporating Vitex into their program, particularly when experiencing extremes of wandering periods. It seems to assist in balancing and regulation, along with many of its other medicinal and traditional benefits. In general if the periods are to be regulated, they will do so with progesterone and/or (Vitex) if you follow your pre pattern prior the erratic changes.

What happens if I do not ovulate or I do not have ovaries?

If your ovaries have been surgically removed such as in the case of a Hysterectomy, ectopic pregnancy, cancer, or Ovarian Cysts / dysfunction then you will not be manufacturing adequate, if any, progesterone required to maintain or oppose estrogen dominance.

If your adrenals and other glands cannot compensate and produce the required amount of sex hormones for the body to maintain its physiological levels, hormone imbalance results, giving rise to other physical problems, e.g. Adrenal Gland Exhaustion.

Other factors that can lead to ovarian failure in a woman's body is tubal ligation. This can often lead to ovarian failure 5-6 six years down the track. Ovarian Cysts, Endometriosis and other factors such as stress and the Contraceptive Pill can shut down the ovaries, thus interfering with the progesterone output, leaving a woman progesterone deficient.

Vaginal Dryness

Vaginal dryness and bladder problems are very common complaints that I hear about, and can affect women of all ages with hormonal imbalances. It is a subject reluctant to be spoken about with Doctors and certainly not a routine question in our quick visits, unless there is perhaps a problem (e.g. Urinary Tract Infection) relating to this sensitive topic.

Vaginal dryness affects most women at menopause (or prior) *due to the decreasing estrogen levels which result in lessened blood flow to the vaginal area.* When this occurs, vaginal secretions can decrease, vaginal walls may become thinner (atrophy) and the tissue less elastic. This can leave women more susceptible to infection and can cause discomfort or irritation during intercourse. Often women complain of dryness that may be associated with itchiness. There are some that say their vagina feels uncomfortable or sore when they walk, particularly if they are overweight. Tissue atrophy and shrinkage of the outer labia does occur in some cases (as reported to NPAN). Visit the section on Libido in my companion book - More Secrets Revealed.

NPAN has always acknowledged that this is where the use of estrogen is important and suggests all women complaining of these problems and/or in her menopausal years, should use Estriol Vaginal Cream regularly (1-3 times a week intravaginally as required and instructed) for maintenance of healthy tissue treatment and prevention of bladder and vaginal irritations. It strengthens up tissue reducing risk of infections and certainly making intercourse more comfortable.

Estriol Estrogen Cream is in a natural safe form and is, in low doses, adequate to treat these all too common problems. There is no need to take estrogen in other forms to address these problems. (Dr. script in Aust.)

Many women have found that with the use of progesterone, phytoestrogen and a natural lubricant, vaginal lubrication and secretions have restored naturally, without the need for estrogen substitution. Some however take Ovestin if they are not in this arena but still suffer Stress Incontinence bouts of Thrush, Bladder infections and irritation.

Balancing the hormones changes the vaginal environment and leaves it less susceptible to Thrush, Vaginitis and infections.

Other Hints

- Use water-based moisturisers or even natural vitamin E, olive oil or sesame oil (natural antioxidants) with healing ingredients and safe to rub around vagina.
- Do not use petrochemical based lubricants or chemical douches (try diluted tea tree oil). There are some very good natural lubricants on the market (with a neutral pH level). Use condoms with a water based lubricant only.
- Avoid underwear that is a heat trapper – change to natural fibres (e.g. cotton/wool) that breathe.
- Avoid usage of tampons. If you do need to use them change regularly (so it doesn't create a warm moist environment for microorganisms to grow in).
- Choose natural tampons and Modess™ pads (chemicals & scents contain irritants that will aggravate a sensitive area.

- Practice meticulous vaginal hygiene. A good thing also is regular intercourse which increases blood flow and improves tissue integrity and lubrication. It also strengthens the vaginal wall muscles.
- Use nutritional backup – high antioxidants (e.g. selenium, vitamin C) and omega oils 3-6 are very helpful.
- Intravaginal progesterone once to three times a week has helped some women or mixes of progesterone and Estriol 1mg. Refer to page 248

Bladder Problems (Stress Incontinence)
Urinary Problems

As with the vagina, decreasing levels of estrogen can lead to the walls of the urinary tract and bladder becoming thinner and less supple.

This may result in urgency – that is the need to urinate frequently or can mean that you may become more susceptible to infections and Cystitis. Weakening of the sphincter muscles around the base of the bladder (the muscles used to stop urine flow) can result in leaking (Stress Incontinence) which occurs when you sneeze, cough, laugh or exercise. Prolapses, obesity and having large babies can also contribute.

Hints:

- Use progesterone & Vaginal Estriol as per instructions.
- Practice pelvic floor muscle exercises (tightening the sphincter muscles then releasing them to a slow count of 20). Regularly try stopping halfway through urination to strengthen and tone.
- Reduce weight if overweight
- Nutritional supplementation, high in antioxidants and phytoestrogens
- Do not sit for long periods
- Do not let your kidneys get cold
- Reduce sugar, caffeine, fruity alcohol intake (e.g. Champagne) high in sugar. Sugar promotes bacterial and fungus growth. Caffeine and alcohol create diuresis and promote an increasing need to urinate. See ANTI FUNGI DIET, Book 2.
- Change the bladder's environment either with daily selenium and vitamin C or cranberry juice (non sweetened). Reduce sugar intake. Reduce caffeine intake.
- Urinate after intercourse (flushes out any bugs that may have entered the urethra). Covered in greater depth in Book 2.
- Drink copious amounts (2 litres) of water a day (flushes and prevents infections and improves bladder capacity). Empty bladder regularly (exercise it!), and on completion cough twice. Sit forward to squeeze the bladder after urination.
- Many women fear wetting themselves so they avoid fluids and become very dehydrated causing the urine to become very concentrated, an ideal environment for bacteria to grow. Use products containing natural fibres, particularly in using panty liners and tampons.

- If you have chronic infections or have a prolapsed bladder seek an appropriate understanding Doctor to discuss options. Try and avoid over use of antibiotics and medications used for bladder control (if necessary short term is advisable).

Hysterectomy
What is a Hysterectomy?

Hysterectomy is defined as the "surgical removal of the uterus" (womb). It is one of the most common of all surgical procedures and can also involve the removal of the fallopian tubes, ovaries and cervix to cure or alleviate a number of gynecological complaints.

Following this operation you will no longer have periods, you will not be fertile and you will not be able to have any more children. How often have I heard "my incubator or oven has gone". This still strikes a chord with me and instantaneously returns me to that moment of truth. A uterus I gave up in desperation and ignorance, unaware of all the facts.

How is a Hysterectomy performed?

There are two main ways to perform a Hysterectomy. The most common way is to remove the uterus through a cut in the lower abdomen either laterally along the pubic line or vertically (rarely done now due to impeded healing because of diminished blood supply to this area of the abdomen) sometimes this route is necessary but check prior.

The second, less common way is to remove the uterus only through a cut in the top of the vagina, the top of vagina is then stitched. Each operation lasts between one to two hours and is performed, in hospital, under a general anaesthetic.

What are the types of Hysterectomy

The type of Hysterectomy that you have will depend upon the condition it is being used to treat (refer website - http://www.althysterectomy.org). Plus for support and information.

- **A "Subtotal Hysterectomy"** removes the uterus leaving the cervix in place. I highly recommend you try to keep your cervix, see my section on Libido. If you have this operation you will need to continue to have smear tests.
- **A "Total Hysterectomy"** removes the complete uterus including the cervix, this is the operation most commonly performed.
- **A "Total Hysterectomy with bilateral or unilateral salpingo-oophorectomy"** removes the uterus, cervix, fallopian tubes and both or one of the ovaries.
- **A "Wertheims Hysterectomy"** removes the uterus, cervix, part of the vagina,

fallopian tubes, peritoneum (this is the broad band of ligament below the uterus), the lymph glands and fatty tissue of the pelvis and possibly one or both ovaries. (performed such as in cancer cases).

What are the real facts about Hysterectomy?

Here are some FACTS as provided by Hysterectomy Education & Resource Service (HERS) (http://www.ccon.com/hers/index.htm), **an independent, national organisation dedicated to the issue of Hysterectomy which advocates for fully informed medical choices by women.**

FACT: Women experience a loss of physical sexual sensation as a result of Hysterectomy. I do not know one who hasn't.

FACT: A woman's vagina is shortened, scarred and dislocated by Hysterectomy.

FACT: Hysterectomy's damage is life-long. Among its most common consequences, in addition to operative injuries are:

- Heart Disease
- Osteoporosis
- Bone, joint and muscle pain and immobility (the uterus is a vital organ for producing prostaglandins - see section on Prostaglandins please.
- Loss of sexual desire, arousal, sensation, difficulty or inability to orgasm, painful intercourse, vaginal damage, displacement, dryness, atrophy
- Displacement of bladder, bowel, and other pelvic organs (loss of bladder tone, temporarily or permanent).
- Urinary Tract Infections, frequency, incontinence
- Chronic Constipation and digestive disorders
- Altered body odour (vaginal secretion changes - reduced, odour alteration).
- Loss of short-term memory
- Blunting of emotions, personality changes, despondency, irritability, anger, reclusiveness and suicidal thinking (my own are in brackets based on my experience and others).

FACT: No drugs or other treatments can replace ovarian or uterine hormones or functions. The loss is permanent. (NHRT can certainly help!).

FACT: Most women are **castrated** at Hysterectomy. The medical term for the removal of the ovaries is castration. (The term Hysterectomy- "hysteria" removed!).

FACT: **The uterus and ovaries function throughout life in women** who have not been hysterectomised or castrated.

FACT: Twice as many women in their 20's and 30's are hysterectomised as women in their 50's and 60's.

FACT: 98% of women HERS has referred to board-certified gynecologists after being told they needed hysterectomies, discovered that, in fact, they **did not need hysterectomies.**

FACT: Gynecologists, hospitals and drug companies make more than 5 billion dollars a year from the business of Hysterectomy and castration (2001 figure).

In the United States 550,000 hysterectomies are performed each year. Up to 60,000 Hysterectomy operations are carried out on women in the UK every year (2001 figures).

In the vast majority of these cases, the indications for surgery are benign, non life-threatening conditions. Only 10% of hysterectomies are performed for cancer.

It can and does help to ease many gynecological complaints, including heavy and/or painful periods, Endometriosis, inaccessible Fibroids etc. It is rarely performed for reasons of saving life, but it **can be a permanent cure for some gynecological cancers.**

No More Hysterectomies, the enlightening and empowering book that has helped thousands of women to make the right choice about their female reproductive health problems. Learn how the male dominated medical profession and insurance industry has sanctioned millions of unwarranted Hysterectomies. Information found on web site (http://www.nomorehysterectomies.com/main_frames.htm)

Dr. Vicki Hufnagel, acknowledged world over as an authority on the subject, candidly explains how you can avoid this often unnecessary procedure. Please research this thoroughly before you sanction it, seek second opinions and find a gynaecologist that is on your side.

I have had a Hysterectomy, since then I've noticed that my vaginal secretions are dry and my vagina lips (labia) and clitoris have shrunk, along with a reduced sexual desire and inability to have deep, satisfying orgasms. What can I do?

This is a common occurrence and complaint amongst women that have experienced a Hysterectomy. The removal of the uterus may bring about an inability for women to experience the deep contractual uterine orgasms that they may have once experienced, and their orgasmic pleasure may be less intense.

Progesterone will, in many cases, help re-establish and normalise vaginal secretions and restore normal pH levels, and often does bring about increased lubrication. However, deficiencies in the sex hormones estrogen and testosterone that have a significant role to play in the changes in the structure of the vaginal wall and the outer vaginal lips can create shrinkage, tightness and pain on intercourse.

So it's advisable to use estriol vaginal cream in conjunction with progesterone to help prevent atrophy of the vaginal walls.

Additional supplementation of minute amounts of testosterone topically applied to the clitoris and estriol inserted into the vagina 2-3 times weekly will return lubrication and restore the tissue integrity. The result is a more comfortable sexual intercourse and longer, satisfying orgasms. I now use a mix of all three hormones intra vaginally 2-3 times a week. Refer to libido in Book 2.

Women also couple this with the use of pH lubricating cream formulas especially designed to balance and 'plump up' cells providing a twenty-four hour lubrication coverage. They contain phytoestrogens discussed in Book 2.

The regular application of these 2-3 hormones usually restores and improves blood flow circulation to the clitoris and vagina thus restoring the capacity for natural lubrication and orgasm. If the vagina has shrunk and it is too small, it needs to be massaged and gently manually stretched using estrogen cream regularly. Regular sex helps increase blood flow, stretch and strengthen the vaginal walls (after you have eliminated pain from dryness and tissue thinning using Estriol). Refer to vaginal dryness, page 244.

I'm suffering bladder problems. Is this connected with my Hysterectomy?

Women often experience bladder problems in conjunction with a Hysterectomy and/or menopause. Conditions include Stress Incontinence, exposure of their urethra, a little bit of agitation or irritation around the urethra, and possibly tender bladder. They frequently complain of feelings of needing to pass urine or difficulty in holding urine during sudden muscle efforts such as sneezing or coughing, known as Stress Incontinence.

This can be brought about due to the fact that Hysterectomy often disrupts the hormone production and creates an early menopause. With the use of hormone therapy (regular application of estriol vaginal cream and topical progesterone), diet, pelvic floor exercise, plenty of fluids, meticulous hygiene, the use of good lubrication and the restoration and balancing of hormones and nutritional status, the bladder will, in time, respond and improve in functioning (may need short term use of stronger topical estrogen).

Thrush seems to partner bladder problems and vaginal changes as a result of hormone imbalance, often in conjunction with extreme stress and a diet high in sugar.

Progesterone has been reported to have a significant bearing in helping to correct women's Thrush and Candida problems, and I believe it's because it helps to regulate the blood sugar in some way. It also helps to restore normality of hormones and perhaps stimulate more natural estrogens which will help vaginal protection and lubrication, and offer a first line of defence. It also assists in U.T.I. management.

Progesterone is also known to be antibacterial in that is helps to improve a woman's immune system **by increasing the immunity globulin factor** which helps protect against dangerous germs and bugs entering the body and targeting organs that could, in turn, create infection and disease (Urinary Tract Infections being common).

What I am saying here is that it's all interrelated (and not in your imagination). Vaginal and bladder hygiene awareness and nutritional support is of utmost importance in women's health but perhaps not often spoken about, much less incorporated in our education.

Women report being advised to stop progesterone at the first sign of bladder sensitivities, infections or even Thrush. These conditions are known side effects of synthetic progestogens. They have absolutely nothing to do with progesterone.

In fact, progesterone, according to our women, many of whom have been chronic sufferers of Thrush and Cystitis, has helped overcome such problems after 12 months use. But don't ever assume your bladder problems are necessarily linked to hormone imbalance. Seek medical advice.

Bleeding Concerns & Menstrual Cycles

My cycles have changed since I'm on progesterone, and I do not know where I should be taking my breaks.

This is very common. Cycles have been known to lengthen or shorten while on progesterone treatment. Generally with women I state that as long as there is a regular cycle occurring with a rhythmic break from cream, then your periods will come and go according to your unique profile, varying slightly by a day or two, here and there.

One woman, let's call her Frances, in her early fifties used to have a 28 day cycle. She stops her progesterone cream at day 26 and has a 5 day break because she suffers very high PMS. Frances has found that when she recommences using cream on day 6 her period arrives on day 6, which ultimately means her cycle has lengthened. Nonetheless, this works for her, and she has maintained asymptomatic (symptom free) estrogen dominance.

Frances is reluctant to take a longer break purely because she really does feel different when she is not on the progesterone cream. This woman has come to understand her body's rhythm and that she will have her period the day she starts the cream. When it's all said and done, your body will find its own cycle. You just need to make sure you have a rest from progesterone cream 5-7 days' every month (12 days break is ideal if you can cope, as it is true to nature's rhythmic pattern, if 5-7 days break is too long adhere to a minimum of 3 days).

In Frances's case, the break from cream is not bringing on her period as she believes. What's really happening here is a 32 day cycle. But this lady has a mindset of a 28 day cycle, and that's the way she wants it to stay. It's also why she suffers from PMS.

Given her real cycle of 32 days, breaking from cream at day 26 when she needs progesterone cream the most to counteract estrogen dominance, makes treating PMS very difficult. If she took her break 5 days later, say day 31, 1-2 days before her period appears, she would be able to cope with a longer break from cream, and perhaps suffer less from PMS.

And she needs to take into account the fact that she is probably entering menopause, and periods will lengthen or shorten until they disappear altogether. Bringing us back to the fact that every woman's bio-rhythms and cycles is unique. You would be very surprised to learn that this lady is a registered nurse, which might explain rigid belief that her cycles cannot be anything other than 28 days!

Another woman, in her thirties, whose periods had stopped altogether, established a regular cycle with progesterone therapy after years of irregularity and heavy bleeding. There was no underlying problem. Her body just needed progesterone.

For those women who find it hard to chart a regular cycle - periods are all over the place or not arriving at all for months on end - I suggest you use your cream 3 weeks out of 4, taking a break from cream for at least 5 days. Longer if you feel up to it (12 days is ideal). You will know when your body is missing progesterone. Sleep disturbance is usually the first sign.

Stopping progesterone cream is not necessarily going to bring on a period if it's not ready to come. However, if your body is primed for a period, it will arrive within 24-36 hrs. Breaks are important - it keeps your cycle mimicking nature, and allows the receptors to up-regulate (refresh).

For women who no longer ovulate or perhaps their periods are winding down, or they are battling severe diseases like painful Endometriosis, severe migraines and/or PMS, Polycystic Ovary Syndrome, or Fibroids, need to use higher doses or stay on cream longer. These high doses will not down-regulate providing you break from cream each month to stimulate cell receptors and your body is, in fact, utilising these levels. **If you do not take even short breaks (3 days minimum) it will render progesterone's work in the body ineffective.** No matter what you are using progesterone for.

I've started using progesterone after using conventional HRT for some time. When I started natural progesterone I wasn't getting any Hot Flushes and my periods were regulated on HRT but now they have returned with a vengeance. Why?

The estrogen and progestogen combination in HRT up until now have carried you over but as they move off the receptors and the levels of synthetic HRT drop, the effects of HRT also wear off. *This is when women suddenly realise they haven't passed through menopause at all.* **Regular periods on HRT are controlled synthetically.**

Furthermore, the introduction of natural progesterone sensitises the estrogen receptors creating Estrogen Dominance Wake Up Crisis. Much of the progesterone sites are still occupied by stubborn progestogens, thus natural progesterone cannot provide full benefits for some months.

The transition period from HRT to natural progesterone can be very discomforting and off putting.

Women coming off HRT find themselves in 'natural menopausal territory', facing symptoms that HRT has perhaps treated but may not have totally resolved, preventing women from making that 'rite of passage' that is gone through menopause. The brain threshold of estrogen has been high signaling the brain that menopause hasn't started. **Stopping HRT tells the body that menopause has begun particularly when the reserves of estrogen in the body drop.** When this occurs symptoms return with a vengeance.   This is the dilemma a good many women face. They cannot cope with HRT side effects, but then they have to deal with the problems of menopause once they stop using HRT.

It's very hard for long-term users of HRT to make that switch to natural progesterone without disruption.. Their body has grown accustomed to strong, synthetic analogues. Maybe their body is overloaded with the remnants of HRT, taken over many years.

Basically, for some women, detoxing from HRT, getting the liver function going again, allowing time for receptors to be available for natural progesterone, then allowing for saturation and response to natural progesterone ... takes personal commitment and an understanding of how the body needs to adjust. *Estrogen therapy is still required if being on estrogen.* **A weaning process in necessary in most.** But *progestins are **not** required in combination with progesterone.* It is a contra indication as you cannot use progestins and progesterone together. Stopping progestins is usually a relief to the body as this synthetic hormone does not match the keyhole remember. Causing undue side effects because of its mismatch.

Coming off estrogen cold turkey is the culprit and can create withdrawal symptoms, which can emerge around 6 weeks or sooner (in thinner women) once the body has diminished its supplies and the brains alarm system goes off saying "not enough estrogen" as it has been used to such high levels. It is likened to instant induced menopause seen and experienced by women who have had their ovaries removed or other causes of destruction and interference of ovarian function ie. Chemotherapy. The brain is shocked! It has not had time to adjust.

The trick is if you are wary/scared of *reducing your estrogen start by halving your dose when starting progesterone* (remember the re introduction of progesterone will re stimulate the receptors and exacerbate estrogen). This in other words will equal what it was used to. *As the levels drop, re introduce small amounts of natural topical estrogen transdermally back into the body to a level it is resatisfied with.* Back off and test, let the body accept the gradual reduction over time. It may take up to 12 months, some less depending on their previous usage and conditioned threshold dosage as well as duration.

For those who have abundance estrogen overload try starting progesterone alone and test your body's compensation mechanisms. You may find you may wish to re introduce a little estrogen, avoid synthetic tablets as they are harsh on the liver and a very high dosage is required to deliver 10% back to the body as 90% is lost and changed in the liver's metabolism breaking this down to form estrogen administration. It is far more effective and safer to use bio identical hormones transdermally.

A few lucky women stop estrogen on commencement of progesterone and never need to revisit estrogen replacement therapy. Liver work, high phytoestrogen, Ovestin may be all they need. Furthermore some women particularly the Gynaeoid body type women store estrogen in their lower body weight.

It is the luck of the game and every woman is individual.

Many women have returned to HRT only to find the need to forever increase dosage to abate symptoms with side effects and breakthrough bleeding worsening. And menopausal symptoms resurfacing despite HRT.

In other words, after 10-15 years, HRT was no longer effective for them, leaving them with little choice but to return to progesterone therapy. To continue with HRT was to put further work on their liver and aggravate weight and metabolic problems (blood pressure, cholesterol, thyroid, insulin resistance), not to mention cancer risks.

It's a difficult process to understand. You might like to read more about 'HRT and NHRT' and weaning off estrogen (chapters 16 & 17). The Doctors often state "It's really a question of the risks as opposed to the treating of unbearable symptoms" coercing their patients to try a newer HRT, promised to be better. The problems will re emerge in a majority of cases and thus the merry-go-round continues.

Please visit Nutrition and strategies in Book 2 'Natural Progesterone More Secrets Revealed', and the importance of phytoestrogens in this book.

I have just started my progesterone cream and I'm have breakthrough bleeding. What does that mean?

It is quite common when a woman first starts progesterone to have a breakthrough bleed and the appearance of another period. This is often the result of cell receptor 'wake up' and influence on the uterine lining and receptor cells therein, such activity bringing on a bleed. Do not to be concerned about this unless it is heavy (haemorrhaging), constant, and/or causing pain that leaves you feeling concerned. It's not unusual for progesterone to do some spring cleaning.

Many, many women report 'wake up' bleeding as being one of the first things that may happen when they start progesterone. It represents positive activity in the body. **NPAN refers to this 'first' bleed as the 'pretend' period**, indicating the positive impact and presence of natural progesterone. A lot of women state their bleed was not "pretend" so I now call this the 'in-between period'.

However, I have heard from women who report too many irregular breakthrough bleeds. They cannot establish a regular cycle and are still feeling quite estrogen dominant with associated symptoms (and increasing dose does not seem to help). Experience has led me to believe that often, unsuitable creams can do this. I suggest that if there is more than one breakthrough bleed and your period becomes erratic rather than stabilising within a four month period, then you seriously need to reassess your cream base (have an ultra sound to ensure no Fibroids for example).

Often the cream has come up on analytical reports as quite suitable and has the correct BP micronised progesterone, but some creams appear to target the uterus specifically. I really don't know why this happens. It's simply my observation. I refer to this effect as 'dumping'. These same women, once they move to another cream, see more favourable results.

Progesterone balances the effects of estrogen on the uterus and it is necessary to produce regular periods, so if these periods are not being regulated, I suspect there is something wrong with your progesterone cream. If in doubt, stop the cream for a month before you try another brand (if all your prior tests are negative, showing no signs of Fibroids, etc and you are not in the pre menopausal dance stage).

Incorporate phytoestrogens into your diet, and always make sure you undergo the appropriate investigations and tests to rule out anything sinister.

You might also like to refer to the section on 'How do I know if the cream I am using is a reliable, high quality cream?' on page 95. Book 2 delves into this also.

My periods are all over the place, light and heavy. I don't know when to start using the cream.

I suggest women try and work out their normal menstrual cycle. Count fourteen days back from the end of the last period to work out when your actual ovulation time would be. Then commence using the cream from that period on day 12 to 26. When you commence the cream because your body is so deprived of progesterone you can comfortably use progesterone continually through the first period without a break. But break on the next due cycle i.e. Days off from where you have established where the periods are meant to be.

Continue this pattern cycle working towards extending your breaks eventually getting to the ideal situation 12 days off 12 days on. Day 12-26. You will be able to align yourself more accurately as the real periods come back on track. The trick here is once you see this then stopping of cream is 2 days prior of each cycle when you know the cycle. For example a 28 day cycle, you break at Day 26. Progesterone is in our body from day 12-26 as in mother nature and starts to decline from the 26th day as does estrogen which brings on the period.

Do this consistently and you should synchronise with some form of cycle in conjunction with the use of progesterone.

Alternatively, many women actually start the cream uninterrupted and find out where the true period falls and recognise where the false period is. Ignore the false pretend period (a break through period) and establish the true period. Within two months uninterrupted I suggest you take a break on what appears to be the truer period and start going cyclic from there. Often you will find that the body will regulate and fall into synchronisation fairly soon thereafter, usually around 4 months.

For women about to start menopause, often their periods are erratic. Progesterone may not help regulate your cycle but it certainly can help reduce the heaviness of your flow. It's rather like the last fling before your periods stop, and periods may vary in patterns for about twelve months. I call this the premenopausal dance which I go into in greater detail in my second book.

Or it may just suddenly stop, and that's the end of your periods for good. Again, herbs and diet seem to help. Progesterone will help carry and support a woman through this erratic time, alleviating many of the associated premenopause and or perimenopausal symptoms.

Erratic periods are commonly reported, and can vary from 3 months on, maybe 3 months off, or perhaps they see a period only every 6 months. Rule of thumb being, if you fall into this category, just rely on a calendar month and 32mg dosage, taking 5-7 days break as symptoms allow. Bleeding irregularities have been dealt with in great depth in book 2.

With hysterectomised menopausal induced women I suggest just take a break at the beginning of each month 3-5 days. It is easy to remember. Fascinatingly my body just knows when a break is needed and is more of my calendar guide than my diary. Often I have forgotten a day or two only to realise it is a new month.

If there is no evidence of hormone imbalance or symptoms present, follow 2 weeks off, 2 weeks on program and you may not need to use much cream (16-20mg). It certainly won't hurt you as progesterone has many multi-factorial benefits throughout the body. Use the 'least is best' principle here. In earlier stages of menopausal years higher doses are usually required and as your body settles you will find you will need less cream in the years to come, when you have fewer symptoms.

To understand and appreciate the complexity of cream usage, please also refer to Book 2 which goes into more detail on bleeding irregularities.

Will progesterone throw my hormone functions out of synchronisation? I'm reluctant to go on progesterone because I'm young and still have regular cycles.

No. Progesterone replacement therapy is employed to treat hormone imbalance, specifically estrogen dominance. If estrogen levels in your body are dominating the hormonal environment, progesterone cream is used to bring levels back into balance.

Hormone replacement therapy does not just apply to women who have entered menopause. There are many women taking natural hormone replacement therapy to treat a variety of symptoms while they are menstruating. It depends entirely on the individual. If diet, exercise, vitamins, lifestyle cannot of itself provide you with hormone balance, hormone replacement therapy may be required to keep you healthy.

If in doubt, get a total hormone profile ordered through your doctor. This will confirm any need for progesterone replacement therapy - make sure your doctor doesn't just check your estrogen levels.

What are some of the causes for heavy bleeding?

Use of estrogen replacement therapy, unopposed by progestogens, leads to build-up and thickening of the uterine lining usually resulting in the need for a curette (scraping of the uterus). Based on observation, curettes do not resolve heavy bleeding. In fact, the procedure may aggravate the situation down the track. And so a vicious circle is established.

Other reasons for heavy bleeding might include uterine Fibroids, Endometriosis, Anaemia, obesity, and exposure to toxins and chemicals (fumes, paints, etc.).

Natural progesterone is of great value in these cases providing progesterone levels exceeding that of estrogen, thus opposing the effects of estrogen. What I am pointing out here is don't fall into the trap of thinking that using high levels of progesterone alone will override these problems. You need to address estrogen dominance symptoms and the underlying causes.

I suggest you read Guidelines of Reducing Estrogen covered in both books.

Should I take my break every time I get a period?

Yes and No, **yes to the real period if it is a "true" period and no to the breakthrough period.** What I mean by this is that often while the body is adjusting and while the hormones are regulating themselves with the introduction of progesterone or the alteration of progesterone dosage, periods can sometimes become haywire and erratic (see the sections on Polycystic Ovary Syndrome and Endometriosis). Period irregularities is addressed in depth in the companion book and when to take breaks.

There are many reasons for irregularities so I suggest you do not break from cream every time a period or spotting appears if it's within the 28-32 days, or what you would consider your normal cycle. If another bleed occurs inside your regular cycle, simply chart it, and work through it continuing on with progesterone usage, taking a break from progesterone cream on your normal cyclic bleed (5-12 days break depending on your situation, problem, time on progesterone therapy, and status of symptoms being treated).

Often women don't know where their real cycle is, so again, I suggest choose the period that is the heaviest, if this is the case, and work on that being the regular cycle. It is imperative you maintain two weeks cyclic use of progesterone (from day 12 to 26 approximately) if you are having regular cycles, and have established balance and you are relatively symptom-free.

NOTE: The start of break time is more important to adhere to i.e. keeping it as a cyclic pattern where the bleed occurs than the starting time back on the cream after the break. I.e. Some women start day 5,6,7 or 12 but always break at period due time. The reason why some women need to resume earlier than day 12 is they do not have good supplies of progesterone reserves and the break uses these up leaving the body quickly depleted, allowing estrogen dominant symptoms to re-emerge. *Each month's breaks allow you to assess how you are assimilating/using your progesterone and coping on breaks.* If you do not miss this hormone (you'll know). Ideally a 10 or 12 day break is perfect and indicates balance. Observation is that many pre menopausal and early menopausal women are in the high territory of estrogen dominance symptoms and cope far better on shorter breaks i.e. the first 4 - 7 months. A too long a break can allow too much estrogen build up on the uterus which causes heavy bleeds. So you need to tailor your breaks and doses to you. The signs of healthy non clotting normal bleeds is your barometer that you are winning this estrogen dominance problem.

If you are menopausal it is not relevant. Basically, a woman needs at least two weeks or fourteen days progesterone in her system every month to mimic nature and periods (menstrual cycles). Most prefer 3 weeks on 1 week off (or less).

Summary

Stopping and starting cream randomly will not only confuse your body's natural rhythm, but will lead to further progesterone deficiency and subsequent estrogen dominance. It may also compound existing problems such as Endometriosis and polycystic ovary syndrome, both of which may present with irregular cycles. Stopping and starting cream can also increase fertility as two of our women have discovered.

In conditions such as Endometriosis and polycystic ovary syndrome where fortnightly bleeding suddenly reoccurs, it is best for these women to return to 3 week progesterone dosage regime to restore their normal cycle or increase dosage usually by 2%.

It's evident that a 2 week progesterone dosage regime often doesn't provide that holding threshold, particularly if they are on lower doses and have had a period of stress (physical or emotional).

Once stabilised, reduce dosage gradually or reduce back to fortnightly regime, both ways have worked effectively.

What happens if my periods stop or are very late?

Get a pregnancy test if you suspect you could be pregnant or if you discover you are pregnant, DO NOT STOP CREAM (see section on Fertility in this chapter).

If you've had a regular cycle and it suddenly goes haywire, continue to use cream as if normal. If you start adjusting cream according to false cycles, your periods won't regulate. If you are nearing menopause and your period stops, chances are you have reached menopause. And a high FSH reading will confirm this (see 'Tests at Menopause' on page 235).

Women become alarmed when their period fails to arrive on time. Some even think they're pregnant. But actually it's not uncommon after 4 – 5 months on cream for a woman's period to become erratic. Assuming you're not pregnant and you've had a regular pattern up to now, stick to your charted regular cycle. Your body will rebalance itself in time.

If, however, your cycle hasn't been regular, this is where charts are relevant. Determine what cycle the body is trying to establish. Then count forward 12 days from the first day of your period, and start using cream from day 12 to 26. Continue this pattern (14 days on, 12 days off) even in the absence of a period; your body will eventually synchronise back into a cycle if you haven't entered menopause.

Don't stop applying cream if a period appears outside the pattern you have established. If you do this, you'll thwart the body's attempts to regulate itself. If you take a break on the tail end of a previous break from cream., i.e. a late period, it will deplete the body of progesterone very quickly. Basically, establish a pattern and stick with it.

If, however, you begin to observe a regular cycle appearing other than the one you are working on, make the necessary adjustment, fall into line with this 'new' cycle which is more than likely your 'true' cycle. Charting here is invaluable in sorting through these ups and downs. *Just make sure you maintain adequate progesterone levels in your body, and your breaks are cyclic.*

There are various reasons why your periods may stop or be delayed. Factors such as stress, death in the family, illness, surgery, diet, weight loss, excessive exercise, fear of pregnancy, certain medications and so. All these things can play havoc on the intrinsic balance of your hormones.

Will progesterone help me with heavy bleeding?

From experience and observation, progesterone will often help with heavy bleeding because it balances the effect of estrogen upon uterus (and breast) thus reducing the amount of menstrual bleeding ... but it is not a quick fix. *Heavy bleeding comes as a result of many aspects* within the body, and often it requires many other treatments such as your vitamins, minerals, *iron* & B12 supplements, diet and stress management, and specific herbs.

Vitamin C, selenium with vitamin E are of great value with powerful anti-oxidants and anti-inflammatory properties. Phytoestrogens have a balancing/regulatory effect on estrogen levels. High levels of *bioflavonoids strengthen capillaries in the uterus and improves vascular healing reducing blood clotting.*

There might be underlying **Anaemia which can aggravate further heavy bleeding** or the possible presence of Fibroids, not forgetting one of the bigger players here - estrogen dominance, whether due to estrogen replacement therapy, progesterone deficiency, obesity, incorrect foods, exposure to toxins or stress. It's advisable to get blood work done and an ultrasound, and other appropriate tests to eliminate all such possibilities.

Progesterone will help over a period of time but usually it requires high doses (7-12 months at least depending on the severity of bleeding and underlying causes), must always be checked by your Doctor, and then a gradual reduction. It takes some time for the body to settle down. I have known women to take between 8-18 months to combat heavy bleeding problems before they've actually found a position of comfort and success with progesterone usage.

Often the doctors will encourage women to undergo progestogen therapy, advise them to have a curette, or go down the path of a Hysterectomy to stop bleeding.

Anaemia causes heavy bleeding, and heavy bleeding causes Anaemia. So get your iron levels and iron reserves checked. If you are low in iron, liquid iron supplementation has helped women with breaking this vicious cycle. Use your progesterone in conjunction with a good diet, exercise and stress management.

There are so many aspects of heavy bleeding. You need to work out exactly what is the cause, whether it is life threatening, and whether it interferes with your lifestyle to warrant clinical procedures (drug therapy & surgery).

If heavy bleeding is actually caused by estrogen dominance alone, you should realise relief from a premium progesterone cream, along with other estrogen dominance reduction measures. Some women suffering estrogen dominance find that just by reducing their weight they are able to reduce their bleeding significantly.

Breaking the rules:

Progesterone use varies here from the normal standard procedures. *For instance, where there is a **sudden appearance of a heavy bleed**, a 'once off' stat dose (immediately) of high levels of progesterone (10%-20%, 100-200mg) has worked dramatically for some women to reduce and control bleeding.*

This approach is adopted in circumstances where heavy bleeding may have started.

Adopting this 'left field' approach has actually brought bleeding under control for some. Worth a try to see if you respond to this approach.

This application is administered at the ONSET of a bleed, adopted purely to see if high doses of progesterone will help control heavy bleeding. Nonetheless, this is a one-off approach, as this cream is actually being applied during a time when you should be breaking from cream if the bleed represents your normal cycle. If the heavy bleed falls in between cycles, do a high stat dose 100-200mg (for 2 days if necessary) then drop the dosage to about 6% and continue application until your next scheduled break from cream.

Note, intravaginal application appears to have significant impact in helping to reducing heavy bleeding problems where topical application at physiological doses has been marginally successful, or they have been successful in controlling their condition and then suddenly find they are facing out of control bleeding.

A couple of months of intravaginal application equivalent to 10% level has been enough to restore normal bleeding patterns (based on easing of bleed, type of bleed, presence or absence of clots), and often women return to topical application of physiological doses of 4%-6% (as experienced by women associated with my Network with heavy bleeding problems). Please refer also to section on intravaginal application, "Creams Used Vaginally", on page 172 and also in Book 2 - More Secrets Revealed

You won't see the true results of progesterone therapy until the period following the one you are currently treating. At that point, if all is satisfactory, you can determine a gradual reduction of dosage, then assess again at the next bleed.

Between these two consecutive periods, you will determine what your baseline dose is. On observation, heavy bleeders range in the vicinity of 4-6% maintenance dose. The reduction program has taken place over a 12 month period, once they have stabilised.

Every woman is individual. Rules vary here. Some women also fluctuate with low doses for months needing to increase for a 3-4 month period then dropping back. Stress and worry are huge players in heavy bleeding concerns.

My observation at NPAN is that many of these women tend to be deep-seated worriers but often give the impression of being outwardly calm and collected. They also strive to please others, sacrificing their own personal wellbeing. Relationships and personal conflict appear to correlate with heaving bleeding issues.

Exercise helps pelvic circulation. If you experience persistent heavy bleeding, haemorrhaging, or you feel concerned for any reason, please seek medical attention and insist on appropriate tests. Too readily a Doctor will suggest progestins and may even be apprehensive in endorsing your continued use of progesterone. Regular tests and persistence (to determine response) and standing firm with Doctors has paid off for many as the progressional results have seen favourable improvement, (and for some avoiding hysterectomies), winning their Doctors scepticism over.

A case always comes to mind here, a fibroid case. Twelve months on progesterone seeing the dramatic improvement and other benefits along with clot free normal periods. At least 13 months she rang in desperation. She had started haemorrhaging with big clots. As advised she went back to her Gynecologist who wanted to do an emergency Hysterectomy. I asked her to get a copy of the recent vaginal ultrasound to determine her fibroid status. On comparison with the previous result, they had actually shrunk. This enforced her determination to not undergo a Hysterectomy (the main reason she came in the first place). On a review we back tracked and discovered she had been under huge stress which compounded 2 months prior (a family crisis) and had become so confidently blasé about her health had abandoned principles. She had given up her phytoestrogen formula, Magnesium and Livatone Plus. Justifying the cost factor and not seeing the need feeling so good. As I pointed out, the emotional and physical cost factor came at a higher price a Hysterectomy was involved and told her that her nutritional program and need to watch her body signals when it called for higher doses of progesterone, was the best investment in health insurance she could spend. Pennies were dropping as I see with so many women, they put themselves last on the family budget and pay the price ultimately.

NOTE: Bleeding irregularities is explored in greater depth in Book 2 'Natural Progesterone More Secrets Revealed'. So many women have continually approached me with their individual cases and inability to grasp usage. It can be confusing.

Metaphysically heavy bleeding means 'lack of or running out of joy'.

Why would I need progesterone if I am having a period every month?

If you are getting a period it doesn't necessarily mean that you are ovulating. A lot of women are of the belief, because they are having a regular cycle that they are ovulating regularly.

Anovulatory periods (not ovulating each month) are quite common especially from 35 years onwards. Again it depends, if you have estrogen dominance symptoms, the chances are you are not ovulating or producing the progesterone required to overcome the estrogen dominance.

That's one reason why you may need progesterone. Just to oppose the levels of estrogen in your body. Furthermore, the adrenals that would normally produce small amounts of progesterone, may not be producing enough for your body to make up for what your ovaries aren't supplying when you fail to ovulate.

The degree of severity of PMS and mood swings are an indication of the need for progesterone supplementation for hormone balance as these are classic symptoms of estrogen dominance, which will vary from month to month depending on whether you ovulate or not, your stress levels, nutrition, sleep patterns, what's going on in your life.

Cancer Concerns
Will progesterone cause and/or promote cancer? If I do not have my ovaries removed will it increase my risk of Ovarian Cancer?

Estrogen gives a cancerous cell the message to proliferate. To divide and multiply. Progesterone, on the other hand, whilst not a cure for cancer, can dramatically decreases cell multiplication rates, providing women with a degree of protection against estrogen-driven cancers. Normal levels of progesterone in the body, therefore, actually help protect you against some forms of cancer. *It will not cure cancer.*

Progesterone deficiency, however, has been linked to an increased risk of cancer. **Most Uterine Cancer, for example, is known to be caused by unopposed estrogen.**

That's why women who have an intact uterus and take estrogen replacement therapy must also be given some form of progesterone to oppose estrogen and reduce this risk. This is generally given in the form of synthetic progestogens, which is not the same molecule as progesterone but is designed to block estrogen effects.

Finally, if you have been diagnosed with cancer, never introduce progesterone therapy without first discussing it with your doctor.

Please read the book 'What your Doctor may not tell you about Breast Cancer' by the Late Dr John Lee.

Can I get Ovarian Cancer without ovaries?

I received the following fax from a client who I understand received this email and I felt it was relevant and helpful to pass this story on.

My Mum sent me this email…she has a friend going through this right now who was NOT diagnosed in time…Patty.

An eye Opener on Ovarian Cancer.

I hope you all take the time to read this and pass it on to all you can.

Send this to the women in your life that you care about.

Years ago, Gilda Radner died of ovarian cancer. Her symptoms were inconclusive, and she was treated for everything under the sun until it was too late. This blood test finally identified her illness but alas, too late. She wrote a book to heighten awareness. Gene Wilder is her widower.

Wanda Deans

KATHY'S STORY: This is the story of Kathy West.

As all of you know, I have Primary Peritoneal Cancer. This cancer has only recently been identified as its OWN type of cancer, but it is essentially Ovarian Cancer.

Both types of cancer are diagnosed in the same way, with the "tumour marker" CA-125 BLOOD TEST, and they are treated in the same way – surgery to remove the primary tumour and then chemotherapy with Taxol and Carboplatin. Having gone through this ordeal, I want to save others from the same fate. That is why I am sending this message to you and hope you will print it and give it or send it via email to everybody you know.

One thing I have learned is that each of us must take TOTAL responsibility for our own health care. I thought I had done that because I always had an annual physical and

PAP smear, did a monthly Self-Breast Exam, went to the dentist at least twice a year, etc. I even insisted on a sigmoidoscopy and a bone density test last year. When I had a total Hysterectomy in 1993, I thought that I did not have to worry about getting any of the female reproductive organ cancers.

LITTLE DID I KNOW. I don't have ovaries (and they were HEALTHY when they were removed), but I have what is essentially ovarian cancer. Strange, isn't it?

These are just SOME of the things our Doctors never tell us: ONE out of every 55 women will get OVARIAN or PRIMARY PERITONEAL CANCER. The "CLASSIC" symptoms seemed to be "abdominal", I went to a gastroenterologist. He ran tests that were designed to determine whether there was a bacteria infection; these tests were negative, and I was diagnosed with "Irritable Bowel Syndrome". I guess I would have accepted this diagnosis had it not been for my enlarged abdomen. I swear to you, it looked like I was 4-5 months pregnant! I therefore insisted on more tests.

They took an x-ray of my abdomen; it was negative. I was again assured that I had Irritable Bowel Syndrome and was encouraged to go on my scheduled month-long trip to Europe. I couldn't wear any of my slacks or shorts because I couldn't get them buttoned, and I KNEW something was radically wrong. I INSISTED on more tests, and they reluctantly scheduled me for a CT-Scan (just to shut me up, I think). This is what I mean by "taking charge of our own health care".

The CT-Scan showed a lot of fluid in my abdomen (NOT normal). Needless to say, I had to cancel my trip and have FIVE POUNDS assure you), but NOTHING compared to what was ahead of me).

Tests revealed cancer cells in the fluid. Finally, finally, finally, the doctor ran a CA-125 blood test, and I was properly diagnosed I HAD THE CLASSIC SYMPTOMS FOR OVARIAN CANCER, AND YET THIS SIMPLE CA-125 BLOOD TEST HAD NEVER BEEN RUN ON ME, not as part of my annual physical exam and not when I was symptomatic. This is an inexpensive and simple blood test!

PLEASE, PLEASE TELL ALL YOUR FEMALE FRIENDS AND RELATIVES TO INSIST ON A CA-125 BLOOD TEST EVERY YEAR AS PART OF THEIR ANNUAL PHYSICAL EXAMS. Be forewarned that their doctors might try to talk them out of it, saying, "IT ISN'T NECESSARY." Believe me, had I known then what I know now, we would have caught my cancer much earlier (before it was stage 3 cancer). Insist on the CA-125 BLOOD TEST; DO NOT take "NO" for an answer! The normal range for a CA-125 BLOOD TEST is between zero and 35. MINE WAS 754. (That's right, 754!.) If the number is slightly above 35, you can have another done in three or six months and keep a close eye on it, just as women do when they have fibroid tumours or when men have a slightly elevated PSA test (Prostatic Specific Antigens) that helps diagnose prostrate cancer.

Having the CA-125 test done annually can alert you early, and that's the goal in diagnosing any type of cancer – catching it early.

Do you know 55 women? If so, at least one of them will have this VERY AGGRESSIVE cancer. Please, go to your doctor and insist on a CA-125 test and have one EVERY YEAR for the rest of your life and forward this message to every woman you know, and tell all of your female family members and friends. Though the median age for this cancer is 56, (and, guess what, I'm exactly 56), women as young as 22 have it. Age is no factor.

A NOTE FROM THE RN:

Well, after reading this, I made some calls. I found that the Ca-125 test is an ovarian screening test equivalent to a man's PSA test prostrate screen (which my husband's doctor automatically gives him in his physical each year and insurance pays for it). I called the general practitioner's office about having the test done. The nurse had never heard of it. She told me that she doubted that insurance would pay for it. So I called Prudential Insurance Co, and got the same response. Never heard of it – it won't be covered. I explained that it was the same as the PSA test they had paid for my husband for years. After conferring with whom ever they confer with, she told me that the CA-125 would be covered. It is $75 in a GP's office and $125 at the gynaecologist's. This is a screening test that should be required just like a PAP smear. (A PAP smear cannot detect problems with your ovaries.) And you must insist that your insurance company pay for it.

Gene Wilder and Pierce Brosnan (his wife had it, too) are lobbying for women's health issues, saying that this test should be required in our physicals, just like the PAP and the mammogram.

In Australia this test is not standard although it is available because it is said to be not reliable enough at this point in time.

Permission to circulate came via my email

Will my ovaries return to normal after chemotherapy?

Understanding and observation is that following chemotherapy, women enter menopause. However, progesterone appears to have enormous value and benefits in these areas, and ought to be considered in a woman's overall treatment when undergoing surgery such as a mastectomy, and ongoing treatment for Breast Cancer.

Many women in my group swear by the use of their progesterone in conjunction with other treatments, and have suffered less debilitating menopausal symptoms such as minimal Hot Flushes.

I have a case which I would like to share with you here. Nancy and her husband came to me after being diagnosed with Breast Cancer and her mastectomy was scheduled in 3 weeks time.

Nancy was referred to NPAN seeking information on natural progesterone by a concerned friend. She began progesterone replacement therapy along with nutritional supplementation with her husband's full support.

Progesterone therapy began immediately on prescription from a local GP without her endocrinologist's consent. This was contrary to any advice provided by NPAN. In fact, I suggested she go back to the doctor whom I knew had written the progesterone script and, incidentally, was operating a women's clinic. It was up to her doctor, in my opinion, to liaise with Nancy's specialist and relay this vital information. This did not happen.

And Nancy was too frightened to open her mouth, perhaps intimidated by both doctors.

Prepping herself for surgery, she started applying progesterone in high doses to saturate her body prior to her mastectomy. She had read a medical article supporting the theory that if women ovulated (producing progesterone) prior to surgery that the likelihood of metastasis would be reduced. Nancy wanted to cover all her options. Following surgery she underwent chemotherapy. Her doctor, however, was concerned because her periods had remained cyclic, with no signs of hormonal disruption after completing her course of chemo. This demonstrated to NPAN the positive impact progesterone was having on Nancy's body under extreme conditions, possibly supporting and/or protecting ovarian integrity.

Tragically, to Nancy's detriment, she did not inform her specialist that she was still using progesterone. In response to this unusual occurrence (of continued cyclic periods), her specialist scheduled Nancy in for more chemotherapy because, in her opinion, and not knowing all the facts, Nancy's periods should have stopped. Her justification for this decision may have been based on the premise that while Nancy continued to menstruate, her estrogen levels were too high which could jeopardise further risk of cancer. This would have been a high probability without progesterone in the equation to oppose estrogen.

Had Nancy been up front with her specialist, or had the GP who prescribed progesterone (who to this date still continues to treat her with progesterone) informed the endocrinologist that she was treating Nancy in such a manner, then perhaps the second lot of chemo may not have been necessary. And subsequently Nancy entered menopause abruptly.

If this information had been revealed at the onset, perhaps the endocrinologist would have been forced to look at the possibility that the higher doses of chemo may not have been warranted. And possibly viewed progesterone's place in Nancy's treatment, recovery and outcome more favourably.

In closing, Nancy is now taking Tamoxifen against her better judgement, (but still in fear of her Specialist) and continues with progesterone therapy in secret. Further, Nancy's doctor continues to keep this information from her specialist. Nancy's case demonstrates the plight of women in Australia. In the past few years since I wrote this, 2000, I've kept in regular contact with Nancy. She has suffered enormous side effects on Tamoxifen, gained significant weight, lost bladder control (has bladder frequency) and has tingling feet also peripheral circulatory blood problems including swollen, tender feet and ankles. She can hardly walk and is also now on antidepressants. The more problems that surface the bigger her cocktail of medications, treating all these side effects and creating in the process, more. Nancy is now looking at her drugs as being a culprit of many of her problems. Now out of control and increased side effects. Nancy is fed up and is prepared to stop looking for the easy way out and is starting to take responsibility for her diet, lifestyle and over burdened liver. She wishes to now get off her Tamoxen and other medications and has been advised by her Endocrinologist that she will be able to do so as she is out of her danger period.

Being in a cancer support group Nancy has concluded that her problems are all too familiar with others on the same treatment, although her Specialist keeps telling her they are not 'side effects of her medications'. Nancy is one of these ladies who is so frightened that she goes along to get along trusting the experts without listening to her body and state of wellbeing. Her husband has been pulling his hair out since her mastectomy and has begged Nancy to start being positive about her health, rather than dwelling on the fear of cancer. She is well and truly clear. Nancy is crippled in this prospect and consumed with all her now additional medical problems.

Most of my efforts have been in vain as Nancy feels guilty spending money on nutritional supplementation or suggested positive self awareness courses. Her husband says 'this is an excuse he would sacrifice all his finances to have a happy, care free, confident, fun wife back'. We have witnessed her lose her self-esteem in obesity and her poor self image. Nancy remains a challenge to me and a committed friend. Sadly my support and closeness to her intercepted listening to advice. I referred her to a Naturopath who has reaffirmed all the things I've been trying to tell her for years and she is now listening.

On the other flip side of this is June. June had the same surgery and chemo but refused to go on Tamoxifen and other medications offered (all of which she researched and informed herself on).

She came to me, well informed about progesterone, then 7 months post mastectomy and having completed her chemotherapy. Her main issue being Hot Flushes, that was 3 years ago. June's Hot Flushes and symptoms were quickly eradicated and her sense of wellbeing restored. She has cruised on healthy productivity and adheres to a good diet, nutrition and exercise. She feels her decision was the best one ever and has what she says is a quality of life and heaps of energy. She does not entertain the thoughts of cancer and views this as a chapter in her life dealt with. She focuses on staying well and living for the now.

Since I wrote this, I received a phone call from June's husband to extend his thanks and convey his sad news. June 6 months ago had died from a massive infection following a cold she could not shake some many months prior. Her immunity system was very low and didn't respond to antibiotics or intensive medical treatment.

How sad I feel even now just writing this and have cried for June. Her husband assured me that she had still up until that cold had been living a full, rich, happy and exuberant life and says he felt the chemotherapy perhaps knocked her immunity system. Who would know, but she did not die from cancer or secondaries (metastasis)

Breast Concerns

I have lumpy (Fibrocystic) breasts. Will progesterone help?

Yes, remarkably so, if it is related to hormone imbalance. Progesterone balances the effect of estrogen upon the breasts (and uterus) and, therefore, has an influencing role in reducing breast pain and lumpiness. Improvement is usually within a 2-3 months once you commence progesterone therapy. HINT: apply directly on breasts daily. Not in breaks.

One very small breasted lady, Susan, a hairdresser, suffered years of chronic Fibrocystic Breasts that were so painful and so inhibiting to her lifestyle and work that she actually 'begged' her doctor to conduct a bilateral mastectomy thinking this would alleviate her pain. Naturally the doctor refused. And Susan somehow found herself in my lounge room in tears, desperate for help.

Within a week of progesterone therapy, her life began to turn around. And within 2 months, all her lumps had disappeared. Such was her pain and discomfort, that Susan was unable to sustain a normal relationship. This all changed once her breast tissue returned to normal. Pain no longer restricted her movements, and with the increased libido and confidence, she could enter a relationship that included physical contact.

I also of course, pointed out to Susan that she needed to avoid contact with toxic chemicals through her skin, (wear gloves lined with cotton) and to work with more ventilation. Xenoestrogens (cell changing chemicals) were clearly having a huge negative impact on Susan's hormonal wellbeing.

Susan is now aware of her chemical environment and takes appropriate measures to protect herself through the use of phytoestrogens and regular liver cleansing, essential fatty acids, Magnesium and, of course, on-going use of progesterone in small doses of 16-20mg 2 weeks on out of 4 weeks as a maintenance dose as Susan does not suffer any other symptoms.

Regardless of the nature, ALL lumps must be investigated. And make sure you conduct regular self-breast examinations. Progesterone will not resolve calcified breast lumps (benign) as some women have discovered. But overall their breast tissue has softened and pain eliminated.

Women often ask me **what's an ideal way to determine their progesterone dosage** and here's my answer. *Breasts are a fantastic barometer to guide you with your hormonal balancing. In fact, many women use their breasts to assess their progesterone dosage.*

If women are using too much progesterone after they have had a period of balance, they may experience itching, tingling, or soreness of the nipples, breast engorgement, a feeling of fullness, a dull ache, or general breast tenderness may be the first indication to reduce dosage. If symptoms are relieved upon reduction of dosage after 2 days, then you know you're on the right track. Don't confuse these symptoms and reduce progesterone if your period is due.

On the flip side, if reducing dosage doesn't help or perhaps increases discomfort, then it indicates the need to increase your progesterone dosage, and pay particular attention to increasing your intake of phytoestrogens to oppose estrogen dominance and the re-emerging symptoms. (If you do not take omegas 3,6,9 I suggest you do).

This situation of estrogen dominance often follows an episode of stress which would account for the shortage of progesterone and the increase of estrogen levels. Drop progesterone back to your previous dose once balance has been achieved and breast symptoms have subsided.

Hint: For quick assessment whether to increase or decrease dosage, apply progesterone cream directly to the breasts to achieve rapid results.

Clearly, your breasts are extremely responsive to hormone fluctuations, some more than others. If you're one of these women, allow your breast messages to help you fine-tune your hormones. Learn to listen to your body.

Protection: Because your breast tissue is so receptive to progesterone, I recommend (for breast protection) you apply cream directly to the breasts 2-3 times a week (not during your break from cream). Unlike fatty areas of the body, for example the tummy and buttocks, breast tissue is extremely vascular (not fatty) and, therefore, progesterone absorbs very quickly into the blood stream and surrounding tissue.

While on the subject of breasts, refer to The Late Dr. John Lee's book, 'What Your Doctor May Not Tell You About Breast Cancer'.

Osteoporosis

I have been diagnosed with Osteoporosis. What does that mean?

Osteoporosis presents itself very subtly in the body and its changes can be marked by dry skin, brittle finger nails, sometimes receding gums and lower back pain. Of course there can be other things like spontaneous fractures or easily occurring fractures, shrinkage in height and, for older women, the appearance of a "dowager's hump".

Osteoporosis means brittle or porous bone. Osteoporosis is NOT a disease of calcium deficiency. It is a disease where old bone absorption exceeds new bone formation. And there are many factors that can help us to moderate this disease. Exercise, vitamins such as vitamin C and D, anti-oxidants help, as do healthy levels of progesterone (for women) and testosterone (for men and women) to promote new bone formation.

Contrary to popular belief, magnesium rather than calcium is a much bigger player and far more important in maintaining bone integrity. It's a fact, Osteoporosis occurs in people who eat plenty of calcium just as well as in people who don't eat much at all. To meet your daily requirement of calcium is quite easy. You only need the equivalent of about 600mg a day, which is a cup of spinach and two tablespoons of cottage cheese. You can look up other calcium rich foods which are listed in the section titled 'Sources of Calcium'. Book 2 covers specific formulations designed for assisting in Osteoporosis found in the nutritional section.

The Late Dr. Lee gives a perfect analogy of the two phases involved in keeping our bones strong. He suggests we think of the two players in bone integrity as 'pacmen'. One type of 'pacman'' is the osteoclasts that move to various parts of your bone to find old bone and dissolve it away (bone resorption).

Once this is completed, the 'pacmen' called osteoblasts move on it to start building new bone (new bone formation). Then your body goes into a resting phase where your bones remain good for a certain length of time before they get old and crystallise and our pacmen get back to work.

Osteoporosis is often referred to as a disease of estrogen deficiency, and is usually medicalised as a disease occurring at menopause. The fact that a female's bone loss starts in her mid thirties when estrogen levels are high indicates that estrogen does not totally prevent bone loss. Estrogen will slow the rate of bone loss by slightly poisoning the 'osteoclasts' thereby slowing down resorption, but it DOES NOT reverse it. What does appear to correlate here is progesterone levels.

When a woman reaches her mid thirties she may fail to ovulate every period leading to a decline in progesterone production. It's interesting that Osteoporosis begins to set in around the time a woman begins to experience a deficiency in progesterone. Further still, Osteoporosis appears to respond favourably when progesterone levels are brought back into balance.

Osteoporosis is presented by the media as a health risk associated with hormonal and/or dietary imbalance that needs medical intervention or correction, depending on who's endorsing the research and/or advertising. Women are understandably driven by fear, fuelled by drug companies and in many cases the dairy industry, in the absence of publicity on the success of reversing, improving or restoring bone re-growth naturally without the use of bone builders (specialised patented drugs), calcium supplements, dairy products, and HRT.

*Natural hormone replacement to promote bone building has **not** been embraced by the medical fraternity. Nor are there any trials at this time to support this approach.* There is, however, very strong evidence of trials using testosterone for bone building, proving there are indeed testosterone receptors on osteoblasts (bone builders). Evidence suggests this is also the case for progesterone receptors, we're just lacking trials.

So many women think that once they have been diagnosed with Osteoporosis it is like a cancer, that there is nothing they can do about it and it is going to lead to further deterioration and visualise premature old age - shrinking height, fractured hips, immobility and retarded lifestyle - relax please.

I have seen women more upset with a diagnosis of Osteoporosis than when told they have breast lumps and possible cancer, and may need aspiration and even mastectomies. Clearly, they panic, perhaps because they are not expecting a diagnosis of Osteoporosis at such an early age.

As stated, there is little positive emphasis put on what we can do to improve and even prevent Osteoporosis. *The good news is if you have porous bone, you have a unique opportunity to fill your bone with new, stronger bone. After all, our bones are living cells that are, like other cells in our body, constantly breaking down and rebuilding.*

Point: The Late Dr. Lee, who had tracked his patients with Osteoporosis over 15 years made the following statement: **"If you add estrogen replacement therapy, you will avoid further loss and pick up about 1-2%** but that's it. If you get yourself onto natural progesterone therapy, you can increase bone mineral density (BMD) by about 15%." And The Late Dr. Lee had the statistics to prove it.

Factors to consider in the overall picture:

- Many younger women are now presenting with a diagnosis of Osteoporosis, possibly because of the fact that there are more women undergoing earlier bone density scanning as a result of post procedure Hysterectomy, voluntary trials etc.

- Overall, an early diagnosis of Osteoporosis means these women are getting an opportunity to do something about their deteriorating bones. In our mother's day, bone readings were not routine. It wasn't seen to be necessary until a woman actually went through menopause, broke her hip, or showed signs of spinal shrinkage (dowager's hump).

- We also have reason to believe we're not making the progesterone our grandmothers made half a century ago. This deficiency in progesterone coupled with our unhealthy diet, our sedentary lifestyle, and even over-use of some medications are leaving many of us exposed to the early onset of Osteoporosis.

- High levels of stress results in high levels of cortisol output, and this cortisol can accelerate Osteoporosis. That's why it's important to learn to manage your stress levels. This is also why cortisone-based drugs will render progesterone therapy ineffective as cortisol competes with progesterone at the same receptor sites.

- Cortisol is basically an anti-progesterone. I mentioned the action of cortisol here in relation to bone building. But I do mention stress levels throughout our book in relation to other situations, and how it interferes with the work of progesterone in the body. Further, taking the drug Cortisone in the treatment of other conditions is likewise mentioned in relation to progesterone.

- If you have started to show bone degeneration, it can be reversed. It CAN be corrected and it can be improved. But I emphasise that it will not improve and reverse by ignoring the situation or using progesterone alone.

- Osteoporosis is multi factorial but it can often be assisted with physiological doses (15-20mg) of progesterone and, in some cases a little dab of natural estrogen and/or natural testosterone for the women who are deficient in these types of hormones. Testosterone information is in Book 2.

- This is where a hormone profile is vital to assess your levels. Request that your doctor, in this case, examines all your hormone levels including progesterone and testosterone which he is not normally inclined to do.

- Just as importantly, weight bearing exercise, diet, vitamins and minerals, lifestyle and stress control certainly play the equally important part as does natural progesterone therapy in treating Osteoporosis.

- Far too many women are embracing natural progesterone for bone building wrongly thinking it's the total solution, without a commitment to long-term lifestyle changes. Be realistic here. Progesterone, while a very important component of the jigsaw, by itself cannot possibly maximise the full benefits without incorporating an holistic approach to Osteoporosis.

Risk Factors of Osteoporosis
Hormonal Imbalance

Progesterone deficiency and estrogen dominance contribute to bone degeneration. It is believed by some that Osteoporosis results because of a lack of progesterone in our body to build new bone once old bone has been reabsorbed.

Body Type/Build

Thin, finer and smaller boned people have a greater risk as they have less bone density and less weight bearing to strength bone. Whereas heavy people unknowingly provide weight bearing to their bones.

Thyroid body types (classified by Dr Cabot) are prone to Osteoporosis.

Antacids

Antacids decrease calcium absorption as they decrease the acidity of the hydrochloric acid factor (found in the stomach, necessary for food break-down). That means that the hydrochloric acid cannot transport calcium to the bone. Decreased acidity increases calcium excretion.

Stress

On the other hand high levels of stress create a blood imbalance. The high level of acidity comes from the outpouring of cortisol and adrenalin from the adrenal glands. Calcium is required to neutralise the acidosis.

Irritable Bowel Syndrome/Diarrhoea/Similar gastro intestinal disorders can also inhibit or interfere with the absorption of calcium and stress often sets off these bowel disorders.

Diets too high in fibre

Vegans need to be careful and ensure they are assimilated correctly with sufficient calcium and Vitamin D in their diet.

Tea and coffee consumption (including caffeine based drinks and health bars containing caffeine!)

Tea and coffee have a diuretic effect so, again, that takes out essential minerals and nutrients like calcium and magnesium, contributing to increasing osteoporotic risk factors. I have heard Oprah say on one of her wonderful shows 'so I am weeing my bones down the toilet'. It certainly made me address the consumption of my coffee!

Family history, diet and lifestyle

People who have very high meat intake which creates acidosis which requires calcium to neutralise the pH levels (high acid levels in the blood); people who drink a lot of Coke (colas), bubbly drinks; smoke. All these things cause the body to draw on more calcium. Excess sugars and refined carbohydrates also can interfere with the blood glucose level and the pH balances. Certain medications and treatments: chemotherapy.

Cortisone

Cortisone increases the risk factor of Osteoporosis because it shuts down and blocks off the receptors and therefore the bone building aspects. Substances abuse and long term drug use can similarly exert a negative influence on bone building.

Chronic stress may cause high cortisol levels in the body that also interfere with bone building.

Read 'What happens when the body experiences stress' on page 295.

Other contributing factors and familial disposition

Tubal ligation, early Hysterectomy, removal of ovaries, Ovarian Dysfunction (Cysts, disease or other), the body's reaction to episodes of stress.

Long term illnesses or disease i.e. IBS (Irritable Bowel Syndrome)

What is a Bone Mineral Density test (BMD)?

A Bone Mineral Density (BMD) test measures the mineral density in the bone by bouncing a dual photon beam of light off the bone, measuring the difference in the density between bone and soft tissue. This shows how porous the bones have become and at what risk you are of having a fracture or degree of Osteoporosis.

Many woman have started to lose bone after age 30 as they are having anovulatory periods and not producing progesterone. This is already detrimental to bone. It is a good idea to have a bone density test quite young, maybe 35, to have a base level to compare with later on and if you are in a high risk factor and a young age you can take steps now.

Should I take progesterone if my bone mineral density test shows signs of Osteoporosis but I'm not showing signs of estrogen dominance?

If you are showing a tendency towards Osteoporosis, then at least you have the ability to take some measures towards correcting this early onset of Osteoporosis that can be correlated with hormone imbalance without symptoms, especially if it is influenced by a history of early menopause, tubal ligation, poor diet, or *use of steroids* or other promoting factors.

Even if you may not show signs of estrogen dominance or progesterone deficiency, the usage of a minimal amount of supplementation of progesterone, correction of diet and lifestyle could make all the difference in rebuilding bone and preventing further deterioration and, consequently, severe osteoporotic problems later on in life.

I've got a good bone mineral density. Should I take progesterone?

If you've got really good bones, taking progesterone isn't going to make better bones. Progesterone seems to be more effective for women who have Osteoporosis mild to moderate, according to The Late Dr. John Lee's work over a fifteen to twenty year period with his patients in his practice.

If you are taking progesterone to prevent Osteoporosis, that is a fifty million dollar question that no one can answer at this point in time. Many women take progesterone for other factors and also it is peace of mind. It won't hurt you but certainly won't add extra bone on to bone if you have good bones.

My doctor wants me to take Fosamax but I don't want to. I want to improve my bones naturally. What is the best plan of attack?

At NPAN I suggest to women to do their homework and research the drugs that have been suggested to them so that they can make an informed decision based on that information. Ask your Chemist for a print out on the drug indication and side effects.

There are a lot of other alternatives and options to rebuilding bone and they say that Osteoporosis doesn't happen at menopause, it happens well and truly before the menopausal years and it is more reflective on the formative years, lifestyle, diet and hormonal and mineral imbalances and healthy history that may have occurred earlier on.

We know that at menopause bone loss is accelerated for a few years because of the estrogen drop which means that acceleration and resorption of bone occurs. After a few years this will plateau out again, things settle, and bone loss may not exceed bone building.

If correctional measures have been adopted, this, in time, with additional support factors, will stop the acceleration and maybe prevent further bone loss. I strongly suggest you read The Late Dr. John Lee's books 'What Your Doctor May Not Tell You About Menopause', Chapter 12, and 'What Your Doctor May Not Tell You About Premenopause', p.197, if you want to look at the options of using progesterone for Osteoporosis, and also to research the bone building drugs, their use and contra-indications. Again, it's up to the person and their own individual choices.

Be aware that bone building drugs can be very harsh on the gastrointestinal tract, so if you have any sensitivity or problems that may **aggravate** your situation, I suggest you think twice about using such drugs without proper research.

I have been on progesterone now for almost 8 years and my bone mineral density has not improved after two separate readings. In fact, I lost 3% in my first 18 months post surgically induced menopause. I am due for my next BMD soon.

I have moderate Osteoporosis and I am resisting my doctor's pressure to put me on the latest designer bone builders for which I qualify (under the current PBS rebate system). I believe it's a time factor, rebuilding new bone will take a committed program incorporating progesterone, some testosterone, phytoestrogens, a premium bone, joint & cartilage formulation, additional magnesium, correct eating, attention to liver detox, stress management, and weight-bearing exercise, for me in the form of gardening.

See 'Suggested Bone Formulation', and nutritional chapter in Book 2. .

I've been on progesterone now for 2 years and my bone mineral density is worse. Help!

As mentioned before, when the estrogen drops there can be an acceleration in bone loss mass in those years. This is because bone loss exceeds bone building.

It is suggested women take 3 consecutive bone mineral density tests with the same machine for 3 years and then make a decision based on those results. Another suggestion is that they take other precautionary factors such as good diet, progesterone supplementation, and avoid the risk factors that contribute to Osteoporosis.

Why it is suggested 3 bone mineral density on the same machine is because there can be slight errors on the machine and if there is a plus or a minus either side, the third one usually shows an average result of the bone mineral density outcome. It also takes more than three years to rebuild bone.

I am are basing our information on The Late Dr. John Lee's work, who was talking fifteen to twenty years with his patients, not two or three years and the studies are only early days at this point in time.

NPAN has observed over a few years women who have reported bone building of up to 15% over 3 years, two cases reported this increase within 18 months. But this hasn't happened with everyone. Perhaps, based on this observation, progesterone works better on some women than others in building new bone. And it's up to the individual to conduct her own investigation as to why this might be. (See 'Risk Factors of Osteoporosis'). Refer to Julie's testimonial.

Other aspects that create a massive bone loss in this millennium is a diet of refined carbohydrates and sugars, fizzy drinks, high sugar, lack of exercise, lack of minerals like magnesium, MSM (organic sulphur) and selenium due to soil depletion, and so on. Interference by drugs can create bone loss, there are *certain drugs that have the ability to destroy bone mass (e.g. cortisone).* Dietary factors play a huge role here and the ability to assimilate nutrition with the introduction of liberal antibiotic use and antibiotic and toxic laced foods. It brings us to the question 'how much are we as a society interfering with our good gut flora?' (i.e. destroying it and affecting absorption capacity).

One would also question 'what is the perfect sun exposure to our Vitamin D manufacturing, are sunblocks interfering or creating further corruption?'

There are so many aspects that it would be foolish to put all your hope on progesterone as being the answer to rebuild bone, especially if damage has already been done.

I have been on progesterone for a couple of years and my bone density has not improved. Why?

If the bone density hasn't improved with a woman on progesterone one would have to ask why. Have drugs and other factors inter-played in the relationship. *Antacids* for example can interfere with re-absorption of calcium into the bone, because hydrochloric acid is required to do this.

Other drugs that can interfere with bone building are cortisone (as well as interfering with many other benefits of progesterone). I will talk about cortisone separately. You cannot use cortisone and progesterone at the same time. One negates the other. *Cortisone actually* **suppresses** *and* **negates** *all progesterone effects as it competes for the same receptor,* unless of course it is natural cortisone, (short term use) which is unavailable here in Australia.

Case History:

I would like to make mention of a case involving a lady who was prescribed cortisone, long term, in the treatment of lupus, and subsequently developed severe Osteoporosis.

When she was in remission, she ceased cortisone and resorted to Calcitriol (form of vitamin D and Calcium combined) and the principles of bone building with no remarkable outcome. However, **twelve months on progesterone in conjunction with Calcitriol and the same principles saw her with a 15% bone improvement, she was in her late 50's.**

My doctor insists that I take HRT to prevent further Osteoporosis. Is this not the same as progesterone?

No it is not. Your doctor may offer you the conventional form of HRT in the form of combinations of estrogens and progestogens, or even estrogen alone. I strongly suggest that you seek out drug information and look into this because the forms of treatment are very different.

Progestogens/Progestins are not progesterone and <u>***do not***</u> ***do the same work in bone building*** as I have already discussed. Estrogen will retard and slow down (resorption) of Osteoporosis to a certain degree but not reverse it. *Ostriol as used in Ovestin has little impact on bone influence (as does the use of phytoestrogens). It is the estrogens, estradiol and esterone that play a greater significance in the effect on bones.* But not the synthetic estrogen from my observation.

Synthetic progestogins, to my knowledge, do not build new bone. In fact, progestogins would **prevent** *any natural progesterone* (produced by the adrenals and ovaries if ovulating) *that may be circulating in the body to enter occupying bone-building receptors (osteoblasts).*

Therefore, any bone-building benefits from real progesterone would be denied to the body while you are using synthetic progestogens, both of which would be competing for the same receptor site.

Progestogens are not prescribed as a form of treatment for bone building. They are prescribed to protect a woman (with an intact uterus) against the side effects of estrogen which, incidentally, IS administered to help delay bone loss.

Progesterone has been shown to stimulate new bone formation, and is a vital link in a chain of multiple factors which together are necessary for good bone building. I suggest, if you want to have the rebuilding aspect, that you use it in a combination that includes natural progesterone, if this is what your doctor insists on some estrogen. Be very clear to him what you wish. You may also qualify for natural testosterone.

And don't be tricked into adopting those 'natural' combination patches now available because while these patches do contain 'natural' estrogen they contain 'synthetic' progestogens. This needs to be understood.

Can I take my bone building drugs such as Fosamax and Raloxifine (Evista) with progesterone?

Yes, you can. **Fosamax** will not effect progesterone benefits for other uses in the body, however, **if you are using progesterone for bone building it will be severely compromised, if not rendered ineffective for this purpose.**

There is no clear data to support other than what I have learnt from the Late Dr John Lee. But I do know from my clients, men (included). Fosamax has a detrimental effect on the gut for those prone to problems such as constipation, heart burn, history of ulcers and IBS to name a few. Elderly are prescribed once a week administration of Fosamax! Many of these elderly people are not eating 3 meals a day, suffering digestive disorder and gastric discomfort so it is prescribed with caution to prevent further gastrointestinal complications. So many daughters have bought their elderly mothers to me. These poor dear old souls with skin dried, thin skeletal problems and digestive disorders and bowel problems. Clearly the Fosamax is disagreeing with them and causing them discomfort, providing little pain coverage for their bones. With the co-operation of the Doctor offering them progesterone assists these people in gaining a good sleep and balance again. Some of these clearly are on mood altering medications such as heavy drowsy inducing medication (sleeping tablets), which in fact increases their chances of falling over thus risking higher incidences of fractures. It makes Fosamax look ridiculous in the bigger picture.

I suggest you consider why you are taking the bone building drugs in the first place and decide for yourself whether it is bone delay that you are seeking or bone building. *Because the bone building drugs are not forming new bone, they are actually stopping and delaying the resorption of old bone.* Age has to come into accountability too. There are many things you can do to build bone rather than to depend on bone building drugs or medication alone. Bone building is a holistic approach.

By taking bone building drugs these can actually block off the action of absorbing old, brittle bone, prevents progesterone moving in to build new bone in place of the old. On X-ray, bone building drugs look fantastic as the bone appears dense, but in actual fact may be quite weak and brittle because the X-ray is depicting 'old' bone that should have been removed and replaced with new.

Slowing bone resorption doesn't necessarily make your bones stronger. As explained above, there are two different actions involved in bone formation, that is taking away old bone and rebuilding new bone.

I cannot make the *decision for you* but I strongly urge you to seek out options, information, and do drug research. Ask your doctor for full disclosure of side effects, benefits, and the test trials, then look at these seriously because at the end of the day, it is your health, your decision, and your body. You might like to visit The Late Dr. John's website to learn his view on bone builders. Articles on his website on particular issues can be still ordered.

There is more evidence suggestive that dietary plant phytoestrogens perhaps have a higher role in bone protection and that dairy is not as conducive as a source of calcium intake as we have been led to believe.

What are some of the substances and factors that disrupt bone formation?

Processed food, smoking, crash dieting, anovulatory periods, salt and sugar, high fat and high protein diet, antibiotics, mineral deficiency, soft drinks, coffee, steroids, antacids, gastrointestinal problems interfering with absorption, stress, lack of exercise, kidney problems, inability to simulate or manufacture vitamin D, lack of sunlight, inadequate omega oils, essential fatty acids, lack of hydrochloric acid, excessive use of diuretics and diet tablets such as laxatives (not natural fibre) and chemical toxins.

Other bone destroyers and factors that contribute to Osteoporosis : lack of weight bearing exercises; abuse during formative years with bad diets, anorexia, bingeing, crash diets, long term use of antibiotics, steroids; unhealthy lifestyle - diet, environment, alcoholism, liver problems, family history of Osteoporosis. *Long term use of contraception - the Pill - is now one of my suspicions to add to this list.*

Will the Contraceptive Pill interfere with my bones? Can I take The Pill if I have Osteoporosis?

There is no evidence that the Pill interferes with, or contributes to Osteoporosis but we do know that the **Contraceptive Pill stops the ovaries from ovulating.** It contains a combination of estrogen and progestins which makes me believe yes.

So it stands to reason that there might be a shortage, or lack of progesterone in the body and, therefore, lack of bone building because of insufficient progesterone levels. So one would have to be cautious in using progestogens (which The Pill contains) if there is a family history of Osteoporosis, or you fall into a high risk category.

What are some of the things I can do to improve my Osteoporosis? Non symptomatic.

You can take progesterone 15 to 25mg if you are post menopause, 3 out of 4 weeks, 5 days off.

For the aged, I suggest, to avoid confusion, use 15mg of cream on a weekday, and break on the weekend where possible. **Anne's mother** who died in February 2004 enjoyed 3 fuller years on progesterone therapy.

Anne was able to have a more enriched short span to enjoy her mother's company, who in that time returned pain free period with full mental faculties and until Parkinson's Disease set in. Her mother died as a result of complications following a fall 3 months after she entered a nursing home, and being placed back on many medications that her daughter felt was unnecessary and perhaps contributed to her losing her balance and falling. Note her hip did not break it was actually a head injury. When Anne bought her gracious old mother to me, she was so miserable and all her medications were causing havoc. Riddled with Osteoporosis and pain Anne's mother eventually ended up on Magnesium and progesterone and a bone joint formulation to control pain and maintain comfort. Her constipation was eliminated and her sleep returned to normal. She brightened up and became more active and involved again. It was a remarkable transformation to witness. I adored her although her Osteoporosis and age was irreversible, this was not the focus or purpose. Anne's mother used to say 'just rub some that cream on my back dear'. It certainly had some impact in her pain management. Perhaps it helped sedate and calm her. She now resides with angels.

Perimenopausal and postmenopausal with hormonal problems, dosage is dictated according to symptoms being treated.

I also suggest:

- Regular bone density check periodically (every 1-2 years, if anxious)
- Saliva-based hormone profile to check that your testosterone, progesterone and estrogen levels are balanced. (The use of natural testosterone also assists bone building).
- Adopt a healthy lifestyle and eating habit as a way of life
- Eliminate things from your diet that are harmful and aggravational (see Risk Factors of Osteoporosis)
- Eat plenty of green vegetables, whole grains and fibre and phytoestrogen foods
- Regular weight bearing exercise
- Reduction of stress (cortisol), reduce gastro intestinal bowel problems
- Fresh air and sunlight (natural vitamin D synthesis)
- Caution with the use of **all** medications
- Take adequate amounts of magnesium (400-600mg) - supplement Calcium if you are not getting enough in your diet.
- Be consistent with your progesterone supplementation (over the years) and follow the Golden Rules
- Take a balanced bone building formulation that is designed to build, strengthen and support the bones, joints, collagen, tendons, ligaments and cartilage.

A good cross section bone building formula would include such ingredients as:

Glucosamine sulfate

Chondroitin sulfate

Calcium ascorbate

Calcium hydroxypatite

Vitamin E

Vitamin A

Vitamin D

Manganese amino acid chelate

Zinc amino acid chelate

Selenomethionine (Selenium)

Magnesium oxide

Copper gluconate

Horsetail

MSM

All these ingredients are in 'recommended formulations' by NPAN and that I personally use. I also use calcium paste sub lingual when my acid/stress levels are high. To prevent calcium being leached from my bones to neutralise my blood PH. I tend to absorb it better in this form as I have bouts of IBS.

In *the post menopausal state, calcium levels in the bone remain the same but magnesium levels drop.* There is more weight and evidence in the value of magnesium more than the value of calcium **but these must be in proportion ratio.**

Also, you need to look at the **type of calcium** you are taking as many will end up in the toilet. It needs to be a calcium in bio available form and absorbable. I talk about calcium absorption and levels required in the section on nutrition in book 2. This is why I strongly recommended that women search the marketplace for a premium formulation that will take the above ingredients into account. Certain Magnesium types have greater impact on the bones as do certain calciums. Suggested guidelines can be found in Book 2 'Natural Progesterone More Secrets Revealed'.

Additionally, other assistors include Vitamin C, sea plants and supplementation in the form of spiralina, soya based food, sunlight and vitamin D, Cod liver oil, omega 3-6 oils (essential oils), weight bearing exercises, eliminate and reduce stress, eliminate all drugs that may be causing a retardation of bone building or impede digestion.

Are there other ways of increasing my daily intake of calcium without using dairy products?

Absolutely. **Milk is not the only source of calcium.** Look to other non-dairy sources such as soy products, green juice drinks like barley grass, wheat grass, seaweed, kelp, brown rice. Calcium is derived from many sources, although the general public believe it is comes strictly from dairy intake. You'd be surprised just how many foods are calcium rich minus the saturated fats (increase cholesterol). Maybe you'd like to visit www.notmilk.com to learn more.

It is true our body needs calcium, especially in the formative years when we are laying down and building strong bones. However, with a balanced diet that includes lots of calcium-rich foods, we are NOT at risk of Osteoporosis should we say "no" to dairy products.

"Sources of Calcium"

Food	Amount	Calcium (mg)
Fish (with the bones)		
Salmon (canned)	1 cup	431
Oysters, raw	1 cup	226
Sardines (with bones)	100 gms (3.6 oz)	300
Tuna (with bones)	100 gms (3.6 oz)	290
Fish (fresh, cooked)	110 gms (3.6 oz)	35
Legumes		
Tofu	112 gms (4 oz)	80-150
Tempeh	112 gms (4 oz)	172
Chickpeas	1 cup (cooked)	150
Tortillas, corn	2	120
Black Beans	1 cup (cooked)	135
Soy milk (unfortified)	1 cup	60
Soy milk (fortified)	1 cup	300
Dairy		
Milk (cows)		
whole	1 cup	288
skim	1 cup	300
Goats milk	1 cup	295
Cheese (cheddar, Swiss)	42 gms (1.5 oz)	300
Cottage cheese	1 cup	150
Feta cheese	28 gms (1 oz)	129
Yoghurt	1 cup	294

Food	Amount	Calcium (mg)
Nuts and Seeds		
Brazil nuts	1 cup	260
Sunflower seeds (hulled)	1 cup	174
Sesame seeds (ground)	3 tablespoons	300
Almonds (hulled)	1 cup	300
Tahini (sesame paste)	1 tablespoon	85
Sea Vegetables (cooked)		
Wakame	1 cup	520
Agar-agar	1 cup	400
Kelp (kombu)	1 cup	305
Hijiki	1 cup	610
Dulse (dry)	1 cup	567
Green Vegetables (cooked)		
Parsley (raw)	1 cup	122
Bok choy	1 cup	200
Spinach	1 cup	178
Broccoli	1 cup	100
Beet greens	1 cup	165
Watercress (raw)	1 cup	53
Rhubarb	1 cup	348
Collard greens	1 cup	300
Dandelion greens	1 cup	147

Supplied & printed with permission specifically for Jenny Birdsey's use from- 'Ask Dr Sandra Cabot Newsletter, Edition 2) Dr. Sandra Cabot & Susie Clift B.Sc.Dip.Ion).

Ageing Concerns
Should my mother or my grandmother use Natural Progesterone?

A lot of women love to see their mother and grandmother on progesterone because they acknowledge there are so many other multi-factorial benefits derived from the use of progesterone. Not to mention protection from more potent estrogens in our environment and food chain.

If nothing else, it can certainly improve mental alertness, sleep patterns, and skin texture, especially with the aged who are prone to very thin skin that tears and bruises easily. Using a dose between 10-16mg daily, breaking from cream on weekends, daughters are reporting fantastic benefits after putting their mothers and grandmothers on natural progesterone cream. See Anne's story about her elderly mother on page 277.

Thrush, Cystitis, Vaginal & Bladder Concerns
I have Thrush. What does this mean? Will progesterone help this problem? I have read that progesterone actually makes it worse.

Most women get confused by the difference between progestogens such as The Contraceptive Pill and Provera, as opposed to natural progesterone. Certainly, there is strong evidence suggesting some drugs, when combined with **synthetic progestogens, have been known to cause problems with Candida/Thrush** (e.g. the pill - OCP).

Over the years with my work I have observed women on natural progesterone supplementation over a period of 12-18 months who reported a marked improvement of their problems. It certainly doesn't become progressively worse.

I have chatted with women who have been sufferers of chronic Thrush and Cystitis for years and years. They're on the anti-Candida yeast-free, sugar-free, refined foods diet and using courses of natural probiotics such as acidophilus and microdophilus all the friendly bacteria, with little effect in killing or combating this chronic problem. Anti-fungal drugs and antibiotics are hard on the liver and kidneys, and certainly can be detrimental long term, and build up resistance.

Progesterone alone will not resolve the problem of Candida, particularly if it's chronic, but it seems to be a missing link in the equation. You need to work in conjunction with a good naturopath or health professional. The most commonly known forms of successful treatment found by women are those that attempt to build integrity of the gut and immune systems through support of the liver. Improve gut elimination by eating high fibres, improving your eating habits and eliminating sugars. Avoid foods containing high bacteria, fungi, and viruses such as processed junk foods, processed meat (deli meat, hamburger meats), and incorporate natural antibiotics such as garlic, ginger root, onion, and radish.

Leaky gut is perhaps the most common contributing cause to estrogen dominance and Candida. *A sluggish bowel is an ideal environment to enhance bad flora growth and fermentation.* So unless the underlying cause is addressed progesterone will have only a band-aid affect on your health.

In conditions such as chronic Thrush, **good hormonal balance begins in the digestive tract and liver.** And if the bowel is suffering leaky bowel syndrome, the body is contaminating itself with toxic xenoestrogens and recirculating fungi yeast.

I suggest women reduce their internal toxicity by working on their liver and cleansing the blood to improve their immunity and elimination systems. This assists the body in the build up of friendly bacteria to optimise gut function creating an environment that bad and harmful bacteria cannot thrive in. *"Olive Life"* has proven in many instances to be beneficial in dealing with this problem as *it appears to have the ability to destroy antibiotic resistant bugs, address fungi and cleanse the blood.* Thus also improving an overloaded immunity system which ultimately disrupts the endocrine system and other bodily functions. (See Chapter regarding Olive Life in the Nutritional section of Book 2 Natural Progesterone More Secrets Revealed).

However, friendly bacteria can quickly become less 'friendly' in poor health and nutritional deficiencies, resulting in hormonal imbalance and estrogen dominance. It is very much linked to stress, bad eating habits and obesity, allergies, poor bowel, gut and liver function. Simply, Candida cannot thrive in a healthy environment.

Candida predisposes women to severe PMS with depression, mood swings and fluid retention. Irregular periods, Infertility and Endometriosishave also been linked to this state of imbalance. So it cannot be over-emphasise enough the importance of taking control and listening to you body. I recommend taking correctional measures in order to bring about a more balanced and healthy environment for the body to function, thus maximising the benefits of progesterone.

Candida presents a constellation of symptoms similar to those associated with liver dysfunction, bowel disorders, and estrogen dominance. And all are inter-related, often masked and undetected due to their similarities. That's why it's important to approach treatment on a number of levels - hormone balancing, detoxification, building gut integrity and immunity. Sufferers of Chronic Fatigue Syndrome (CFS) often fall into this category.

Progesterone dosage is in accordance to estrogen dominance symptoms, the average dose being 32mg from day 12-26; menopausal 3 weeks on, 1 week off. If there is severe estrogen dominance due to weight problems and diet, a *strict estrogen dominance reduction program must be adhered to,* otherwise progesterone will have minimal benefits on Candida. ***Candida appears to thrive in an estrogen dominant environment, promoted by a sugar and high carbohydrate diet.*** A diet low in fibre also contributes to this problem. Improving these factors will improve the assimilation of progesterone in dealing with this problem.

You may wish to visit website www.health-truth.com and section covering Bladder Problems, Stress, Incontinence and Hysterectomy.

Skin & Hair

Will progesterone make my hair fall out? I was on the Pill once and this is what happened to me.

Be aware, the body does not react to synthetic progestogens contained in the Contraceptive Pill in quite the same way it reacts to natural progesterone. The alterations to the molecule to render it a synthetic progestogen means The Pill has the potential to cause undesirable side effects in the body.

Loss of scalp hair is one such side effect when a progestogen is combined with estrogen. However, the molecule used in the manufacture of natural progesterone cream has not been tampered with, giving it a significant safety margin.

Low progesterone levels, month after month, can trigger hair loss. This can be halted by bringing the body's progesterone levels back to normal. New growth occurs, in most cases, within approx. 6-12 months, hair will have stopped falling out in 90% of women within a 3 month period on progesterone. Women reported improvement of hair thickness and texture whilst on progesterone over a 12 month period.

Nails

Falling into this category also, certainly not mine, I haven't derived benefit from progesterone with my nails but nearly every other woman I see has. Often complaining that they have to cut them back because they grow too fast. This is a demonstration of how progesterone is so individualised and not every person will obtain the same benefits reported by many people.

Will my varicose veins worsen or my broken blood vessels on my face get worse with the use of progesterone?

Reports from women suggest the opposite. Women who reported a reddening of the face later described as fine, broken capillaries were able to restore or halt progression with the use of progesterone.

Progesterone, when continually applied to the affected area, has been reported to relieve aching, throbbing varicose veins. It seems to restore tone and vascularity at that particular section in the body and helps normalise blood clotting, reduces swelling, and tenderness.

It's phenomenal just how many women report exceptional (pain management) results when progesterone cream is applied directly onto the area causing pain (in a variety of situations).

Broken Face Capillaries :

Until I revisited the update of this section I had forgotten myself that I had started to experience broken vein capillaries on my face which I had noticed whilst travelling to the U.S.A 15 years ago. I looked in the plane mirror under the fluoro light only to discover broken face capillaries which were exacerbated by dehydration on flying these progressed there after and were a concern for me at the age of 30. I had never worn a foundation but was considering using one to conceal this problem. A beautician told me they were irreversible and that I would have to take extra care with my skin. Interestingly since commencing progesterone these broken capillaries are no longer evident and I still don't use a foundation nor a sun screen. I have only used as a moisturizer being an aqueous cream with Vitamin E and Olive Oil (cold compressed) which my husband makes for me. As a child I have always suffered dermatological problems (skin) and suffered many bizarre face reactions and allergies. Especially around certain trees in springtime. My father being a Dermatologist never advocated the use of antibiotics or cortisone but insisted on water sealing it with a moisturizer to protect my skin from further exposure and dehydration. I am convinced without a doubt the use of bio identical hormones all these years has retarded skin aging progression, enhanced my skin, improved its elasticity and texture.

Women constantly report the improvement of their skin on their face and body when using progesterone and the disappearance of many odd markings (even skin tags).

Usage of Progesterone for Skin Care: (as a moisturiser for cosmetic usage)

Providing you do not have Chloasma, or a history of it in pregnancy. Chloasma is often referred to as the 'butterfly pregnancy mask' which is a dark and blotchy brown facial pigmentation which appears with women when they become pregnant or severe acne with open sores, then I suggest you can apply progesterone to the face once a week sparingly i.e. physiological dose.

I had a situation where a lady with Chloasma (who wasn't pregnant) actually experienced a flare up and the existing pigmentation darkened after administering generous amounts of progesterone to her face on a regular basis. This lady failed to understand that her cream should not be used so liberally. I pointed out that progesterone cream is not a moisturiser as such, but rather a steroid to be respected. If you have experience any such conditions please err on the side of caution if using progesterone as a face moisturiser or for its cosmetic properties. It is at this point I would also like to point out that whilst progesterone is a wonderful hydrator and fantastic skin restorer it should not be used liberally on the face, once a week is what I would recommend if you are apply progesterone as a intensive hydrating facial (adding natural Vitamin E in this treatment will also be of great benefit). The exception to this if you are suffering from specific ailments that are covered in the book where it is suggested to apply otherwise. E.g. sparingly on a regular basis for example skin tags and dry gritty eyes to address specific problems.

NOTE: It is not wise to use a steroid cream such as natural progesterone and expose your face, once its applied, to the sun. Therefore it is recommended that

you apply this facial treatment at night on a clean skin before retiring (once a week only). For maximum benefit.

Summary

Progesterone appears to aid repair and hydration, and is a fantastic anti-ageing, revitalising cosmetic secret. Even sensitive skin seems to tolerate progesterone cream when applied as a moisturiser. The skin will derive rehydration benefits, even if cream is not applied to the specific area.

Reports from women support that progesterone helps reduce blotching, dry spots, and wart-like lesions on their face, and improves elasticity and absorbability. Women report that their foundation / makeup goes on smoother, skin glows.

It has also been observed that acne rosacea has improved and disappeared with the use of progesterone over many months however it can become worse before it gets better.

Progesterone has been reported to help strengthen skin texture, and skin is less inclined to bruise and tear (especially in elderly).

Arthritic swelling, oedema/edema and inflammation in the targeted tissue area of these women responded favourably, perhaps because progesterone helped relieve fluid retention which, in turn, improves circulation.

About Acne Rosacea:

What is Acne Rosacea - it is a chronic skin condition affecting the face consisting of redness often accompanied by red lumps, pustules and dilated capillaries which causes a flushing of the skin. Areas most often affected are over the nose and cheeks. This condition from what I have come across appears to worsen with hormonal imbalance in peri menopausal and menopausal women. Progesterone has been of great benefit and combined with liver work. MSM and Selenium, frequently clears within a 12 month period. Women are ecstatic after suffering years of this affliction.

Dry Gritty Eyes:

You may dab minute amounts of progesterone under eyes nightly until this problem is corrected. (Usually only a couple of months).

Weight Issues
Will progesterone put on weight? I have been on other forms of hormone replacement therapy in the past and have experienced weight gain.

Progesterone will not cause you to put on weight. In fact, it will do the opposite. One of progesterone's jobs is to **convert fat into energy.** However, it may initially exacerbate estrogen dominance symptoms such as fluid retention which can have the appearance of weight increase which is usually only temporary. Natural progesterone eventually opposes the sodium influence exerted due to estrogen dominance. Progesterone inhibits this process in time assisting in controlling blood fluid balances and preventing intracellular oedema within the cells.

Progestogens, on the other hand, which are used in HRT usually do put on weight that, many women find it very difficult to shift. This may be due to incorrect dosage or combination HRT (estrogen) for the individual's body type, or because HRT overloads the liver. *Also one of estrogens jobs is to convert this hormone into fat (as seen at puberty and menopause where women put on weight in their thighs, hips and stomach).* One of estrogens messages and functions to the body is to divide and proliferate thus at puberty the changes to appearance and body shape and development of breasts. Another message of estrogen is to convert this hormone into fat as seen at nearing menopause. *This increased weight gain at menopause is mother nature's way of compensating for the changes to come when the ovaries cease to produce high levels of estrogen.*

Also being a natural diuretic, progesterone assists weight loss by regulating sodium imbalance within the body, correcting fluid retention and thereby assisting the elimination of excess fluid from the body. Using natural progesterone is not a means to lose weight. Weight loss will only come about as a result of balance of all the hormones and correct metabolism. *Initial weight loss when commencing progesterone is usually due to the diuretic effect* (I lost 1/2 a stone initially, but this was only fluid).

Some women actually stop using their progesterone cream after they gain a little weight thinking, incorrectly, that it was the progesterone creating the weight gain. They failed to understand the other factors that contribute to weight gain once progesterone is introduced.

Dr Sandra Cabot recognises four (4) different body types, all with their own unique hormonal and metabolic characteristics.

So how do these body types relate to progesterone and weight?

Understanding these body shapes will explain why you are over weight and have difficulty losing it. And you will also learn why *some hormones will actually aggravate your weight problem or assist.*

One thing I have come to understand in my work with hormonal balancing is that progesterone is the common denominator to all four body types, and where hormone imbalance exists can play a vital part in assisting with weight loss and balance. This is particularly relevant to the Android and the Gynaeoid body shapes.

Android women have an anabolic (builds muscle) metabolism which leads to a body building tendency, so strength, both physical and mental, are prominent characteristics. They tend to produce more male hormones than do other body types, which add to the muscle building tendency and often male-like features. Weight gain occurs in the upper part of the body and on the front of the abdomen so that an apple-shape may develop. Progesterone and phytoestrogens are important in 'feminising' this body shape and rebalancing the huge testosterone dominance ratio imbalance. They can still be estrogen dominant even with high levels of testosterone.

The Gynaeoid body type tends to have a predominance of the female hormone estrogen which targets the uterine region, the hips, thighs and breast. An excess of estrogen results in estrogen dominance. Excess estrogen promotes fat deposition in the lower body around the hips, thighs, buttocks, with cellulite. Progesterone opposes estrogen dominance and assists in the treatment of symptoms.

Book 2 Natural Progesterone More Secrets Revealed extensively covers body types, their hormonal compatabilities or incompatabilities, weight issues and hormonal and metabolic constitutions of each body type.

Understanding your body type and its specific hormonal and metabolic constitution is one of the greatest keys in successfully mastering hormonal balance and knowing your personal unique needs. Getting your hormones stabilised assists correct metabolism and weight loss becomes a reality - one without struggle, desperation, starvation calorie counting or fad diets. Sounds too easy doesn't it! I've proved it with myself as have many others and believe me I'm not into deprivation and self discipline (I'm human). When I had my Hysterectomy I accepted weight shape change as what I believed was part of the deal. I used to refer to myself as the 'spayed look' like female dogs who undergo sterilisation. It was another gripe and regret on my endless list of post Hysterectomy complications and non satisfactory results. Weight gradually kept creeping on and my petite size 8 figure became unrecogisable. When Dr Cabot sought me out and approached me to adopt her weight loss program incorporation with my work, flying down personally in her jet, I told her I wasn't interested.as 'I'd never seen a program that worked long term and my experience of women who had done all the yo yo diets and weight loss programs were deluded and miserable. I did not want to be placed in a situation whereby women were coming back dissatisfied and feel responsible for their misery. Sandra persisted and how grateful I am that she did, as are many other women who have now reaped this knowledge. Since that time I have combined my 2 hour consultancy which incorporates weight control, their body type to fine tune their hormones. Sandra relentlessly went on to give me a crash course inspite of my scepticism, resistance, explaining where the missing jigsaw puzzles fitted. The pennies were dropping at last after 5 years I was getting the answers I was seeking on the million and one dollar question. Why women were failing to lose weight on progesterone and in many instances gaining? Thus taking themselves off progesterone blaming the hormone.

I had always known the liver and phytoestrogens were some of the keys to balance and had adopted these principles very early in progesterone usage and having stumbled in the search for the best phytoestrogen formula started in 98 using Femme Phase and Liva Tone Plus, Health Directions products designed by Dr Cabot. As I stated to Sandra when she questioned my high usage that it was because they worked not because of who she was. I even went on to tell her I had never even read her books prior to our first meeting. Following that encounter I expressed to her my need to always be an independent operator, not a Dr Cabot puppet, and my passion lay in progesterone advocacy not weight loss. She respected my stance with admiration. We have always been independent operators respecting each others work, honesty and humour.

The Thyroid, Android, Lymphatic and Gynaeoid body type share one thing in common in the use of progesterone. All four body types can successfully take progesterone in assisting hormonal imbalance particularly if this is one of the factors interfering with weight loss or inability to shift weight from various areas.

However the **Gynaeoid body type** (lower body weight storage, pear shape). *Should be very wary about taking estrogen as she is already an estrogen dominant.*

The Android body type (upper body weight storage - apple shape) should be very *wary about the usage of testosterone as this is already her predominant hormonal constitution especially if already overweight.* It could compound her problem. I suggest to these women if they require testosterone for libido only after progesterone is not addressing this problem and given 4 months to assessment, use testosterone with minimal doses with caution.

If she has had a Hysterectomy chances are she will still need testosterone but will resonate on smaller amounts that the lymphatic, gynaeoid and thyroid type.

The Lymphatic body type has a problem with sluggish metabolism. So testosterone needs to be used with caution. If seeking weight loss as *testosterone can be sodium retentive and the last thing this poor lady needs is extra fluid, thereby adding to her sluggish metabolism.* On the positive, testosterone assist energy and can often get her up and running. It is balance.

Summary of factors that need to be taken into consideration with weight gain:

- Your metabolism (which is controlled by the liver, thyroid gland and adrenal glands)
- Incorrect eating (which adversely affects your liver function, immune system, right levels of insulin and hormones)
- Behaviour patterns and eating habits
- Your body type and hormonal constitution
- Dysfunctional or fatty liver - you might also like to read the section on 'Why is the liver so important in hormone balancing?', liver principles and liver detoxification in Book 2 Natural Progesterone More Secrets Revealed.
- Stress and excessive amounts of cortisol (hormone made in adrenal glands).

Excessive levels of cortisol produced by prolonged stress levels can cause fluid retention weight gain (neck and trunk moon shaped face).

Please read question 'Why does stress upset my hormones and weight issues' (page 295) and visit www.weightcontrol.com .There is a questionnaire on this web site to help you determine your body type. If you are unsure there is email online support available at this web site address.

My association with Dr Sandra Cabot and WHAS (Womens Health Advisory Service)

Many people ask me what my connection is with Dr Sandra Cabot and the most common questions asked are:

Do I get paid by her/commission?

Am I part of the WHAS organisation?

Is Dr Sandra Cabot American?

Does she live in Australia?

How old is she?

Is she married?

Has she got children?

I do not get paid by Dr Sandra Cabot. A small percentage of my organisation's income comes from the sale of products that so happen to be Sandra Cabot's simply because I am truly impressed with them. I have witnessed fantastic results using them in women's regimes.

Dr Cabot and myself are two very different women, operators and organisations.

What we share in common is our passion and quest for a common goal to inform, educate and help women. Our incorporated work in women's health and books compliment each other. Sandra has over the years been a great mentor and support infrastructure to myself. She has encouraged and offered to me so much moral and personal support and advise in my times of troubles and doubts. (Thus being the strength beneath my wings, spurring me on, to continue running NPAN when I felt some despair). She has given me inspiration sharing some of her own personal and financial battles with me. She has become a fantastic sound board, colleague, teacher and friend (her humour never fails to amuse me and she is a walking encyclopedia). What you see with this amazing women is what you get. A down to earth kind woman who knows, accepts and likes herself. She has thousands of followers and is a household name. She is famous for the top selling book 'The Liver Cleansing Diet'. She has been publicly crucified by media Doctors alike and still rises above it and holds her own. The unsung heroine , a pilot with her own uniqueness and a beautiful and caring human being who is not frightened of herself, her views and beliefs or to share her wealth of knowledge (or her wealth) with anyone. She is very often wrongly judged and unfairly criticised. She is not American she is Australian and trained for her medical degree in Adelaide. She is a Doctor with enormous experience who specialises in nutrition. Her age and private life obviously are not for me to comment on.

After that day in my lounge room, I decided I had nothing to lose (except weight) and everything to gain from this woman who flew herself down to meet me. So I followed the Liver Cleansing principles, increased my protein, stopped carbohydrates, gave up dairy reluctantly - it took me 5 months to knock off the milk in my morning cup of tea which led to the final step in my reduction in bust size returning to my perfect cup size bra, I now had the perfect figure and I was back to size 8 (not size 10-12 and still 3 years on remain so) and wearing designer outfits and evening wear (20 years on from my hospitality reception centre when I was aged 22-30 years when I'd collected a lot of evening wear) that I was too stingy to throw out. I have since been a true size 8 and have remained that for 3 years. My figure has returned to when I was in my early 30's (others may disagree!!!) I live a non deprived (maybe a little hectic, stressful and sleep deprived) life. I love my food, good wines and have an addictive nature. I am 4'10", an Android body type and did have the beginning of Syndrome X.

So do yourself a favour and read Sandra's books and visit her website to gain a wealth of knowledge from her 30 odd years in medicine as a Doctor and nutritional expert. She has currently updated "Hormones Don't Let Them Ruin Your Life!"

How do I know what nutritional supplementation, diet plan or eating plan I should follow when I am on progesterone?

This is a very good point that is often raised by so many women who approach me at NPAN with questions on calorie control diets, blood type diet, nutritional supplementations and herbs. Perhaps they have sought herbalist or naturopathic advice, which may often create confusion on what is best to use or which diet to follow.

Throughout my books I repeatedly mention nutritional supplementation, vitamin regime, diet plan, exercise and lifestyle. All are very important if you *want to maximise the benefits and the outcome of progesterone therapy, and to derive optimum hormonal balance* and vitality.

From my experience with our group meetings, and in the earlier days when we were all having a variety of problems with our locally compounded creams, the women went on a crusade in search of things that could perhaps help us.

We all had our own naturopaths, herbalists and other alternative therapies, so we brought back to our group meetings in my lounge room, an infinite wealth of knowledge on products. Some women would be taking mixed phytoestrogens, some would be taking wild yam supplements, others specific herbs, or vitamins and/or minerals, and some were simply taking progesterone. In other words we experimented on ourselves.

This broadened our knowledge while giving us a unique insight into the role products play in conjunction with progesterone cream. It was like uncontrolled studies conducted by ourselves.

Some enhanced progesterone cream action within the body, others impeded performance. What we found in common through all the various sources of information, and trial and error, was that certain products and lifestyle changes resonated with the women using progesterone cream.

We went in search of the best phytoestrogen in the marketplace. We wanted value for money on minerals and vitamins. We followed all sorts of professional advice from our naturopaths, iridologists or doctors, or books that we'd read, or Internet research. I came up with what I believe are sound guidelines. Which I expanded on and fine tuned them and have been working with certain products and principles since those days all these years, which I share and elaborate in Book 2 Natural Progesterone More Secrets Revealed in the Nutritional section. As women have been insistent over the years asking me exactly what I use and why, I have listed my favourite and most popular used products by myself and so many other woman. It also offers guidelines for comparatives so you can choose other similar products and formulations of your choices. I have also included formulas and principles in hormonal balancing in conjunction with nutrition.

When Jessie Hanley and Virginia Hopkins' revised new book came to Australia in conjunction with The Late Dr. Lee's book, "What Your Doctor May Not Tell You About Premenopause", we were somewhat let down because we were looking for new revelations beyond what we'd already discovered. However, we were very proud of ourselves as a group of women (intelligent, resourceful women that we are), that we'd worked it out for ourselves and were on the right track.

This is not to imply we did not appreciate or learn something new from this publication. It simply affirmed that women have an innate intuition that they ought to follow more often. I suggest you to get a copy of this brilliant book to expand your knowledge.

So, in answering the question, "How do I know what is best and what to use" in amidst all these different opinions and ideas, and people peddling particular products, say "Value for Money". It must be a formulation that resonates with your body. Given nutrition is expensive, shop around but rule of thumb is usually you pay for what you get. Learn to read ingredients, compare dosage strengths, (the level at which they work efficiently) and recognise natural products versus unnatural. e.g. Vitamin E is natural and not synthetic another example if you are using probiotics (good gut flora) make sure (in my opinion) they are live enzymes which should be stored in the fridge, the Vitamin C is natural/ascorbic and CoEnzyme Q10 studies show most effective levels are at 100mg and less than this may not be providing you with optimal benefits. Also if it is in a phosphate base it will be far more effective. This is extensively explained in Book 2 Natural Progesterone More Secrets Revealed in the Nutrition section.

If you're using a phytoestrogen, don't just rely on soy or believe absolutely all the marketing hype. Use one that offers multiple phytoestrogens incorporating vitamins and minerals where possible, for there are some wonderful, varied phytoestrogenic herbal formulations for women. Specifically, formulas that offer a cross section of multiple vitamins and herbs designed for women's concerns.

I compare formulations that are available in the marketplace, regularly with an open mind. I also check whether they are filled with packers, glucose or gluten-free, contain preservatives or any harmful derivatives. Refer to section on 'Supplement with a PREMIUM phytoestrogen formulation', (Femme Phase) as a guide.

So what I suggest to women is to do your homework. Check your comparative lists, research it and see what is best value for money. You might find cheap products such as cheap forms of vitamin E, but they might be synthetic. You might find cheap forms of magnesium but there might be only one component of magnesium. Speaking of magnesium, I have discovered from observation that certain types of magnesium operate quite differently depending on the combination. I recommend a 'complete' magnesium because it is exceptionally absorbable and the results are quite phenomenal.

An ideal synergistic magnesium combination that I use in my regime with hundreds of other women now contains 4 magnesium compounds being: Magnesium orotate, Magnesium aspartate, Magnesium amino acid chelate and Magnesium phosphate. This product is Magnesium Complete a Dr Sandra Cabot formulation. The women have proven its popularity.

If something is not working for you, try something else. Your body may respond much better. You might be on the right track ... just on the wrong product. Horses for courses. Also you body may become resistant or complacent to certain products so often it is wise to change and try other things.

Reducing estrogen is not about crash diets; that will send you absolutely ballistic and, besides, it's not intelligent or very wise to risk further chemical imbalance that might result in increased appetite, depression or mood swings.

Instead, increase your essential fatty acids omega 3-6 oils such as evening primrose, lecithin, flaxseed/linseed which are the building blocks for hormones and cells. Reduce or cut out fats completely. (Oil you body don't grease it). *Eliminate dairy products because they have the potential to be hormone disrupters.* Take calcium in supplementation form or eat foods rich in calcium such as seaweed, nuts, etc. (See sources of calcium rich foods). Cut out bad yeast's and avoid or reduce drastically the consumption of sugar and refined carbohydrates (especially highly refined and bleached white flour products), particularly women who have leaky gut and suffer Candida. Combine these modifications with progesterone supplementation and you're going to see an incredible result!

Guidelines in reducing weight and assisting hormone balance using, complimenting and supporting products are strategies I address in Book 2 Natural Progesterone More Secrets Revealed.

Women have been insistent over the years in asking me exactly what I use and this is why I have listed my favourite and popular products used by myself and so many women. It also offers guidelines and comparatives so you can chose other similar products and formulations.

Too many women come to me distraught, dismayed, disillusioned because they've been on these special diets, special herbs, special this and that, always without seeing results. It's because they haven't combined it properly, or there's a missing link. That link tends to be in the way it's formulated, the way it's pieced together.

What you've done in the past may not be wrong. In fact, it's probably been very beneficial to you. It's quite possible you would have been worse without it, but try it again this time with experience, reintroduce a product or herb back into the picture and reassess it. Give it another go, along with your new-found hormonal knowledge.

I myself was one of these skeptics disillusioned with years of unsatisfactory nutritional supplementation and was very anti-liver cleansing, purely because of my exposure and experiences, (no one ever explained to me the principles and purpose behind the liver in healing and health) in a 30 year quest for health and to resolve my problems with Endometriosis, there was always this comment passed by alternative therapists that "It's your liver". No one ever stopped to explain to me why the liver is so important and I just assumed it was the latest craze. Therefore I didn't realise the importance to detox to improve immunity, to reduce estrogen levels, to assist my metabolism, increase energy, balance my hormones and so on. Therefore I thought it pointless, believing it to be a trend with naturopaths of the day. (Just another fad).

As sceptical as I was, I began a liver cleansing with powders and really felt quite ill. Again, it wasn't explained to me that this was a detoxifying period. That my liver was dysfunctional through years of abuse, of codeine dependency, heavy analgesic use, heavy smoking, drinking alcohol, eating very badly, looking for quick fixes just to keep myself going, and being on The Pill. Little wonder then that I had a hard time getting through detox, not very much 'enjoying' the sensation of liver cleansing, but I persisted. It was a frightening experience because of the lack of information provided.

Myself along with others have learnt not to be so negative or close-minded because of past bad experiences. Adopt a different approach. Incorporate processes, strategies, nutrition with your progesterone cream and you will find incredible results and perhaps you might surprise yourself that these things, had they been combined with hormone balancing and an understanding of your particular body shape type and your metabolism, in the past would have been a different outcome. Good news, it's not too late!!!

At NPAN, I advise women to listen to their body. Check your charting, assess your progress, get better at interpreting what does work and implementing them more often. Move away or eliminate altogether the things that don't work for you. One could argue that most of the methods, up until now haven't worked, or your eating plan, or way of life has not served you well. Reassess it.

In Summary: You don't have to change dramatically overnight. You just need to change your awareness and perspective, and adopt strategies that serve you.

Move away from the things that are harmful to you. Move towards things that are more conducive to your goals. Make a fair assessment and even more preferably 6-7 months to see even better results and the bodies response to new strategies and nutrition adopted. Being methodical and consistent will bring about change. I always tell women it takes a 120 days approximately for a new blood cycle. So it is important not to abandon a program before one complete blood cycle. To give a fair assessment. A lackadaisical approach will give the same results. Don't settle for less than optimal health whatever your current state of health is. It can be improved with a dedicated commitment. I have been on nutritional supplementation and liver principles daily for 3 years. I do not compromise what I call my health insurance. I consider it to be the financial premiums of my health. Nutritional costs and eating organically is a necessity not a luxury as I used to view it. My husband and I have modified our thinking and budget and spend less time and money in the supermarket buying quick packaged expensive pre cooked meals and comfort foods. This way of thinking and our previous mind set (based on negative past results) has changed over a number of years and did not happen over night for us. In fact my husband a Clinical Pharmacist used to say "you do not need nutritional supplementation if you eat a health balanced diet" however he too has come to realise the need to take supplementation because of the depletion of vitamins and minerals in our soil and encourages his cardiovascular patients to do the same along with dietary and lifetime changes in conjunction with their cardiac medications. *He is also more opposed to the usage of estrogen in large doses having seen too many women come into hospital with heart problems following estrogen administration of increasing doses in cardiac conditions.*

I have been on a diet and cannot lose weight. Why would this be?

One of the greatest complaints I receive here at NPAN and the cause of untold frustration is women's inability to lose weight. They have reached a point where, for the first time in their life, weight suddenly increases around the hips, tummy and thighs.

Their breasts may increase in size, and they're becoming quite flabby, gaining cellulite and a fatty liver roll. They go to the gym, exercise as much as they've always exercised and yet have not witnessed any degree of weight loss as they have in the past.

Some may join a weight control centre offering weight control diets but, again, cannot sustain the svelte body shape once they abandon such control measures. The weight creeps back on again. These women 'yo-yo' from one diet to the next, often getting fatter with each episode, causing enormous despair and suffering, without a hint of the underlying problem.

When I explain to women that perhaps the weight problem, or the inability to lose weight is hormonally connected, there is a sense of relief, joy, perhaps a ray of hope. It's almost like that dark cloud hovering overhead begins to break allowing light to shed on this sinister, life-disrupting problem that is absolutely consuming their life, causing untold heartache.

It is also important to note that if *you are on hormone replacement therapy, natural or synthetic, and it's the wrong hormone regime for your body type and metabolism, you will continue to put on weight. Particularly if you are eating the wrong foods for your body type.*

There is a condition emerging in Western industrialised countries known as **'Syndrome X'** as identified by Dr. Sandra Cabot which refers to a metabolic disorder characterised by high blood levels of the hormone insulin. (Insulin resistance).

These people also have abnormalities in blood fat levels. They may also have elevated blood levels of uric acid. Syndrome X is very common in societies where fast food and refined carbohydrates (white flour & sugar) are easily available. This condition can affect people of all ages, and is not rare in adolescents. A fatty liver and steroid hormone imbalance are commonly associated with Syndrome X. As Sandra Cabot has personally trained me in Syndrome X Weight control and body shaping I have included this in hormonal balancing in Book 2 Natural Progesterone More Secrets Revealed.

Books that I recommend to assist with weight problems are Dr. Sandra Cabot's book, 'The Body Shaping Diet'. This book guides you into the specific foods suited for your body type and will guide you to achieving your metabolic and hormonal constitution according to your body type. Eating the correct foods for your body type will not only balance your hormones but will assist in correct weight loss.

Likewise, Dr. Cabot's Healthy Liver and Bowel Book, The Liver Cleansing Diet will target these major organs that actually contribute to hormonal disruption and weight gain and her book "Can't Lose Weight? You could have Syndrome X" addresses the specific chemical imbalance that makes women and men store weight.

I have incorporated Dr. Cabot's theories into my own work with women with some outstanding results!

Women are flocking to progesterone and to the potential benefits progesterone has on their health and life generally. NPAN seeks to educate, empower and share, imparting discoveries and truths.

These wonderful discoveries have been helping women put into place the missing links so that everything falls into place for them. They come to realise the long term benefits of weight reduction, and they obtain renewed hormonal health and energy.

Stress

What happens when the body experiences stress?

Five things happen simultaneously:

- Sugar is released into the bloodstream. If more sugar is released than is needed, a disharmony occurs.
- The thymus gland contracts. This large gland is in the centre of the chest behind the breastbone and is related to the immune system in adults. Sustained contraction inhibits the production of blood cells and adds to the feelings of anxiety.
- Muscles tense. Sustained muscle tension will cause cells to break down, toxins to accumulate and oxygen and nutrient supplies to diminish, causing a lack of oxygen at the cellular level.
- Capillaries dilate, under sustained tension, lymph movement is slowed down and plasma and proteins accumulate between the cells, causing a build-up of toxins, pressure and swelling, as well as inhibiting the cells' supplies of nutrients and oxygen.
- Cells release toxins. Our cells are releasing toxins all the time as a natural part of their regular activity. Under stress, their activity increases. The natural process is for these toxins to be washed clear by the plasma and carted off by the lymph system to be discharged through perspiration, respiration and elimination.
- When sustained tension inhibits the cleansing of the toxins they build up locally, poisoning the local cells and finding their way into the bloodstream through different capillaries, where they can effect the brain and the glands.

(Source of this information is unknown).

Why does stress upset my hormonal imbalance?

The corticosteroid hormones are made from progesterone. *Therefore, stress forces progesterone to be used in the body in a different way, taking the hormone down another steroid pathway* (see the Hormonal Cascade diagram), thus depriving the body of it's usual supply of progesterone and cascading benefits.

High cortisol production which occurs with stress of any kind, including trauma, inflammation or inflammatory diseases, emotional and even chemical stress, can induce high levels of cortisol and this *leads to significant reduction of progesterone, resulting in estrogen dominance.*

While there are high levels of cortisol, the cortisol is actually taking over the progesterone receptors, thereby competing with progesterone.

Over time, repeated triggering of stress hormones (corticosteroid hormones) can deplete your body of energy and progesterone and leave you less able to respond.

Stress can be a factor in the development of *Cardiovascular Disease, hypertension, cancer and many auto-immune disorders such as lupus, multiple sclerosis and perhaps Endometriosis. Additionally, stress can contribute to irritable bowel syndrome, Osteoporosis, chronic fatigue syndrome, polycystic ovaries, thyroid dysfunction, headaches, sleep disturbances and many skin conditions. Chronic stress depletes many nutrients from the body, including most B vitamins, antioxidants, zinc and other minerals necessary for immune-system function and the optimal functioning of adrenal glands.*

Clearly, long term stress and constant output of cortisol causes nasty consequences to the body. I make mention of the importance of stress management in maintaining hormone balance throughout both books.

In recognising **extreme stress,** be it high pain levels, chemical, illness, or emotional, **always accommodate by slightly increasing your progesterone dose** to cater for the body's need for additional progesterone supplementation to assist in the manufacture of this stress hormone, and help compete for access to the progesterone receptors.

Try an increased dose for a cycle then return to your normal dose. Use symptom re-emergence as your guideline to accommodate the need to increase progesterone doses in times of stress. Your body will signal the need for additional support in progesterone as it has been robbed to be used for the survival hormones. Adding more helps the body compete for the same receptors, assists the body to calm down thus lowering stress thereby making the receptors once more available for progesterone to occupy and work effectively once again, other than converting it to the corticosteroid pathway. You can now see why it is so easy to fall out of synch and become hormonally imbalanced after a period of stress and why the body has no reserves left in its fuel tank (storage - fat cells.) Chances are they have all been used up and utilised in the corticosteroid production. It does not take long (I suggest a cycle at double the dose of what you have been on) to restore the reserves. Your break will indicate if you are back on track. If you are not coping on your break it is a sign that you have not got enough adequate reserves behind you yet. In this case continue at higher levels until the next break and recheck. Doing your charts (the Estrogen dominant progesterone deficiency chart) will help guide you and support you in keeping an eye on your symptoms. Sleep patterns are a great barometer. Restored sleep indicates progesterone is beginning to work efficiently.

Estrogen Dominance Wake Up Crisis and the reasons for the return of has been addressed extensively in Book 2 Natural Progesterone More Secrets Revealed.

Symptoms of Adrenal Gland Exhaustion/Adrenal Exhaustion

- Morning fatigue and depression, which improves as the day goes on
- Low blood pressure
- Dizziness and faintness
- Low blood sugar levels
- Increased allergies
- Increased aches and pains
- Chronic fatigue syndrome

My Observations:

- Hormonal imbalance (often deficient in some hormones)
- Lowered immunity and susceptability eg. To colds, infections, Thrush.
- Often depressed
- Sleep disorders insomnia
- Anxiety disorders
- Possible lack of response to nutrition and hormone supplementation (sluggish or non responsive cell response)

Thyroid Concerns

Will progesterone help my thyroid?

Providing you do not have a recognised thyroid problem requiring thyroid supplementation, progesterone has been noted to help many women improve their thyroid function.

Nearly every woman who has come to NPAN has indicated thyroid dysfunction and has been sent to have their thyroid tested, all reporting back with clear results. Evidently estrogen dominance has a negative impact on thyroid performance, lethargy, fluid retention and weight gain. A few months to 18 months on progesterone has reversed all their apparent 'thyroid' symptoms (if hormone induced). Read page 323.

If you have been diagnosed with a thyroid problem, and you are on thyroid medication, and now want to incorporate natural progesterone into your regime, there's no reason why you can't providing you do so under the strict supervision of your treating physician. Your thyroid dosage, however, may require regular adjustment as progesterone exerts an influence upon the thyroid gland.

NPAN has seen many women who have ceased their estrogen therapy and replaced it with natural progesterone have a remarkable improvement on their existing diagnosed condition of hypothyroidism (low thyroid function).

And over a time requiring a reduction of their thyroxine medication. Interestingly it *is believed estrogen binds up the hormone thyroxine (protein bound) thereby rendering it inaccessible thus causing symptoms of low thyroid* (such as cold hands & feet) or increasing the severity of existing hypothyroidism. This is why many women who are estrogen dominant and have a thyroid function test find that their results are normal.

The thyroid gland function can be improved with trace minerals such as selenium, iodine, zinc and manganese. *Selenium is very important as it is required for the conversion of T4 into the active form of T3.* A diet rich in kelp and iodine is also beneficial. Seafood, green leafy vegetables come into this category.

If you are unsure whether your thyroid is functioning optimally (this can be characterised by an inability to lose weight, puffy and swollen body appearance, lethargy, muscle weakness, dry skin, hair loss and constipation), I suggest BEFORE resorting to progesterone to fix these problems you might be well advised to ask your doctor to order the appropriate tests.

This includes blood profile to measure the levels of both thyroid hormones, T4 and T3, and also TSH (Thyroid Stimulating Hormone). A shortage of T4 would be administered in the form of thyroxine tablets. In the USA, thyroid replacement therapy is available in cream form by way of natural thyroid hormone replacement using bio-identical hormones. (Containing both T4 known as armathyroid, there is a website, and T3 hormones in balanced amounts). T3 known as Tetroxine, is administered in Australia in medication form which is not bio identical. A special license is required to prescribe this in Australia. Bio identical thyroid hormones can be compounded by the same method as natural progesterone with a script from the Doctor only Specialising Doctors in bio identical hormones would be familiar with this. One centre being Dr Sandra Cabot's clinic in Sydney.

Fibroids
What are Fibroids?

Fibroids are tumours which grow within the normal muscle of the uterus (womb). Single or multiple Fibroids may be present and may vary in size from a grape (1cm) to a grapefruit (10 cm) or even larger. Fibroids are usually benign (not cancerous).

What causes Fibroids?

The cause of Fibroids is not known. It is known however, that the female sex hormones estrogen is involved in fibroid growth as are a number of other growth factors.

Who gets Fibroids?

Fibroids occur during a woman's reproductive years and affect at least 50% of women over the age of 35. With the decrease in production of estrogen at menopause, Fibroids stop growing and symptoms tend to disappear. more of the following symptoms:

Heavy Bleeding

This is the most common symptom and may vary from bleeding for a longer period of time, passing clots, episodes of "flooding" or irregular periods.

Will my Fibroids turn into cancer?

Some women fear that Fibroids may turn to cancer. This is no longer thought to occur. Cancerous Fibroids (leiomyosarcomas) begin as cancer and these account for only one in 2,400 women with Fibroids.

What are the symptoms?

Most often, Fibroids cause no problems at all. However, for some women Fibroids produce troublesome symptoms which may leave them feeling tired and lethargic and cause disruption to lifestyle and relationships. You may experience one or

Pain

Moderate to severe period pain may be experienced which may feel sharp, cramp-like or may produce a constant dull ache in the abdomen or lower back. This last type of pain is related to the Fibroid placing pressure on the surrounding organs within the pelvis. A dragging down feeling may be experienced.

Pressure Symptoms

Fibroid uterus is placing forward pressure onto the bladder. Difficulty passing bowel motions, constipation or feeling as though you need to open your bowels more frequently may also indicate that there is backward pressure onto the bowel.

Bladder frequency or difficulty in passing or emptying the bladder may be experienced. Many women have continual lower abdomen swelling which worsens prior menstruation. Some may even have an appearance of pregnancy which is and can be very embarrassing especially when comments are passed like 'when are you expecting'. I have been guilty of this myself and have felt extremely embarrassed also. How can you retract such a comment!

Infertility

Infertility, or failure to achieve pregnancy may occur when certain types of Fibroids block the fallopian tubes (preventing the sperm and egg from meeting) or distort the cavity of the uterus (interfering with the embryo embedding in the lining of the uterus) Fibroids in the wall of the uterus (intramural) may also cause Infertility and some of the symptoms resulting from Fibroids i.e. excessive bleeding or pain may also reduce the chance of conceiving.

Types of Fibroids

Submucosal

These Fibroids protrude inwards into the cavity of the uterus. They may grow on a stalk, which if long enough may protrude through the cervix. These are called fibroid polyps.

Intramural

These begin as little lumps in the muscle of the uterus. As they grow, the shape of the uterus becomes distorted.

Subserosal

These vary greatly in size and may be multiple. They grow and protrude outwards from the uterus, sometimes on a stalk, which may twist and cause pain.

Cervical

Some Fibroids (about 2%) occur in the cervix.

Some more facts:

Most women with Fibroids do not require treatment.

The presence size and position of Fibroids should be confirmed by a gynecologist before beginning any treatment.

Shrinkage of Fibroids by drugs, embolisation or surgery may avoid major surgery in women, particularly those over 40.

Myomectomy (fibroid removal) can usually be done laparoscopically or from the vagina and is most suitable for those wishing to become pregnant or and wish to retain their uterus, avoiding a Hysterectomy.

Second opinions are important before consenting to major surgery.

The choice of a specialist gynecologist may provide surgery with a shorter stay in hospital and a decreased risk of complications.

In Australia, we have the some doctors who specialise in the treatment and removal of Fibroids. These practitioners endeavour to help women preserve their uterus wherever possible. They are skilled surgeons.

SOME OF THE INFORMATION PROVIDED IN THIS SECTION WAS FOUND FROM MFC'S WEBSITE TO ASSIST YOU IN YOUR SEARCH FOR RELIABLE INFORMATION - http://www.melbfibroidclinic.com.au

I must mention here that the Clinic does NOT incorporate natural progesterone as part of their treatment plan but rather incorporates synthetic progestogins. This shouldn't sway you from visiting their very informative website.

Since updating this book I believe this clinic does no longer operate in Melbourne but the website information is still available to date.

Will progesterone help with Fibroids?

Is it the heavy bleeding that creates the Fibroids or the Fibroids that create the heavy bleeding? In my work with this all too frequent problem, and from observation, NPAN has found that many women who suffer fibroid problems come to me as a last resort before a Hysterectomy. And with serious management, progesterone use and a commitment to their health and patience, the Fibroids usually come under control. It can be a persistent and diligent journey to combat.

If you look at it another way, when a woman goes through menopause and her estrogen levels drop to the degree that her periods stop altogether, her Fibroids will naturally shrink (atrophy). That is, unless her estrogen levels remain elevated by way of synthetic hormone replacement therapy, obesity. or other factors.

Fibroids are almost a direct result of estrogen dominance so in order to minimise the effects of your Fibroids you have to get your estrogen dominance down in control.

Your aim, therefore, is to reduce your body's estrogen levels so that the Fibroids will not continue to grow. Women associated with NPAN have successfully used progesterone to assist and bring about this effect. Further, they reduced their estrogen dominance in the body through diet, particular attention being given to increasing intake of fibre, exercise, reducing refined sugars, a combination of herbs and vitamins high in antioxidants, stress management and lifestyle changes and liver detoxification.

This is where phytoestrogens can play a major part in protecting the body against the more potent estrogens that can be responsible for 'driving' fibroid growth, thereby blocking receptors with weaker plant estrogens, but still providing the body with estrogenic benefits.

Far too often women with Fibroids have a history of taking some estrogen as well. I find that therein lies half the dilemma. They usually have a history in taking some form of estrogen supplementation - I have even seen women in menopause - get Fibroids which has perhaps caused and contributed to Fibroids (one can only conclude here!). There is a vicious circle that goes on. If women want to try this option it does take persistence, time, tolerance, understanding and patience. It is not an instant fix and it may not be the answer for a lot of women. A lot of women will often go and have their Fibroids removed and leave the uterus intact. That has been a very successful option for some. Microwave surgery has also proven successful in others and certainly halted bleeding problems.

It's my observation that many 'Gynaeoid type' body shaped women suffer Fibroids because these women tend to store lower body fat rendering them estrogen dominant. You might like to refer to 'The Weight Control Doctor' website (http://www.weightcontroldoctor.com) for more information on Body Shape.

So it's important for these women to eat correctly avoiding fats and sugars which increase the body's sensitivity to estrogen which, in turn, will reduce weight and estrogen dominance, dramatically assisting in the successful outcome of fibroid management. Please read page 363 "Reducing Estrogen Dominance naturally".

Whilst progesterone therapy has proved successful for a majority of the women experiencing heavy bleeding associated with Fibroids, there has been a couple of cases reported where Fibroids have not responded to progesterone therapy. They, in fact, grew in size.

One lady required a Hysterectomy because excessive bleeding was interfering with her lifestyle. The Hysterectomy was necessary due to the location of her Fibroids. And another lady had her Fibroids successfully removed leaving her uterus intact, and continues in good health, maintaining her hormonal health with progesterone at 32mg, 2 weeks on, 2 weeks off.

'Mary' is a case in point. She managed to reduce her heavy bleeding subsequent to Fibroids (and migraines) using progesterone at 64mg but was advised by her doctor to drop to 32mg. Her doctor believed her dose was perhaps too high.

She was fine for 2 months, then suddenly episodes of migraines and renewed heavy bleeding re-emerged which led to a deficiency in her iron. She was referred to a gynecologist who recommended a Hysterectomy. Fear stricken and in a state of panic, she phoned me at NPAN. I suggested she get another ultrasound which was scheduled anyway.

Two days later she called me back, ecstatic, stating that she'd retrieved the second test results from her doctor and, when compared with her results 12 months prior, realised that her Fibroids had shrunk considerably.

This affirmed to Mary that she was on the right track. Her body, particularly her Fibroids, was responding favourably to progesterone. She just needed to return to the procedures that were working successfully for her.

Mary went back to a 64mg-100mg dosage for a few months to stabilise herself, using her headaches as her barometer, and once she had her bleeding under control, gradually reduced her dosage to between 40mg, or 50mg when under stress which provides Mary with a good buffer.

NPAN has always encouraged women to do their own detective work. To make sure that whenever they have tests conducted, whatever they may be, to insist on a copy for their own records. This approach empowered Mary, but more importantly she was in a position to bring together two ultrasound comparative results which were in two different doctors' records.

But not all stories that find their way to NPAN are happy ones. For Fibroids may disguise problems of a more insidious nature. 'Bernadette' insisted on a Hysterectomy upon being diagnosed with Fibroids. Bernadette had lost a girlfriend to cancer who had been diagnosed with Fibroids and awaiting a more thorough diagnosis and elective surgery. Bernadette didn't want to take the risk.

NPAN's message: always make sure you have regular check-ups, appropriate tests, and remain under the supervision of your specialist. And if you're not comfortable or satisfied with your treatment and outcome, get a second opinion. Having your own copy of your test results will assist your treating physician, and gives you the freedom to go elsewhere. Make your own informed decision. NOTE: Doses as high as 200-400mg have been used with success by some women and reports of intra vaginal application have been even more promising but it is still early days and NPAN women and myself are on a learning curve.

Endometriosis
What is Endometriosis?

Endometriosis is defined as the presence of normal tissue in an abnormal place. The endometrium (lining) of the uterus spreads to the pelvis through the tubes and settles most commonly in the pelvis.

Like the lining of the uterus, the endometrium grows under the influence of the major female hormone estrogen. The most common sites in the pelvis are on and below the ovaries, and deep in the pelvis behind the uterus, called the Pouch of Douglas. Here the Endometriosis grows on the ligaments behind the uterus and on the vagina and rectum. It also may grow on the bladder, appendix, abdominal wall and even sometimes in the upper abdomen.

It is a disorder in which the *endometrial cells* (cells found within the endometrial lining and confined inside the uterine cavity) find their way outside the uterus to other parts of the body such as the abdomen or the pelvic cavity. They can also be scattered throughout the body.

Endometriosis usually results in severe pain during or prior to menstruation. The cause is unknown although it is often referred to as an estrogen driven disease and familial and is believed may be linked to an auto immune disorder.

YOU MAY BENEFIT FROM VISITING THE 'ECCA' WEBSITE FROM WHICH SOME OF THIS INFORMATION WAS FOUND: http://www.ecca.com.au/.

What causes Endometriosis?

Although the exact cause is still unknown, there are a number of factors which influence the development of the disease. The most likely explanation is that women menstruate backwards through the tubes into the pelvis and the cells of the uterine lining then implant and grow.

Although 70% of women do menstruate through the tubes, only 10% develop the disease so this is only a partial explanation of why it develops. The majority of women have a natural defence, killing the cells of the menstrual fluid before they implant.

Women who develop Endometriosis have reduced ability to kill these cells or a reduced ability to stop their growth after they implant in the pelvis. These defence systems involve the immune system.

Sometimes the disease will develop in the absence of the uterus and this must result from normal cells lining the pelvis changing to the same cells that line the uterus and thus forming Endometriosis.

Factors increasing the risk of Endometriosis

Early onset of menstrual periods

Heavy periods

Painful periods

Prolonged periods

Hormone imbalance

Allergy (e.g., foods, eczema, hay fever) autoimmune problems

Obesity

Family history of Endometriosis e.g., mother or sister

Prolonged stress

Insidious, unknown origins - Auto Immune Disorder.

Ovary dysfunction and anovulatory cycles

Estrogen dominance

Diet high in estrogen chemical fed steroid laden chickens, fodder.

Low fibre intake

Sugar laced foods and soft drink

High exposure to xenoestrogens

Inadequate production of progesterone upon ovulatory output.

Hereditary factors

Unknown - auto immune disorders, Ovarian Dysfunction and reasons for failure to ovulate. Estrogen dominance for unknown causes.

Environmental toxins are also a possible cause of the disease such as the chemical/toxin dioxin (which has shown to cause disease in a factory where it was used excessively and also has been shown to cause Endometriosis in monkeys.

Endometriosis is very difficult to treat and can be very debilitating. It's one of the most painful afflictions a woman can experience. The symptoms of cramping and abdominal pain result from the islets of endometrial tissue which migrate out of the uterus and scatter throughout the pelvic area and attach themselves to the ovaries, the intestinal walls, the bladder wall and even membranes in the abdomen, and between the uterine muscle wall (ademyoses).

When a woman's body responds to her monthly surges of estrogen, these tiny islets become swollen with menstrual blood at the same time the uterine lining sheds bringing on a period. These endometrial islets also shed blood, but because it has nowhere to go, it creates local tissue inflammation in the pelvic and abdominal regions, resulting in significant scar tissue.

This internal bleeding and chronic inflammation creates congestion, the internal bleeding needs to be reabsorbed back into the body, again putting a lot of stress and workload on the body.

Many women suffering Endometriosishave experienced adhesions of organs as a result of many years of internal bleeding.

It is not life threatening and it is not related to cancer (although cells proliferate as such, driven under the influence of estrogen not malignant). This disease is very debilitating and often leads to other complications such as compromising a woman's auto-immunity, and left untreated long term often leads to chronic fatigue and Fibromyalgia, and other difficult to treat conditions that compound.

Diagnosis is difficult and often delayed. It will not show up in x-rays and often it is very hard to detect because these little islets can be scattered throughout the body, often hidden. Exploratory surgery will reveal the evidence of Endometriosis.

Factors reducing the risk of Endometriosis

Aerobic exercise of 5 hours per week which in two studies has shown a 50% reduction in the risk of recurrence. (Sometimes unrealistic achievement due to high levels of pain and a restriction of activity).

Childbearing reduces the risk of recurrence by about 50%, due to a 9 month state of pregnancy whereby the absence of bleeding (menstruation) prevents   further spreading of the disease. Perhaps high levels of progesterone have a major play here.

Smoking also reduces the risk of Endometriosis, I don't know why it helps, although it is obviously not a reason to start or continue smoking. One Naturopaths view on why smoking may assist in reducing estrogen driven disease is because smoking reduces natural estrogen production however you need to take into account that it also creates high toxic xenoestrogens. Many smokers claim that it assists in pain management. But remember cigarettes also contains lethal poisons - xenotoxins and can bring about more serious diseases - all of which are publicly drummed into society now. I suggest you seek alternative stress pain management if possible.

Eat whole foods free of chemicals - organic where possible

Avoid foods high in chemical estrogen, i.e. chicken

Eat regularly, don't skip meals or use stimulants to keep you going

Avoid caffeine - disorients the endocrine system and leaches your bones

Keep very high roughage in your diet to speed up the elimination process, shortening the life span of excess toxins in the bowel which can be reabsorbed back into the body mimicking xenoestrogens.

Find a good masseur who will assist in lymphatic drainage and cell oxygenation which helps reduce the pelvic inflammation and pelvic congestion, and stress.

High use of anti-oxidants and anti-inflammatory and nutritional supplements (vitamin C, selenium, MSM and essential fatty acids, oils such as vitamin E, evening primrose, linseed and lethecin have proved beneficial in facilitating healing and boosting the immune system, including amino acids and B group vitamins). See section on Prostaglandins, understanding the importance of omega oils in the role of anti inflammatory, anti thrombotic - in Book 2 "More Secrets Revealed".

Address fatigue and exhaustion

Learn to handle stress (whereby reducing high levels of cortisol)

Learn to drink at least 8 glasses of pure water a day

Positive attitude (find positive support and an understanding doctor in this disease).

Rest and recreation

Reduce estrogen dominance (page 363) and triggers

Most importantly (in my opinion) use progesterone therapy. This has timelessly proved invaluable in bringing this disease and pain into control in a very short time span.

From observation, other factors that reduce or help control the progression of Endometriosis is early diagnosis, this includes looking for the disease in young menstruating girls. Too often they are placed on the contraceptive pill to Band-Aid 'period problems' without thorough investigation or being offered alternative treatments in management. Whilst the OCP/Pill will control pain by reducing and synthetically controlling periods, it comes with a big price tag especially for the young. Their bodies are still maturing. Their pituitary gland (the hormone regulating centre) not fully developed must be disrupted to a certain degree (in my opinion and my observation), not to mention the pill is turning the ovaries off, telling them not to ovulate and these are the bodies most vulnerable prime years. Mother nature is working towards preparing the body to be in ultimate optimal balance and health, ready for reproduction. Surely then why would we want to throw a spanner in the works, disrupt mother nature and eliminate one of the most vital hormones - progesterone. If the periods are not right it is mother nature telling us something is wrong. Chances are diet herbs and essential fatty acid a little progesterone where required can assist the body's normalisation and balancing aiding it to get back on course naturally. See information on the Pill, pages 283, 346.

Granted, this disease is difficult to diagnose, but managing symptoms rather than looking for the underlying cause is the approach I would NOT recommend. I would like to say here that while the oral contraceptive pill has assisted many young women in pain management it is really delaying sorting out the true problem and it is denying the body of real progesterone, due to it preventing ovulation.

What are the symptoms of Endometriosis?

- Changes in bowel, bladder, sexual or menstrual function of a cyclical nature
- Changes in menstrual pain: increasing severity or duration of pain, pain not responding to drugs such as Ponstan or Naprogesic, pain which interferes with normal daily activities or employment
  - Bowel symptoms of pain, constipation or diarrhoea (or both) prior or at time of the period sometimes blood or mucous may be passed from the rectum
  - Frequency and pain when passing urine, pain when the bladder is full in the morning. Sometimes blood may be passed in the urine

- Menstrual changes including heavy bleeding, prolonged or shortened periods or periods which stop and start (may be light then heavy or vice versa).
- Spotting before the period
- Premenstrual syndrome including heavy bleeding, prolonged or shortened periods or periods which stop and start
- Tiredness, depression, symptoms of adrenal gland exhaustion
- Pelvic pain
- Low back pain
- Infertility
- Ovulation pain
- General body & muscle stiffness
- Fatigue & exhaustion due to pain stress
- Mood alterations & atypical behaviour / attitude swings
- Pain with sex, felt deep in the pelvis which is worse before and during the period and may alter with change of position. A similar pain may be felt during pelvic examination when the doctor places pressure behind the uterus.

My Observation Additional List:

- Contraction period pains/cramps
- Pain associated with nausea
- Attacks of irritable bowel syndrome and/or diarrhoea
- Inexplicable nervous irritability or anxious energy. Can be uptight, always on the go with surges of energy and adrenalin releases
- Often very thin or poor eaters
- Excessive and obsessive working or cleaning habits and cycles correlating with hormones
- Perfectionist traits, controllers, workaholics
- Bouts of sheer exhaustion and collapse versus hyperactivity
- Can resort to stimulants in replacement for food and nutrition
- You may wish to read my observational profile of an Endometriosis woman.
- Usually Android type, very muscular, strong, steroid constitution, but all body types can be prone

Why is progesterone effective in treating Endometriosis?

It is thought that Endometriosis is an estrogen driven disease. We know that when a woman falls pregnant, often Endometriosis will disappear, only to return again after pregnancy.

There is some very strong correlation between the two. This suggests that the sex hormones are involved and that high progesterone levels produced in pregnancy play an important part in controlling this disease.

That's why progesterone is recommended from days **5 to 28** or whenever your normal menstrual cycle ends. *This mimics a pseudo-pregnancy state, and facilitates healing.*

Higher than normal doses are required which appear to be well tolerated. In fact, levels around about 54-60mg are usually required for pain management. Most women will find that they can reduce their dosage of progesterone after 7-12 months, however, attempts to go below say 4% (40mg) progesterone often allows symptoms to creep back in.

I don't believe progesterone cures Endometriosis but I certainly know that it plays a major role in controlling its distressing symptoms. I am also convinced that Endometriosis women can always be prone to a resurgent/flare up. In March 2003 upon lifting a heavy item incorrectly (in a squatting position) I ripped my internal bowel ligaments. At the time it was excruciating internal contractional pain which felt like an elastic band twisting and untwisting. It was likened to labour and did not let up for 3-5 minutes. While lying on the ground wondering to myself what I had damaged as I had nothing there, in other words my uterus was gone, I just got up and went on my merry way. Two days later my stomach flared acutely and I ended up in Casualty with Peritonitis and had a stomach of a 7 month pregnant women. Nothing was found on scan however following that my Irritable Bowel Syndrome, Candida and symptoms of Endometriosis raged. I had excruciating pain in the back ligaments, the uterine like bearing down feeling which I used to experience and all the other associated back pain that I experienced with Endometriosis. Whilst I cannot confirm this diagnosis of Endometriosis flare up, I believe that given the right environment Endometriosis can resurge itself as was my case. I lost control of my progesterone and became severely estrogen dominant so no one is exempt. It took me several months to gain control, bring back my balance, eliminate Candida and settle my Irritable Bowel Syndrome. This was the first time I had ever experienced Candida and the unquenchable need for sugar and I now empathise totally with women that experience this condition. Ironically once I sorted this out my husband felt *I needed a break* and took me on a second honeymoon to Vanuatu where I broke my arm the first morning, strolling down the beach. Again the Irritable Bowel Syndrome flared under the stress but not the Candida. So much for 2004.

We have had great success with the usage of progesterone and the treatment, or maintenance of Endometriosis, particularly for pain control. Usually there is a great swing around within 7 months.

I get quite excited when I see young girls approach NPAN presenting symptoms that look suspiciously like Endometriosis. Treated early with progesterone, their symptoms disappear. Many of these young girls actually get well enough to no longer require progesterone therapy.

Chronic Endometriosis

Women who have been long term sufferers of Endometriosis and undergone years of chronic pain and various treatments often leading to chronic fatigue syndrome (CFS) and other complex health issues, I've found that the progesterone does not respond in the same way as those with an early diagnosis of Endometriosis. Progesterone therapy and recovery is slow. Hormone imbalance is not the only issue at play here.

Women who have had any form of surgery - a Caesarean Section, Appendectomy, Tubal Ligation - and present with symptoms of lower pelvic backache, particularly before period, muscle stiffness, estrogen dominant symptoms, period irregularity or period problems, I suspect that perhaps Endometriosis may be involved, despite unconfirmed diagnosis.

Often women intuitively know there is a hormonal link to their problems even though their doctor fails to find anything wrong with them. They present with randomised, non-specific symptoms that may persist for many years. These women are often made to believe they are hypochondriacs.

A delayed diagnosis after numerous years of medication and synthetic hormone cocktails often leads to liver dysfunction, Adrenal Exhaustion, and chronic pain/fatigue. Progesterone therapy is valuable and contributes towards overall improvement, however, it requires a consistent, persistent effort in conjunction with nutritional and often psychological support.

It is a very long haul back for women who have suffered say ten to twenty years of Endometriosis undiagnosed, with perhaps a lot of medical mismanagement as a result of an incorrect diagnosis. Some women also have had a lifetime of synthetic HRT which really does compromise their body and liver in the long run.

I have witnessed some very odd cases involving women with chronic Endometriosis.

One woman in her 40s complained about lactating for years outside pregnancy and without any underlying sinister causes such as a tumour on the pituitary. This in itself is a huge indication of hormonal imbalance and perhaps progesterone deficiency in her own unique way. To this day, doctors have not be able to determine why this is occurring. But this woman, a trained nurse, has great faith that progesterone is one of the missing links in treatment, and her long-term healing. (Progesterone inhibits the hormone Prolactin. Prior delivery the progesterone manufacturing then around 400mg a day drops dramatically so that Prolactin can bring on lactation).

I encourage these women to go step by step. It is simple by the inch but hard by the yard. (Refer to Stress, Adrenal Gland Exhaustion on pages 295-298).

It takes endurance, patience and commitment and often I recommend that they seek out a very reputable herbalist and/or naturopath who will also embrace progesterone therapy. At this level of the disease there are many compounding problems which usually accompany chronic Endometriosis and many holistic approaches need to be incorporated and embraced. It is important that you feel comfortable with the various health professionals you are working with. You also need to be aware that chronic Endometriosis is a slow path back to healing and wellbeing.

Profile of an Endometriosis woman

These are my collected thoughts from observing and compiling a profile of an Endometriosis woman and common characteristics and mannerisms.

Compiled by Jenny Birdsey©

Generally speaking, women with Endometriosis can display some very common behavioural characteristics and personality types.

My observation is that they tend to have a very strong mental constitution, be high achievers, and usually very competitive with themselves. They can hold high profile positions which demand much of them physically and mentally. Even though they may be unwell and suffering chronic pain, they are able to draw on their adrenals to continually push themselves forward as if 'superwoman'.

They appear to have this phenomenal energy that can override pain and fatigue. The adrenals over-compensate and this continual cortisol output can aggravate the disease even further (because it is denying the body of any progesterone that may be available in the body). This may explain why these women often find themselves dealing with chronic fatigue, Adrenal Exhaustion, and further auto-immune conditions.

This 'fight or flight' mechanism designed to be used only for emergencies or life-threatening situations is being overused by the body constantly, creating burnout (Adrenal Exhaustion) and hormone imbalance.

These women 'get off' on this adrenal rush, and actually depend on it for energy (which is a false energy). The body's production of this 'fight or flight' hormone draws on andrenous energy (male/yang) whereby creating imbalance.

A woman's body is not designed for this constant pull of this particular steroid pathway. One of the consequences of this action can be to shut down ovarian function (lack of ovulation and progesterone production), promoting further estrogen dominance which, as we know, drives Endometriosis.

Interestingly, often 'endometriosis women' choose careers that demand perfectionism, competition, excellence, long hours, heavy workload, huge responsibility. You often see them in the upper echelons of large corporations which tends to suit their personality traits. They operate from a position of control and order.

This control orientation, sense of order and perfectionism is reflected in their personal life as well. Women with Endometriosis go to great lengths to have things done 'their way', expecting others to conform to their set of rules (like putting things away in their proper place). Do as I say not as I do was my motto as I have observed with other women.

Ironically, these women can tolerate their own untidiness, but not when exhibited by their partner or children. It's as if there is a need to control others and their environment because they have no control over their disease. The more out of control they are in their own body, which can vary from month to month, the more they exert pressure and control upon others, and drive themselves harder at work (perhaps an unrecognised antidote to their pain) and others in the process holding high and unrealistic expectations of other peoples performances.

If these women stopped and listened to their body, they would collapse because ultimately these women do collapse because the adrenals become exhausted. They don't know how to get off the merry-go-round.

Metaphysically Endometriosis is often referred to as "the running away disease", perhaps running away from themselves and their femininity, although they can present as immaculately feminine in makeup and dress. They are also noted to run away from taking on responsibility (nurturing) of themselves. They do this by keeping busy and living a high pressured lifestyle and will often be over responsible for their families, friends and job.

Often this femininity presents as a liability, a vulnerability, and it challenges them to new belief systems. It's easy for these women to be 'out there' and responsible for others (carers, nurturers, approval seekers, workaholics) so that they can avoid (unknowingly) being responsible for themselves. Or to face up to the need to be self-nurturing and embrace their 'Ying' energy. This feminine energy would bring balance back into their life and go a long way towards helping them resolve their diseases. The dilemma is how to go there without compromising their performance level and sacrificing the driving force behind their male driven energy. (This is mentioned only as food for thought and comes from my own personal experiences and observations of common characteristics displayed. Obviously, not all 'endo' women fall into line with, or concur with this description.)

This facade of strength and responsibility and match of masculine physical and mental strength often comes about because a woman with Endometriosis believes herself to be weakened by her disease. In reality she has turned herself into 'superwoman'. She is able to do the things she does because she has a high pain threshold and quite courageous, yet she sees herself as very weak. She is also often an Android Body Type and can work and lift equivalents in strength of a man. She very often threatens men because of her strong mental and physical constitution. They can also display characteristics of hyperactivity and can be quite thin due to the fact that their body is running on so much adrenaline and cortisone with her high pain causing the body to produce survival hormones which she rechannels to perform her super tasks and gives this woman the ability to exceed normal pain thresholds.

Her frustration and anger is perhaps her driving force. Sadly, though, this negativity impacts the energy field perceived and messages that she gives off to others. And this can affect her relationship with people, making her more resentful of her condition.

In all this, there's this hurt and pain that she's being misunderstood and unsupported. Maybe this is what drives her to seek out approval, acceptance, recognition, self-worth perhaps via her performance, achievements and overall perfectionism and super capability/coping power. This profile is almost the opposite to that of Fibromyalgia and Chronic Fatigue.

Progesterone - the feminine "essence hormone" - brings about this transition naturally, and restores hormonal balance. This is why I see so many women enter a new phase, and reacquaint with a part of themselves they have pushed aside for such a long time when they introduce progesterone back into their body. It may also create a sense of strangeness and a period of adjustment. Coming off the adrenal pain pathway can bring the super energised women with 'false energy' into a state of real energy. It is then she may realise how tired she really is and how hard and long she has pushed her body. This is the time for her to rest and become reacquainted with herself and not feel so responsible keeping the whole world going. It is a time for her to nurture herself and reassess her values and beliefs, to rest and heal her often burnt out, self abused body.

I sense that there will be many women that relate to this profile and it is with hope that I have shed some light on your life if you are one of those women. I was.

Often women ask me where I get this 'stuff' from. I say 'from LIFE' and I am just a student passing through. In other words life is our teacher.

I suggest you read my belief regarding 'The Spiritual Side of Progesterone'.

Can you be suffering from Endometriosis and Fibroids at the same time?

Often women will come here with diagnosis of Fibroids coupled with other symptoms such as pain and bowel problems prior to their periods which leads me to believe there is Endometriosis lurking in the background. The very fact that such a woman responds so well to the progesterone in reducing pain is a positive indication for me, even if it has not been officially diagnosed.

I suggest that they use their progesterone according to alleviation of pain and bleeding concerns. Usually after about 7 months women are able to start reducing back to a physiological dose, but again, I tell women that it is an individual thing according to their symptom management.

Every woman's pain threshold is different and her need for progesterone will vary, averaging between 54-64mg for 4-7 months is quite common. With the confidence and knowledge their disease is under control, women can start relaxing and incorporate normal activities back into their life such as exercise. This, in turn, will promote further healing and sense of wellbeing. If 64mg is not alleviating pain you may need to go higher in dosage until this is under control (higher doses if coupled with Fibroids). Don't forget to rub over areas of pain particularly back ligaments. Refer to pages 298-300.

Will progesterone cure Endometriosis?

I am sure by the reports that it doesn't get rid of the disease because it has been found that women who had stopped for a few months felt great for a while and then suddenly the disease will re-flare itself. Most women stay on progesterone for maintenance, and adjust their dose when necessary, increasing when indicated such as in times of stress and reducing to maintenance least is best when in maintenance. Younger women (teenagers) are the exceptions. They can successfully continue without progesterone (12 months on progesterone recommended) if they have taken reduced steps to change dietary and lifestyle aggravators and their ovaries are ovulating and menstruation is pain free and normal.

Some have returned for short periods to progesterone but overall a young healthy body repairs quickly and given the right nutritional base strategies will restore equilibrium and normal physiological functioning.

Will a Hysterectomy cure Endometriosis?

Not necessarily. The aim of a Hysterectomy is to remove the uterus to stop periods, thereby reducing blood loss thus slowing down progression of the disease and further migration of endometrial tissue.

However, if the endometrial islets that escaped to other regions of the body and have not been removed by surgery, they can continue to grow under the influence of estrogen. Please refer to page 246 on 'Hysterectomy'. Also to Book 2, "Specific Problems".

I have seen women who had hysterectomies as a result of severe Endometriosis and one particular lady who comes to mind was sent home on estrogen patches to help prevent her from going through the discomforts of Hot Flushes once she had had her Hysterectomy and ovaries removed.

Sadly, 12 months later that woman ended up back in hospital with kidney problems and, on investigation, they found that the Endometriosis had actually almost encased her kidneys and severed her ureter's (the two long narrow tubes that convey the urine from the kidney to the bladder). She had to have kidney tubes put in to allow the urine to pass through.

This is just so sad because any woman who has had Endometriosis will probably know that estrogen is not a good thing for her body and would try and steer clear of it at all costs. Progesterone works wonders for controlling post-hysterectomised symptoms without the danger of Endometriosis re-emerging under the influence of estrogen replacement therapy.

I have also found that women who've had very severe Endometriosis long term require an average of around about roughly 4–6% which is between say 40-60mg of progesterone, varying of course, but again it depends on how the body uses it.

And this is where charting is very important. Because these women work at high stress levels and have a background of pulling on the corticosteroid pathway, they tend to use every bit of the 4-6% without ever running the risk of overdosing.

I never ever ridicule a woman for her choice of treatment. A woman will choose a treatment which is right for her at the time, regardless. If she finds me, then this is where she is meant to be. But I do encourage women to do their research and to look at options and to do it diligently and ask for guidance.

Tubal Ligation
What is a Tubal Ligation?

It is the surgical procedure known as surgical sterilisation in which the fallopian tubes are cut and tied. There are several techniques of Tubal Ligation. The fallopian tubes may be cut & tied, pinched closed by the use of plastic rings or clips, or severed using laser treatment which 'burns' tube endings.

A Tubal Ligation prevents fertility because the egg released from your ovaries during ovulation cannot travel down the fallopian tubes to be fertilised by the man's sperm.

Will a Tubal Ligation affect my hormones?

Usually "yes", it's just a matter of when. I have spoken with a number of women who reported a variety of problems subsequent to a Tubal Ligation. Irregular, heavy menstrual bleeding, for example, that has, on occasions, resulted in a Hysterectomy.

These women reported increased period pain, longer periods, pain during intercourse, severe PMS. Even Endometriosis has been known to occur after "surgical sterilisation".

These women post Tubal Ligation often go into early menopause, or experience perimenopausal problems such as Hot Flushes, sleep disturbances, anxiety attacks and all the estrogen dominant symptoms that are commonly listed (due to decreased progesterone output by the ovaries).

Of the women who contacted NPAN, I have observed some common characteristics. Overall, these women reported hormone imbalance 6-7 years after their Tubal Ligation. However, occasionally, a woman reported insidious side-effects virtually the day after she had surgery.

I have listened and empathised with many women who, soon after their tubal ligation surgery, abruptly entered menopause. The reason why women suffer hormonal imbalances is unclear. Perhaps blood supply to the ovaries has been interfered with, or severed, which compromised the performance of the ovaries. Perhaps the messages from the brain to the ovaries is more complex than is understood. The mind-body correlation cannot be understated here.

Some women do escape significant hormonal problems while others experience extreme perimenopausal or menopausal symptoms. The degree of hormonal problems is dependent upon the damage to the ovarian blood supply and the state of the woman's health in general. The production of progesterone by the ovaries is likely to be compromised dramatically.

Additionally, estrogen may also be compromised as it needs a greater supply of oxygen for the many steps necessary in its synthesis by the ovary. Progesterone output, on the other hand, may be dramatically reduced even though you can continue to ovulate. (Many women are not ovulating regularly regardless).

In other words, the quantity and quality of progesterone is not what it once was, and a ratio imbalance between these two hormone results. You may be short on both hormones, but there is a greater likelihood that your progesterone levels will be lower than that of estrogen, accounting for estrogen dominant symptoms that arise subsequent to a Tubal Ligation.

After a Tubal Ligation, women often enter the circuit of 'doctor hopping' in search of answers for their failing health.

They cannot put their finger on any particular cause, and are subsequently fobbed off with demeaning comments like, "That's just the way it is", "You're getting older", "Just get an interest", "It's all in your head", "Just learn to live with it". Round and round in circles they go.

These poor women - the casualties of Tubal Ligations - suffer in silence and isolation because they ought to be healthy. They look healthy enough, or rather tests proved unremarkable. Yet, incredibly, they're all experiencing severe menopausal and perimenopausal symptoms, minus any semblance of sympathy or recognition by the medical fraternity.

Often they are told they are too young for menopause and that it can't possibly be linked.

So, what are these poor women to think? That they are hypochondriacs? It's all a state of their confused mind? Undiagnosed and untreated for years on end, they arrive at our doorstep very angry and disillusioned.

Often casualties of medical misrepresentation or medical neglect because the doctors simply failed to recognise the connection between Tubal Ligation and the presentation of gynecological and psychological problems that, in some case, do arise as a result of surgery.

Ironically, women who opt for a Tubal Ligation, believing it to be an easy form of sterilisation, often end up with a Hysterectomy which really negates the reason why they chose a Tubal Ligation in the first place. Because it's touted as a relatively risk-free, permanent form of contraception.

Many women feel very angered, ripped off and downright annoyed when they make the connection between their health problems and that particular surgery. The resultant complications to their health and emotional wellbeing is understated.

These women claim, time and time again that, had they been given more information, they certainly would not have journeyed down the path of a Tubal Ligation. They also feel that had they known how it was going to affect their hormonal balance and *in many cases libido*, then perhaps they would have looked at other forms of contraception.

Most women agree they would have suggested their husbands or partner undergo a vasectomy rather than put up with the havoc hormone imbalance is now having on their wellbeing and their marriage/relationship. Contrary to what Health Professionals may allow men to believe or the myths surround Vasectomies, men will continue to ejaculate (minus the sperm which is still produced and reabsorbed) and will not become impotent or cause premature ejaculation. Their libido's will not wane as they will still produce testosterone. This surgery is a relatively simple procedure and can be

315

performed under a local anaesthetic if elected this may be done in the Doctor's surgery. There are less reported post operative complications than with women undertaking sterilisation (Tubal Ligation) and certainly less hormonal disruption. Healing is quick and pain and discomfort is temporary (not a lifetime) as they would have us believe. A lot of men have huge fears (pain and the psychological impact on their sexual performance around sterilisation). So many women become angered with their partners for even refusing to consider this option and find the least line of resistance by taking it upon themselves to undergo Tubal Ligation. Contraception is a joint responsibility and certainly one that should be looked at more fairly, weighing up the pros and cons. Ultimately Tubal Ligation may have an impact on their sexual relationship, as often reported by women who have experienced lowered libido post Tubal Ligation, so perhaps men should become more informed to the possible consequences involved with this procedure to help and support the women they love. Furthermore Vasectomies have been successfully reversed with more success than with Tubal Ligations if a couple wishes to try for more children.

Since my first released book, so many women have written and thanked me for enlightening them of other women's Tubal Ligation regrets and have gladly not undergone this procedure. Instead their husbands having a Vasectomy.

How can the problems after Tubal Ligation be treated? Can progesterone help?

It certainly can. Largely because progesterone can oppose estrogen dominant symptoms such as PMS, pelvic congestion, bowel problems, mood swings, irritability, sleep disturbance, depression, generally all those disruptive health concerns associated with hormonal imbalance.

The reality, however, may be that the ovaries are becoming dysfunctional. Progesterone also helps modulate and balance the estrogen fluctuations and surges occurring as a result of ovarian failure due to the diminished blood supply and tissue scarring around the ovaries.

However, the hormonal output from the ovaries is similar to that found typical to a woman in her late forties who is approaching menopause. This ultimately means you may need hormone replacement therapy. It is advisable that you assess your estrogen, progesterone, testosterone and DHEA levels on a regular basis, particularly if progesterone alone is not resolving your symptoms (eg lowered libido).

Some women may in fact require a little bit of natural estrogen and natural testosterone replacement therapy. It pays to check your levels with saliva assays and blood profile.

Because these post Tubal Ligation women can enter menopause earlier than nature intended, it is recommended you schedule yourself in for bone mineral density (BMD) test to assess the state of your bones. See if you are predisposed to Osteoporosis.

If I reverse my Tubal Ligation, will my symptoms go away?

No, unfortunately not. Sterilisation by Tubal Ligation is as good as permanent. The surgical interruption to the blood supply that damages the ovaries is irreversible.

Even if surgeons could microscopically re-establish the blood flow to this area, it is not going to reverse the situation. Your symptoms will not disappear without addressing the resultant hormone imbalance.

I have had two cases in the past 2 years where women were moderately symptom free from their Tubal Ligation performed years ago and have reversals for reproductive purposes. Both successfully conceived however still ended up in my lounge room with toddlers and an earlier than usual list of pre menopausal symptoms and problems.

In my consultancy work and my observation over the years is that the women who had undergone early surgical techniques 10-15 years ago have gained better mileage out of there ovaries (7-10 years) than the women who have undergone sterilisation in the last 5-6 years. I question that this may be because they were exposed to less endocrine disruption, or was the formative techniques used 15 years ago less traumatic and less disruptive to ovarian blood supply?

Does Tubal Ligation work for any particular woman?

Based on observation, **women who have a history of heavy bleeding or Fibroids, even Endometriosis, PMS and nasty Postnatal Depression should take their existing hormone imbalance into consideration when considering a Tubal Ligation.**

Furthermore, I have observed women with a history of heavy periods discovered that their Tubal Ligation often increased their problems and a Hysterectomy was necessary to treat such a severe haemorrhaging.

Tubal Ligations do not sort out hormonal problems. It is a procedure performed to prevent pregnancy, and provide a permanent form of contraception.

Any woman that has a history of hormone imbalance and associated gynecological problems should consider alternative options for contraception such as suggesting her partner undergo a Vasectomy instead. I remind here that this will not render him impotent or affect his libido (as a Tubal Ligation may effect a woman), erectile function or his ability to ejaculate (minus sperm).

Memory Loss / Mental Faculty

I'm having memory loss and I can't concentrate, focus and recall. Will progesterone help?

Diminished mental acuity with underlying depression, anxiety and subsequent sleep deprivation is a tremendous concern of women who contact myself at the Natural Progesterone Advisory Network.

Their inability to concentrate, focus and recall, especially women in high profile jobs and demanding careers (teachers, nurses, IT consultants, company and corporate executives, etc.), triggers alarm bells that things are definitely not as they should be.

These symptoms, experienced by women of all ages, are all correctable with progesterone, at least in cases that tend to be associated with hormone imbalance.

Progesterone clears foggy thinking, helps you sleep better, clears the confusion in your head, helps you collect your thoughts, and think more clearly and rationally. It likewise relieves agitation and the tendency to over-react. It basically calms the brain down and assists in copper and zinc balance. The peripheral distractions, too many things going on in your head, can be associated with these imbalances especially before menstruation when you could murder, yell or cry. Progesterone has a calming effect on the brains chemistry allowing clarity of thought and focus to return.

It's usually within two months of using progesterone that women make comments such as, "My fuzzy head has cleared", "I can think clearer", "I'm not as forgetful", "My memory has improved" or "I'm no longer over-reacting". I can articulate again and make precise practical and logical decisions. Thus bringing order and control back into their lives again.

Very few women take progesterone solely to treat foggy thinking or memory loss. Rather, they find relief of these common but accepted complaints very quickly once starting progesterone therapy for hormone imbalance. These wonderful 'benefits' result after commencing progesterone therapy. It also allows women to look at there problems more logically and get into the too hard basket with a more practical approach.

Musculoskeletal
Will progesterone help with my arthritic problems?

At NPAN I have observed that many women experience increased intensity of joint and muscle pain at some stage of their progesterone therapy.

One such case is myself, I experienced significant discomfort around the seventh month. In those early days when I understood very little about the side effects of progesterone therapy, I went racing off to my rheumatologist who wanted to put me on cortisone-based anti-inflammatory drugs which would have counteracted progesterone benefits long term and perhaps impaired my hormonal health.

I now believe, based on women's input, that *the incidence, or exacerbation of joint and muscle pain while taking progesterone is a result of receptor activity (a wake up which is often delayed) in those areas.* And when women complain of this insidious yet common theme, I encourage them to bear with it because it is an experience a good many women connected to NPAN have gone through.

It occurs on different levels at various stages (7-8 months average), however, more importantly, the incidence of pain and increased discomfort does not appear to be suggestive of progressive degeneration of any pre-existing disease.

Rather, I have to conclude based on our experiences that it's an indication cell receptors are waking up; in most cases, a sign the body is responding favourably.

Many women with arthritic or inflammatory problems find, after about 2 years on progesterone, they are reporting significant joint and muscular mobility, and their pain has dramatically reduced, allowing them to resume physical activities that were once restrictive or beyond them. Many have reported remission of their arthritis with no further progression 3 years on.

There seems to be a very fine line between stress, diet, nutrition, lifestyle and hormone balancing. As in my situation, I know the minute I am out of balance because I experiences intense, deep right hip pain and my index finger becomes arthritic, painful, and loses mobility. This can be corrected within 36 hours of re-balancing my hormone profile. Adding progesterone on the joint also helps.

Only one joint is now effected by arthritis where prior to progesterone therapy all my joints were involved, causing swelling and disfigurement of all my knuckles. My finger joints are no longer 'shiny'. I have returned to knitting and fine embroidery these past 8 years whereas before progesterone therapy even weeding the garden created excruciating pain.

I believe progesterone has had a huge impact on my auto-immune system at various levels, and likewise observed the dramatic improvement in her hearing (having 50% loss in both ears from a childhood virus). I occasionally resort to my hearing aids particularly following flying which affects my hearing dramatically. My son tells me to wear them more often as I tend to speak very loud (mother's love to be heard regardless and kids hate to listen).

CHAPTER 15

Charting Recommendations and Guidelines for Journal Keeping

- *Is it important to keep a chart?*
- *Subtle Changes*
- *Share your charts with your doctor*
- *Which Chart Suits You?*
- *Monthly Score Sheet to Determine Progress / Effectiveness of Progesterone Usage*
- *Suggested Dose Guideline for Monthly Score Sheet*
- *How to interpret your score and use it to Guide your progesterone dosage requirements*
- *The importance of this chart*
- *How to Interact*
- *Health Observation Calendar for Monitoring Hormone Balance*
- *Calendar-style Notation of Symptoms*
- *Quick Tick Chart - Spreadsheet*

- *How to approach your Charting*
- *Addressing Questions to Assess your progress*
- *Gynecological Symptoms*
- *Menstrual Cycles*
- *Skin & Hair & Ears*
- *Breasts*
- *On-going Chronic Conditions, Ears Nose and Throat (including Auto Immune)*
- *Pain Disorders*
- *Reproductive*
- *PMS*
- *Muscular-Skeletal*
- *Other Pain*
- *Pain Considerations*
- *Bladder*
- *Gastrointestinal*
- *Sleep Patterns*
- *Sex/Libido*
- *Metabolic*
- *Cardio Vascular*
- *Fertility*
- *Muscular, Skeletal & Nerves*
- *Vision*
- *Concentration Memory Performance*
- *Headaches*
- *Emotional WellBeing*
- *A time for reflection*
- *Taking control*

Is it important to keep a chart?

This is entirely up to you. I suggest that you do keep your own chart to better understand how your body functions and to tune into your needs. Charts help you become aware of the day to day changes in your body. They help you interpret symptoms that may be relevant to your hormonal balance and general well-being. Symptom relief is an important barometer in your hormonal well-being, and acts as a guide to using the least amount of progesterone required to maintain balance.

When you first begin natural progesterone therapy, it's always advisable to go through the list of estrogen dominant symptoms and mark off what applies to you and date it. Add to this list anything that is unusual or is idiosyncratic to your hormonal profile. Don't, whatever you do, judge what you put down believing it to be totally irrelevant. Write it down anyway because it's guaranteed somewhere along the track your 'peculiar' symptom may actually correlate with other women's stories of hormonal imbalance. Women become so conditioned to discounting themselves and undermining their problems, especially if they have been long-standing. We are told to ignore ourselves and get on with it! Not so, don't trivialise!

Make no mistake, you are not alone in this struggle with this new emerging condition - estrogen dominance. Women who approach my Network seeking help are invariably surprised to learn that their constellation of symptoms have absolute relevance within the context of determining and balancing estrogen dominance. Comments like "I can relate to that" or "the same thing happens to me" tells me at NPAN that women out there continue to suffer in silence, year in, year out, unable to compare and validate their experiences with other women.

NPAN is essentially about empowering women so each can, in time, resurrect herself from the 'hormonal' abyss she finds herself. And in order to do this, she needs to get in tune with her own hormonal persona so to speak.

For your convenience I have listed all these aspects of your overall health in sections. Be aware of them. You may find your own amongst these to include in your charts. These questions below make you aware of your own body, particularly before using progesterone, and how you are responding once you've started using progesterone.

This is an on-going journey, and things will change in your body, over months and over years. Often women abandon progesterone when they are well again. Nearing 8 years of my work I often get a phone call from the women stating they are feeling second hand again. The first question I ask is 'are you still on progesterone?' the answer invariably is 'no'. I then ask why? 'Oh, I didn't think I needed it anymore'. My comment is 'I think you have answered that for yourself as you wouldn't be ringing me'. They agree. I then say 'why on earth would you give up something, a natural hormone your body needs, with multifactorial purposes that you continue to reap the years of benefits from, not to mention protection from our severe exposure to estrogens in our environment, stressful lifestyles and poor eating habits. And why would you jeopardise your possibility of maintaining healthy bones'.

I explain that this is a journey, not a quick fix and combined with nutrition will provide enormous rewards, not to mention slowing down aging skin and tell tale signs.

My belief is least is best and I tend to agree with the Late Dr John Lee - review of 99.

Subtle Changes

To become aware of changes over a period of months, you need to ask yourself the questions below, or at least those that apply to your condition. Month to month, you probably won't realise the subtle changes. It's only when you reflect over a period of 12 months that you realise you have found alleviation from so many minor symptoms. Symptoms that add up to a significant health problem when left untreated.

Along with hundreds of other women, I have learned to identify with the use of charts when my hormones are imbalanced. Particularly being post Hysterectomy (now 8 years in January 2004) with surgically induced menopause. My hormone imbalance triggers uncharacteristic behaviour leading to aggression or even depression. My body retains fluid, particularly around the ankles. I use to suffer gastric pain and cramps in the stomach, coupled with bowel irregularity. An early warning to hormone imbalance in the earlier years, less now is deep right hip pain that constantly aches, an arthritic finger that flared, and bladder sensitivity which can lead to Cystitis. Basically, I learnt to track my symptoms with the use of a chart to help me immediately identify and address estrogen dominance. Over the years of awareness and formative years of charting I now recognise triggers and symptoms and can heed immediately to take control before imbalances get out of hand.

A case comes to mind of another woman who told us how she's learnt to recognise when she's heading towards estrogen dominance. Acne, fluid retention, nasal congestion, sinusitis, and headaches tend to be her first indicators. Mary was diagnosed with an enlarged thyroid and yet tests proved normal. Following 18 months of progesterone supplementation, her thyroid is back to normal. But, interestingly, her *neck size changes, indicating thyroid interference when she has allowed estrogen dominance symptoms to go unaddressed.* It just goes to show you how important charting is in the bigger picture. Mary wouldn't have recognised these subtle changes as being associated with estrogen dominance had she not tracked her progress.

Julie, however, has very few indications of estrogen dominance other than a sense of apprehension. An inability to cope and interact harmoniously with her surroundings and her loved ones that, if left unchecked, can manifest as panic attacks, withdrawal into herself, dark feelings of doom and gloom, and apathy.

Joan's first sign is disturbances in her sleeping pattern indicating more progesterone and going back to basic correctional principles. Joan has been on her progesterone 5 years and was too scared to use more than 16mg, by her Doctor's advice. She is 68 years of age by the way.

After reading my book she realised she was not reaping the full benefits and has become more confident to add more in times of stress (she is in an unhappy relationship) and now realises she won't overdose herself. She returns to her 16-20mg once on track.

Therefore, not surprisingly, NPAN strongly urges women to keep charts. **Learn how to monitor your health to better identify key elements to your predominant symptoms, and learn to monitor the signals of the start of estrogen dominance.** Use your charts to identify your own personal formula for quick correction. I tackle imbalances by increasing my progesterone and estriol creams vaginally, using a small amount of testosterone, addressing my stress, nutritional and diet plan, particularly phytoestrogens, and incorporating liver cleansing principles. Mary, like Julie, ups her progesterone dosage that month, looks at reducing her refined sugars and stress levels, increases her phytoestrogens to tone down her estrogen receptors, and revisits her charts to determine patterns and triggers.

My point here is, simply, *imbalances can occur at any time, but once you set-up a hormone 'template' by charting for the initial 7 months, you have the blueprint that you can always refer back to.* Many women are actually staggered at the value of charting when they may need to revisit them 2-3 years down the track. And it may only take a small adjustment to get themselves back in balance ... because they already have the roadmap! *Whilst many of the symptoms may never reoccur because progesterone has actually corrected the problem, there will always be a persistent 'weakness' that you will, in time, come to see is idiosyncratic to you.* That can be an indicator you need to start listening to your body, and implementing whatever strategies are required to maintain continued health.

Through these charts you will learn that symptoms can be quite insidious. They creep up undetected and are easily overlooked, particularly if a woman is out of balance or preoccupied. If you understand these patterns and realise the connection, you can quickly get on top of it. Take action to correct the problems before they compound.

This is particularly true for women who suffer joint pain, arthritis, Fibromyalgia, hypothyroidism (low thyroid function), high blood pressure or bladder problems, sinusitis, and headaches. They tend to be unaware their symptoms all fit together like a jigsaw puzzle.

To appreciate the benefits of progesterone and to fully recognise the positive effects, you have to stay on the cream and monitor your progress, long term. If you do this, then results can be truly astounding. *What you end up with is a charted record of your body's rhythms; in itself a template for future references.*

Share your charts with your doctor

Your doctor will appreciate your efforts because he can use the data you have meticulously collected to better assess which way he would like to go with treatment and monitoring. Similarly, your charts will help him better understand progesterone, how it is all interrelated, and that all these years you weren't imagining things. Your symptoms were very real.

By charting and gaining confidence about your own body, the vibration level at which you deliver your information to your doctor is such that it comes across with conviction.

Even if he says it is a placebo (an imagined response) you can retort, "Well it's a damn good placebo!" Hopefully, by this stage of your journey into improved health, you won't feel the need to storm out of his surgery, to justify, or discount your needs. If, however, your GP fails in his duty to appreciate and respect your physical and psychological well-being, then perhaps it's time to seek out a more understanding doctor.

By taking these charts to your doctor, he will be able to assess - hopefully with your active involvement - which way he'd like to go with on-going treatment and monitoring. Particularly when it comes to other medications that you may be taking which could require adjustments due to positive responses of progesterone. An example of this would be women on blood pressure tablets. Often women find they require less simply because their blood pressure has reduced after using progesterone.

This will also help him to understand progesterone, how it's all interrelated, that progesterone is multifactorial, and that all these things you have been complaining about over the years were not imagined, nor were you the hypochondriac that you may have been led to believe.

You might want to visit the section on 'Approaching Your Doctor' (chapter 7).

Please refer to Chart samples off the website www.npan.com.au (you can also print them) or use your own and decide which one to use.

Which Chart Suits You?

Monthly Score Sheet to Determine Progress / Effectiveness of Progesterone Usage

Charting should be conducted monthly to assess reduction / flare-up of symptoms. Your monthly score should be reducing each month. I commonly use a 7 month time frame as a fair gauge to work in, although most symptoms will start to disappear around 4 months if it's a progesterone deficiency / estrogen dominance problem. *If some symptoms persist you would need to look at possible physiological cause other than hormonal,* i.e., depression that is not alleviated by progesterone.

If your score is not reducing over 4-7 months, it indicates that your progesterone cream is not being assimilated by the body effectively. This can be for various reasons (see also 'Cream Usage & Guidelines' chapter 9).

Most women who are estrogen dominant present with a score average between 26-36 (out of a possible 45). And within 4-7 months I have observed most women's total score drops to under <10, after following my suggested guidelines. Nonetheless, it's important you maintain yours charts for a minimum of 7 months, at which time stability would have been established.

Suggested Dose Guideline for Monthly Score Sheet

How to interpret your score and use it to Guide your progesterone dosage requirements

High Score:	(dosage initially >10% or 100mg)
Moderate - High Score:	(dosage between 4%-6% or 40-60mg)
Moderate Score:	(dosage between 3%-4% or 30-40mg)
Low Score:	(dosage between 1%-2% or 16-20mg)

You may need to increase slightly yourself. Always try an extra 10mg and assess in 36 hours. Before increasing more. You need to trust your intuition and be confident.

The Importance of this Chart - Estrogen dominance/Progesterone deficiency

This score sheet determines estrogen dominance progesterone deficiency. It is perhaps the most important chart of all and this is the one I refer to the most in determining your dose requirements according to your score, and progress. For this reason this score sheet appears here and also in the back of the books.

This score sheet will:

- Help you assess your response to dose adjustments
- Help you acertain your physiological progesterone dose requirements where you remain asymptomatic
- Help you to recognise insidious problems reimerging so you can activate proticols and strategies to address
- Will guide you in recognising Estrogen Dominance Wake Up Crisis
- Give you an appreciation of your improvement over time
- Teach you to become 'tuned in' to your hormonal health and wellbeing
- Assist you in distinguishing hormone problems, as opposed to other health issues
- Help you recognise triggers
- Will be a template for your progesterone journey

Charts can be printed off websites: www.npan.com.au
or www.natural-progesterone-advisory-network.us

MONTHLY SCORE SHEET TO DETERMINE
PROGRESS / EFFECTIVENESS OF PROGESTERONE USAGE

**Symptoms of Oestrogen dominance / Progesterone deficiency
for a MENSTRUATING woman**

Below is a list of the most common symptoms, please rate them as follows:

0 = Never;   1 = Rarely;   2 = Occasionally;   3 = Frequently or daily

Symptom	MONTH 1 Date:.............. Rating Pre Menses	Post	MONTH 2 Date:.............. Rating Pre Menses	Post	MONTH 3 Date:.............. Rating Pre Menses	Post	MONTH 4 Date:.............. Rating Pre Menses	Post
Heavy &/or irregular periods								
Fatigue or lack of energy								
Breast swelling / tenderness								
Loss of libido (sex drive)								
Weight gain-unexplained								
Bloating or fluid retention								
Generalised aches & pains								
Headaches/Migraines								
Sleep disturbance								
Hot flushes								
Night sweats								
Irritability or mood swings								
Confusion / disorientation								
Lack of self esteem								
Craving for sweets								
TOTAL SCORE								

Other symptoms, please tick any that you experience:

☐ Inability to lose weight
☐ Panic attacks / palpitations
☐ Crying for no reason
☐ Alienation or guilt
☐ Thrush
☐ Cold hands & feet
☐ Cold buttocks
☐ Foggy thinking / vagueness
☐ Irritated eyes – dry/gritty
☐ Acne Rosacea / skin problems
☐ Urinary tract infection/stress incontinence
☐ Breast Cysts / lumps, ropiness

☐ Allergy symptoms, ie asthma, hives/rashes, sinusitus
☐ Anxiety
☐ Memory loss
☐ Depression
☐ Mouth ulcers
☐ Hair loss / thinning
☐ Facial hair (upper lip, chin)
☐ Excess body hair
☐ Restless Leg Syndrome
☐ Inability to orgasm
☐ Vaginal dryness / pimples

NATURAL PROGESTERONE ADVISORY NETWORK (NPAN)©

MONTHLY SCORE SHEET TO DETERMINE
PROGRESS / EFFECTIVENESS OF PROGESTERONE USAGE

Symptoms of Oestrogen dominance / Progesterone deficiency for a NON MENSTRUATING woman

Below is a list of the most common symptoms, please rate them as follows:

0 = Never;   1 = Rarely;   2 = Occasionally;   3 = Frequently or daily

Symptom	MONTH 1 Date:	MONTH 2 Date:	MONTH 3 Date:	MONTH 4 Date: ....
	Rating	Rating	Rating	Rating
Fatigue or lack of energy				
Breast swelling / tenderness				
Loss of libido (sex drive)				
Weight gain-unexplained				
Bloating or fluid retention				
Generalised aches & pains				
Headaches/Migraines				
Sleep disturbance				
Hot flushes				
Night sweats				
Irritability or mood swings				
Confusion / disorientation				
Lack of self esteem				
Craving for sweets				
TOTAL SCORE				

Other symptoms, please tick any that you experience:

- ❏ Inability to lose weight
- ❏ Panic attacks / palpitations
- ❏ Crying for no reason
- ❏ Alienation or guilt
- ❏ Thrush
- ❏ Cold hands & feet
- ❏ Cold buttocks
- ❏ Foggy thinking / vagueness
- ❏ Irritated eyes – dry/gritty
- ❏ Rosacea, pimples
- ❏ Urinary tract infection/stress incontinence
- ❏ Breast Cysts

- ❏ Allergy symptoms, ie asthma, hives/rashes, sinusitus
- ❏ Anxiety
- ❏ Memory loss
- ❏ Depression
- ❏ Mouth ulcers
- ❏ Hair loss / thinning
- ❏ Facial hair (upper lip, chin)
- ❏ Excess body hair
- ❏ Restless Leg Syndrome
- ❏ Inability to orgasm
- ❏ Vaginal dryness, spotting

NATURAL PROGESTERONE ADVISORY NETWORK (NPAN)

Health Observation Calendar for Monitoring Hormone Balance

This chart suits the methodical person who likes to record keep in symbols, and who is very involved in her health agenda. It probably wouldn't suit the lady with a busy lifestyle who's on the go. (Download from www.npan.com.au)

Calendar-style Notation of Symptoms

If you are a woman looking to record 'unusual' symptoms and may not be recording in-depth details, this chart gives you a guideline of where / what may be happening at certain times of the month. The charts can then be used as a comparison, month to month. Patterns can be determined using this method. It's always important to note dosage of cream on all charts, to correlate dosage versus symptom relief.

(Download from www.npan.com.au)

Quick Tick Chart - Spreadsheet

This is a very popular chart because it's so user-friendly. All you need to do is tick the appropriate columns each day as they apply. It doesn't require lengthy reporting, just helps you acknowledge how you're feeling, and what's going on. Perfect to stick on your refrigerator.

(Download from www.npan.com.au or use chart on page 419)

How to approach your Charting

I have already provided you with a ideas of charts and pointed out the benefits of each style. Now, for your convenience, I pull together all the aspects of your overall health in sections so that you can be aware of them. I present you with the questions that you may wish to ask yourself, month to month, to gauge how progesterone is influencing your particular problem and life. Choose the sections and questions that apply to you. Many of these questions have been completed from my own consultancy (phone and in person) profile techniques used invaluably for personal assessment. You can apply these to yourself. Addressing questions to assess your progress.

Addressing Questions to Assess your progress
Gynecological Symptoms

- Is there incidence of, or changes in Thrush, vaginal irritation, itchiness?
- Has vaginal lubrication improved?
- Is there evidence of a discharge? Note type, colour, odour. Any changes?
- Is sex less painful?
- Is vaginal tissue strengthening, not feeling as dry and fragile with intercourse?

- Is pelvic comfort improved overall, i.e., no dragging or bearing down feeling or back ache, less restricted?
- With hyperplasia, has the next Pap smear result become normal (are the cells showing positive normalisation after a few months on progesterone)?
- Has vulva acne disappeared (do not confuse with herpes)?
- Is sexual libido (sex drive) fluctuating or stabilising or improving?

Menstrual Cycles

- Have your periods improved?
- Are your cycles regular? Or are they wandering?
- How long do your cycles go for? What is normal for you?
- What sort of menstrual cycles do you experience (heavy, light)?
- Is there a pattern of bleeding, i.e., spotting, heavy, light, stop/start. Are you having in-between periods?
- Are there clots? How often, small or large? With every period?
- Is there pain, cramping, nausea or bowel irritability with your period, prior to, or both? What sort of pain is it duration/location?)
- With Fibroids, have they shrunk (by scan results), is there less haemorrhaging or less bleeding and clotting?

Skin & Hair & Ears

- Have you observed changes in your skin, i.e., texture, blemishes, unusual growth/lesions (skin tags), pimples, dryness or scarring, is there evidence of psoriasis or less psoriasis? Are these problems lessening?
- Does your skin feel creepy, crawly, itchy, the feeling of mites or bugs running all over? If so, is this diminishing?
- Is your complexion clear or muddy?
- Are there black rings under your eyes?
- Is there a tiredness about your skin and/or dehydrated?
- Is skin elasticity and vitality improving?
- Does your moisturiser sit on the surface and not soak in readily? Or is absorption improving?
- Does your skin appear full of fluid, dimply?
- Is there acne? Is it cyclic? All over or specifically facial 'T' zone?
- Is your head dry, scaly, do you suffer from dandruff? Do you have dry limp hair, greasy hair, tight feeling in skull?
- Has your hair stopped falling out or are you losing more? Is your hair volume thickening?

- Is your skin overall more subtle and hydrated, less scaly?
- Is your skin less prone to bruising or tearing?
- Do you have any body rashes? If you have shingles or impetigo is it improving? Is the pain lessening?
- Are your wrinkles softening?
- Are your broken face capillaries improving?
- If you have, has it improved?
- Is a butterfly mask appearing?
- Are your ears less itchy? Sensations of ringing or foreign bodies lessened?
- Have you noticed an increase in body and facial hair or a decrease of growth?
- Has pubic hair loss lessened and is it increasing in volume?
- Is there a noticeable difference in the amount of grey hair appearing?

Breasts

- Are the breasts less lumpy?
- Have lumps gone altogether? Are fibrocysts diminishing in size & discomfort?
- Is the breast tissue softening and more subtle?
- Are the nipples more sensitive and not so itchy, less tenderness, less swelling, less fullness, less pain, and not burning as much?
- Is there less breast engorgement overall?
- Monitor the presence of hairs around the areola.

On-going Chronic Conditions, Ears Nose and Throat (including Auto Immune)

- Any sign of congestion, phlegmy or dry throat? Is it cyclic?
- Is there any associated teeth or facial pain? Is it cyclic?
- Are you experiencing flu-like symptoms, blocked ears & nose, cranial pressure, aching eyes? Are symptoms frequent, and do they follow a pattern? Any improvement noted?
- Has sinus conditions improved? Is there less congestion and pain? Is it pronounced prior to period?
- Have your allergy symptoms improved or gotten worse?
- Any inflammation present such as arthritis, joint & muscle pain or burning? Is there an obvious change to the patterns, duration, intensity?
- Have you recently been diagnosed with an auto immune disorder? Lupus, for example. Is it in remission or has it accelerated?

- Have you had less need of Ventolin and Asthma drugs? Is your Asthma problem improving? Is it more predominant just prior to periods?

Pain Disorders
Reproductive

- Is there pain on ovulation?
- Is there pain in the region of your ovaries, i.e., spasmodic, constant, cyclic? Type and intensity? Any phantom pain after ovaries that have been removed?
- Any pain in the back area or in either groin?
- Any pain present prior, during, or after your period?
- Less bearing down feeling? Less muscle spasms?
- Any pain associated with sexual intercourse? Improvement with different positions?

PMS

- Is this improving? Have you less sugar cravings?
- Are you less irritable, less emotional, less out of control?
- Are you retaining more fluid or less?

Muscular-Skeletal

- If you have arthritis has the pain improved?
- Are you suffering a chronic pain condition such as Fibromyalgia that has improved?
- Increased joint pain or less?
- Increased muscle pain or less? Is it worse morning or night, or following activity?
- Has your sciatica or hip pain improved?
- Has back pain improved?
- Are your legs and feet less achy, particularly your feet in the morning?
- Are your heels less tender or less burning sensation?
- Are your knees less painful?
- Restless leg syndrome improving?

Other Pain

- Are aches and pains more obvious at certain times of the month or are they all the time?
- Have your migraines / headaches improved? Less intense or a change in character?
- Chronic depression can masquerade as a pain disorder.

Pain Considerations

- Is your pain threshold improving, meaning are you able to tolerate pain at higher levels?
- Is the nature of your pain changing in character / location / intensity?
- Are you finding you're able to cope and are less stressed, your body more relaxed?
- Is your mental attitude towards your pain strengthening?
- Are you using less analgesia to control pain?

Bladder

- Are you going to the toilet more or less frequently?
- Is there better bladder tone and are your able to empty your bladder more completely?
- Is there more bladder control and less incontinence?
- Is the bladder able to hold more fluid?
- Is there less occurrence of bladder infections or burning sensations? Does your bladder feel less sensitive?
- Is the urine colour changing, less concentrated? Has the odour changed?

Gastrointestinal

- Have your gastrointestinal tract symptoms improved (digestion & elimination)?
- Are there less stomach digestion problems, wind, burping, heartburn, bloating, indigestion and less sugar cravings?
- Have your bowel movements become regular, less constipation, less diarrhoea? Are these patterns cyclic or diet and stress related?
- Is your elimination process moving through the bowel much quicker and have your bowel patterns changed for the better?
- Is there less bloating and stomach distension, less discomfort on eating?
- Are you naturally choosing to eat more whole and healthy foods?
- Are you experiencing any nausea or has it lessened?
- Is there an improvement if you are suffering from Colitis, Irritable Bowel Syndrome, Crohn's Disease, or other related conditions?

Sleep Patterns

- Do you have a better quality of sleep (deeper, more revitalising)?
- Do you have better sleep overall (more relaxing)?
- Are you waking less or more? Can you go to sleep faster?

- Do you feel rested on waking or do you feel worse?
- Are you less tired?
- Are you having better dreams?
- Are you getting up to go to the toilet less frequently during the night?
- Are your patterns of wakefulness settling?
- If you wake up, are you less anxious or preoccupied with worry? Are you experiencing less obsessional thought patterns and/or anxiety panic attacks?
- Do you have the need to nap in the day? What time?
- Are your night sweats less severe, and reducing in time, duration, and occurrence?
- Are you less over-heated at night time? Is your body odour (sweat) changing?

Sex/Libido

- Do you find yourself anticipating sexual intimacy? Is your libido improving?
- Are you finding yourself preoccupied with thoughts of sex?
- Is sexual intercourse less painful and more enjoyable?
- Are your orgasms improving in intensity?
- Is your sexual satisfaction greater?
- Is your emotional intimacy improving?
- Have your vaginal secretions altered in odour and texture?
- Do you have less vaginal dryness, better lubrication?
- Are your sexual needs changing?
- Are you experiencing erotic / colourful dreams?

Metabolic

- Any weight loss or weight gain? Where?
- Are you less cold this month, particularly hands and feet, even buttocks?
- Is your body over-heating? Or is your body temperature more regulated?
- Are you aware that your metabolism has increased (energy)?
- Have you got the ability to burn energy better (possible weight loss)?
- Has your blood picture, your electrolyte profile improved, (e.g. increased B12, stabilised blood sugar, improved iron readings)?
- Have you more even levels of energy, rather than bursts of energy followed by exhaustion?
- Are you looking for less sugar fixes, not relying on sugar for quick energy?
- Do you have less need of stimulants for energy, such as coffee, fast-foods, refined sugars, fizzy drinks?
- Are there signs that your liver and adrenal function are improving with evidence of more efficient elimination of body waste and toxins through bowel, bladder and skin?

Cardio Vascular

- Are your varicose veins throbbing as much?
- Has your blood pressure improved or normalised?
- Have you had any incidents of vertigo, fainting spells, or dizziness?
- Are you less fluid retentive, particularly in the hands, legs, ankles, are your rings fitting better?
- Are your extremities warmer (feet & hands including cold buttocks) indicating better circulation?
- Have you had less headaches?
- Less palpitations?
- Less Hot Flushes/night sweats?

Fertility

- Are you aware that you have ovulated this month?
- Are the follicle stimulating hormone (FSH) and luteinizing hormone (LH) readings within normal range?
- Do you have fertile mucus (is there a presence of a clear, egg-white like, stretchy vaginal discharge, appearing around the middle of your cycle)?
- Is there a return of regular cycles? Is there a pattern emerging?
- Have you conceived? If there's a possibility, please do NOT suddenly come off your cream. Get a test to confirm your condition.

Muscular, Skeletal & Nerves

- Are your overall general aches and pains improving?
- Is your head and neck less tense? Souls of feet less tender?
- Are muscle spasms, cramps, 'busy legs' particularly at night time lessening?
- Are your joints more mobile, flexible? Less arthritic evidence?
- Has nerve pain improved (e.g. facial neuralgia, sciatica)?
- Are your noticing an improvement to your discomfort and generalised pain?
- Are your joints more flexible, and is there less stiffness particularly of the spine and lower pelvic region?
- Is there evidence of improvement of symptoms such as eye lids twitching, muscle spasms/cramps?

Has your hearing slightly improved, such as less Tinnitus (ringing or roaring sound in the ears)? Less muffled or swishing sound? Less internal fuzziness?

Vision

- Are your eyes less tired?
- Has your vision improved or is it blurred? Has visual adjustment improved?
- Do your eyes feel less dry and gritty?
- Are the eyes more lubricated?
- Are your eyes sensitive to light?
- Do you feel pain or pressure at the back of your eye sockets?
- If your eyes have been watery, are they improving?

Concentration Memory Performance

- Has your concentration span improved?
- Are you able to easily make decisions without procrastinating?
- Are you more confident in your own judgement?
- Are you more systematic in your approach to tasks?
- Are you able to take on multiple tasks once again?
- Are you less forgetful?
- Are you less dependent on your diary to retain, recall, and organise?
- Are you able to put things away and not lose them?
- Are you able to remember your children's names, and not confuse their names with that of the your dog!
- Is your head less foggy?
- Is your thinking faculties and general awareness improving? Is there more clarity of thought, better recall?

Headaches

- Are your migraines diminishing?
- Are normal headaches less frequent or have been eliminated entirely?
- Are you taking less medication for headaches?
- Are you more relaxed, less stressed?
- Do you have less neck tension contributing to headaches?
- Are you able to control your headaches before they become migraines (recognising triggers).
- Has that tight head-band/tight scalp pain behind the eyes and temples disappeared or improved?

Emotional WellBeing

- Are you still fluctuating between high and low moods, or are you stabilising?
- Do you feel good about yourself?
- Are you more confident?
- Can you interact better in a social situation, do you feel less vulnerable and fragile?
- Are you more assertive, particularly where your own needs are concerned?
- Has your moodiness improved?
- Do you still feel old, redundant and full of self loathing?
- Do you continue to sabotage, discount, or dismiss yourself?
- Do you feel more energised?
- Are you willing to take risks?
- Are you willing to tackle new projects?
- Do you feel less sluggish?
- Are you coping much better with general exercise, do you feel inclined to be more active?
- Are you able to maintain and use energy better?
- Are you still experiencing panic or anxiety attacks? Are they less frequent, less intense, more controllable?
- Are you coping better, not freaking out or over-reacting?
- Do you behave less erratically, less inclined to flee from situations, or behave inappropriately?
- Do you feel less disorientated, or did you lose your way, perhaps got lost on the most common route to work that you have travelled for the last 20 years?
- Do you find yourself incapable of making 'small talk', feeling inadequate or can't be bothered in social situations? Or are you feeling more sociable and confident?
- Have you lost the art of entertaining, and find yourself floundering without reason?
- Did you forget someone's name that you should have remembered?
- Are you feeling less agitated or anxious?
- Did you yell at the kids or hubby/partner less this month?
- Are you more easygoing, more patient, loving, tolerate?
- Are you more settled in your relationship, not so obsessed with faults? 'Nit picking?'
- Has your self worth improved?
- Are you happy and comfortable with yourself, and experiencing a sense of completeness and wellbeing, inner contentment and calmness?
- Are you having more positive inner dialogue or are you still hard on yourself?
- Are you negative about yourself, feeling alienated against the world?

- Are you still wearing the 'should do' label that is causing you to feel guilty?
- Are you easily brought to tears?
- Are you feeling depressed or weepy for no reason, or dipping in and out of depression? Or are these episodes improving?
- Are you more loving and lovable, more dependable?
- Are you less co-dependent, looking for other's acceptance and approval?
- Do you experience a feeling of well-being and renewed independence?
- Do you feel strong and resilient emotionally?
- Are you feeling more spiritually connected?
- Are you coping better with situations/problems?
- Does the world look brighter to you now?
- Are you feeling more creative?

All these things can be monitored on a monthly basis, and give a general indication of your progression and response to progesterone. Become your own detective! But please don't over analyse and beat up on yourself when things go wrong. Be patient with yourself and mother nature.

It truly is a rewarding experience to put the effort into your charts. Often women will stick their chart on the fridge at home and tick off daily. Other women chose to reflect of an evening in the privacy of their bedroom. The main point here is that your charting is convenient and designed to suit you. It is like a road map back to you, and the way to discovering rewarding results.

A time for reflection

Most women, when asked to refer back over their lists of twelve months ago, are quite shocked to see how many symptoms were on their original list (to discover more they were not aware of). So, for this reason, I ask you to continue your journey. Be patient and persistent. What you put in you'll get back in improved health. In other words, discover what works for you, get good at it, allow it to become a habit and way of life that, in time, sustains good health, vitality and inner equilibrium.

Women have submitted to NPAN charting guidelines and templates. They vary from very complex to very simple. I offer you here some guidelines only. Pick the one that suits you. Or using these guidelines, create your own. You are free to make up what works for you. And at the same time of each month, I encourage you to not only tick off what symptoms still exist and how many negatives or unusual symptoms you have reported for the month, but to list all the things that have improved. *The score sheet is ideal for putting together a quick summary that indicates the effectiveness of progesterone for that month. Stay focused on a positive outcome.*

The main thing to remember here is that these are your charts, more or less a diary of your journey and validation of who you are. For very busy women, fasten the Quick Tick Chart to your refrigerator and you can be sure if you forget to fill it in your husband

and kids certainly won't. NPAN often hears women report that their charts have been completed by their kids and husband for the month!!

Clearly, in some cases, the family are more tuned in than women realise. And these charts have served as a positive support infrastructure because the family starts to see patterns emerge from a different level of comprehension. Certainly women report they get more hugs and support. More so some women have been unaware to this point, how much their hormonal imbalance, has negatively impacted on their loved ones.

So many times I have heard the comment 'progesterone saved my marriage'.

Your monthly journal and list of all the positives are so important because so many women have been conditioned to expect a negative cyclic experience. Two examples would be Migraine sufferers and women with Endometriosis who suffer pain that incapacitates each month, sometimes for days. These women tend to be focused and fear-driven by ingrained negative belief systems based on past experiences. Charting can help break such cycles and re-program their belief system, thus inducing the healing process. When documented proof of improved health is evident in their charts, it can dramatically alter their perception.

This is especially important since we tend to, as human beings, focus on what's not right with our body forgetting to acknowledge and give thanks for that which has improved our quality of life. For to get well and be healthy you need to focus on the best possible outcome, not the worst. *Good health is, after all, a synergy of mind, body and soul. Our positive attitude, commitment, and love of ourselves fuels the body's power to heal. What you change in your thinking is how your body responds! Progesterone can be the catalyst.*

Taking control

It's gratifying to watch a woman take control of her situation, adopting a more positive approach to hormone imbalance. In so doing, she discovers that cyclic hormone headaches are not normal. That she no longer has to feel anxious and apprehensive, and plan her month around the two days she is going to be bed-ridden, throwing up, incapacitated with pain or bleeding heavily. That all the things she'd been told, taught or come to accept as normal are, in fact, abnormal. She sees, feels and experiences a sense of well-being she has not known for a very long time. There is this renewed level of joy and enthusiasm in her life. More involvement and an ability to commit to activities she may have avoided at that particular time of the month. **Ultimately, she rediscovers her freedom.**

Break the cycle of pain and incapacitation with progesterone therapy and you see women who have failed in previous attempts to help themselves begin delving into their 'too hard basket', gravitating towards lifestyles changes that positively effect their health and their family.

Charting helps women become aware of things and situations that have, in the past, upset them and triggered an immediate need for 'comfort' food, a hit of caffeine and/or nicotine, drug dependencies such as analgesics.

I suggest women use their charts to reformulate their own life to make it work for them.

It's my belief that I've based my organisation NPAN on and my work on, that if you give a woman back her missing hormones, some genuine understanding, empowering knowledge, and formulas for self-help, she will go on and do the rest.

Once there's a 'shift' - a conscious state that is arrived at through charting - women suddenly realise that they have considerable control over their health (by established, proven strategies). They then choose to move away from lifestyle habits and triggers that can contribute to their health problems, no longer seeing the giving up of these things as a state of deprivation.

I just want to remind you that you ARE already magnificent. Keep this in mind as you review your charts and progress. Be patient and gentle with yourself. And remain committed. *For I do not doubt your ability, no matter how difficult you may believe it to be, to accomplish the kind of results that you feel good about. Thousands of women have already proved this.*

You might want to visit my section on 'The Spiritual Side of Progesterone'. And don't forget **progesterone usage is a health journey not a quick fix.**

CHAPTER 16

Hormone Replacement Therapy (HRT) and Natural Hormone Replacement Therapy (NHRT)

- *Is natural hormone replacement therapy (NHRT) addictive and will I be able to come off it?*

- *Is HRT the same as NHRT?*

- *Is NHRT safer than HRT?*

- *Possible risks and side effects of The Pill and HRT:*

- *More serious effects of The Pill and HRT:*

- *Possible risks and side effects of natural progesterone:*

- *Types of HRT regimes that might be offered by your doctor:*

- *How is conventional HRT usually taken?*

- *How is NHRT usually taken?*

- *Alternative therapies*

- *Women who are considered low risk and possibly do not require any hormone replacement therapy are women that:*

- *Regarding hormone replacement therapy, about which form of hormone replacement therapy I should use.*

Is natural hormone replacement therapy (NHRT) addictive and will I be able to come off it?

No it is not addictive. The aim of 'hormone replacement therapy' is to put back into the body the hormones that are either missing, or the body is not producing in adequate amounts to offset hormone imbalance. And women requiring hormone replacement are discovering that bio-identical hormones, like natural progesterone, that are physically and chemically identical to the hormones made in our body, appear to be safe, free of side effects and non-addictive if used wisely and in moderation.

Do women experience any side effects coming off NHRT? Based on observation, "no". Women who stopped using natural progesterone cream were not bothered by drug-related 'withdrawal' symptoms. Rather, they reported a resurgence of their estrogen dominance symptoms indicating their body genuinely required natural progesterone supplementation to support their hormone balance. (The side effects are not those as such as withdrawal from a drug but a deprivation of the body's need of this hormone).

Synthetic HRT is another story entirely. I have seen women seek out other doctors who will surgically insert a replacement estrogen and/or testosterone implant long before replacement due date. They claim that as time went on, their implants became less and less effective, and they experienced withdrawal symptoms even though blood tests indicated normal to high levels. It is suspected the medical profession recognises the potential to become addicted to, or reliant on implants of high levels.

Women who withdraw from HRT do experience very distressing side effects as a result of estrogen levels dropping and the brain being conditioned to what I at NPAN refer to as "an estrogen conditioned threshold". The body appears to be conditioned to these high levels of estrogen, and variance appears to trigger a re-emergence of symptoms with a vengeance. Depression and anxiety surfaces, often peaking at around 3 months after discontinuing estrogen. Women can become desperate and very distressed.

This is one reason why long term estrogen users need to 'wean' off estrogen slowly in order to allow the biofeedback mechanism in the body to adjust, and allow for adequate time for natural progesterone to saturate the body and to buffer this huge ratio difference. Women who go off estrogen therapy 'cold turkey' find it a very uncomfortable experience, and may return to HRT despite all their previous side effects purely because they are unable to cope with the inevitable withdrawal and associated menopausal symptoms which appears to be far worse than those faced by women going through a difficult menopause 'naturally'.

Interestingly, many women who stop taking synthetic progestogen tablets after experiencing negative side effects usually feel instant relief, especially if they replace progestogens with natural progesterone. I have not seen evidence of progestogen withdrawal symptoms other than the thickening of the uterine lining, **particularly if estrogen is continued.** This is where my work, at NPAN, advocating natural progesterone gets a bad name (Read the article on the Reference page 'Progesterone

Absorption'). Doctor's do not trust natural progesterone or have the confidence that it has the same ability as progestins to oppose endometrial lining build up and are partially correct. The natural progesterone doses need to be extremely high to be equivalent to synthetic progestins and its designed action to prevent endometrial hyperplasia whilst a women is supplementing with estrogen.

Whilst a woman continues to use estrogen therapy, estrogen will dominate the hormone environment allowing the potential problem of uterine build-up to occur whilst that woman is being weaned off estrogen. This is when initial high doses of natural progesterone administration (10% or equivalent intravaginal dose 4-5% based on estrogen dosage) needs to be higher than estrogen until there is a balanced ratio between estrogen and progesterone and where progesterone can oppose estrogens affect.

A reduction program of progesterone is required in accordance to the reduction of estrogen levels in the body. And it's only when a woman has totally weaned off estrogen and is asymptomatic for 4 months will she then be able to establish her true physiological dose of progesterone (around 20-32mg). In cases where, after 4 months, symptoms have not abated, very small doses of natural estrogen are required to be reintroduced. Use hormone blood profiles to ascertain levels. Along with symptom observation and charting (your score sheet).

It's important to make sure that your progesterone is actually opposing uterine build-up. So work closely with your doctor, and have the required tests that keep a check on this.

Note: while weaning off estrogen you must take a break at the same time you take a break from progesterone. Otherwise estrogen dominance will reside, potentially causing uterine problems.

It is also vital in my opinion to work on the liver during this time (suggest use Liva Tone Plus) and use a premium phytoestrogen formula. Also get regular checkups on your uterine lining thickness.

Is HRT the same as NHRT?

No, that's why chemically-altered hormones can shut down or reduce our production of natural hormones. Because the molecules have been changed, the synthetic hormones used in the Contraceptive Pill and HRT do not have the same effect on the mind and body as our natural hormones do. In fact, many of the effects of synthetic hormones are the exact opposite to the natural hormone they so ineptly replace.

One prime example of HRT's 'unnatural' molecular makeup is in the case of medroxy-progesterone acetate, a synthetic progestogen. If used during pregnancy, this progestogen has the potential to cause birth defects. Natural progesterone, however, being bio-identical to the body, is routinely used in fertility clinics around the globe to help sustain pregnancy in high-risk situations.

Another 'advantage' of NHRT is it's deliverance system. Transdermal creams, like natural progesterone, that are applied directly to the skin, actually bypass the liver and gut to get taken up by the blood stream. This means, in most cases, using the transdermal route you only need introduce 1/10 that of an oral dosage (in pill form) to deliver the same amount of hormones into the body. And, because it goes straight into the blood, it's bio-available much quicker. Many women with a fatty / dysfunctional liver often cannot cope with potent doses of hormone replacement therapy as it overloads the workload of the liver. And this can actually aggravate weight problems and obesity. They do well with natural progesterone transdermal cream.

Is NHRT safer than HRT?

From a woman's viewpoint, it can go both ways. Some women clearly do ok using synthetic hormone replacement therapy. They do not consider these drugs to be a danger to their health because they have not experienced the debilitating side effects of HRT that pushes women to seek out alternative options. I rarely see at NPAN these women who do fine on HRT, therefore, I am not in a position to comment on balanced statistics. I mainly see those women who've had bad experiences, and have nowhere else to go. They have exhausted all their options or intuitively do not want to pursue synthetic HRT. With so much evidence appearing on the risks of HRT. More and more women are approaching me seeking alternatives.

The internet is jam-packed with publications and websites containing information posted by the medical profession and laypersons for and against both forms of hormone replacement therapy. You want to be very aware, however, who is actually funding the research of the data and the trials that are being put forward (Sherrill Sellman expands on this in her book 'Hormone Heresy').

NPAN is self funded and remains free of all funding other than that of sales of my publications, my consultancy and some product sales. I have adopted this very strong stance in order to remain neutral and try to maintain an unbiased voice in this debate. As desperate as I am for funding to enable me to reach more women, I choose to retain my freedom from any ownership (censorship), to say what needs to be said. To be the watchdog for women. To decipher my way through the clever advertising campaigns which are, in my opinion, no more than 'smoke screens' thrown out into the public domain by pharmaceutical companies fiercely competing with each other to confuse and capture the attention of the huge number of women approaching menopause.

But the confusion does not merely lie with synthetic HRT. The term 'Super Hormones' is used in the USA to describe the group of anti-aging hormones that are becoming increasingly popular in the post-war baby boomer generation to rejuvenate flagging endocrine systems. The hormones that belong to this group are natural progesterone, testosterone, estrogen, pregnenalone, DHEA, thyroid hormone and melatonin in the form of creams, capsules and lozenges/troches.

To load further inconsistency upon women who are searching for answers and some objectivity to arrive at an informed decision, mostly we are bombarded with words like 'precursor', 'natural', 'bio-identical', 'from natural sources', 'wild yam', 'diosgenin', 'saponins', 'plants steroids', 'phytosterols', 'phytoestrogens' and the constant interchanging of the word progesterone and progestogen/progestins in the same paragraph. Here's an example of a push for HRT taken from one reputable pharmaceutical company website:"Fact - Progestogens are hormones similar in action to the progesterone produced by the ovary." Similar does not mean 'the same'. If this were the case, why do progestogens cause birth defects whereas progesterone does not?

Some drug companies DO include natural-to-the-body estrogen in their HRT, usually combined with a synthetic progestogen. How do you know the difference? This is usually the scenario that catches women off guard because the drug companies CAN advertise their HRT drugs as 'natural' because PART of that combination hormone may contain natural-to-the-body estrogen. What they omit to state is that the combination progestogen IS NOT natural-to-the-body, although originally derived from 'natural' plant sources.   Interestingly I have noted of late, drug companies are using the word progesterone less and less when they are talking about progestins, in the drug information. They are tightening up their act and perhaps because too many women have tripped them up on this and perhaps educating their Doctors who are in return questioning the drug representatives pushing these forms of HRT.

Natural estrogens are estrone, estradiol and estriol (also spelt as oestrone, oestradiol and oestriol). Premarin which most women are familiar with is not a natural estrogen. Actually the drug **'Premarin'** comes from **<u>PREGNANT MARES URINE.</u>**

Learn to familiarise yourself with the words that are going to be constantly thrown at you via crafty advertising or confused Doctors. Then learn to be more discerning. Just remember, the body sees as 'natural' that which has the same molecular configuration (bio-identical).'Natural to the body' is what you need to regard as most important when you are contemplating hormone replacement therapy. Any altered molecular structure to that of our body's molecular structure will alter the message! Drug companies in order to be able to own and patent a hormone must alter the molecular configuration of the techniques of deliverance *(as with natural estrogen they have patented the patch).* Many women ask me 'why then don't they patent a progesterone patch?' Good question. The reasons are several. Progestins are far stronger and specifically designed to prevent Endometrial Hyperplasia. When combined with natural estrogen studies with progesterone did not oppose this action (so mega doses would need to be administered), secondly progesterone works more effectively transdermal and in my opinion intra vaginally. I also have found another reason why natural progesterone does not exist in a patch as does natural estrogen. This I explain in my companion Book 2. It is due to absorption results, medical attitudes and drug companies not convinced of profitability.

A progesterone (natural) gel has been created. It is the deliverance (gel) that has been patented. There are no satisfactory controlled studies to warrant the use of progesterone other than in fertility, as there are no drug companies willing to spend billions of dollars on a hormone everyone can own. It is not viable.

Estrogen based on a false premise has been the focus all these years and has reaped substantial financial rewards. Being so heavily prescribed being the hormone that promised all (sadly based on a few trials - these now proving to be wrong as more evidence surfaces).

It is time they woke up, fast, there would be money in progesterone given that women are demanding this hormone. If only they would listen and look. Estrogen has reaped nearing to the top in records the highest sale in the drug industry, drug profits and I believe progesterone would surpass it placed in the medial arena.

(See section Medical References chapter 22, page 420).

Possible risks and side effects of The Pill and HRT:

- Allergic reactions
- Birth defects
- Breakthrough bleeding
- Decreased immune system function
- Disturbances in liver function
- Eye disorders (double vision, swelling of optic nerve, contact lens intolerance, corneal inflammation)
- Facial and body hair growth
- Fluid retention and bloating
- Fungal Infections and Tinea
- Infertility increased with The Pill
- Irritable Bowel Syndrome
- Hair loss
- Hay fever, Asthma and skin rashes
- Loss of Libido
- Lumpy and tender breasts (Fibrocystic Breasts)
- Migraines and headaches
- Nausea
- Nutritional deficiencies especially zinc, B6 and magnesium
- Psychological and emotional disorders, depression, mood changes
- Secretions from breasts
- Skin discolouration
- Higher rates of suicide
- Weight gain
- Systemic Candida infection
- Urinary tract infection
- Venereal Warts

- Vaginal discharges (increased incidence of vaginal Thrush)
- Fatigue

More serious effects of The Pill and HRT:

- Disturbance of blood-sugar metabolism (contributing to Diabetes and hypoglycaemia)
- Increased incidence of thrombosis (stroke)
- Increased incidence of hardening of the arteries and high blood pressure
- Increased risk of blood clots
- Increased risk of Gall Bladder and Liver Disease
- Increased incidence of cancer of the breast, endometrium, cervix, ovaries, liver, lung and skin
- Increased risk of heart attacks
- Increased incidence of MS (my thoughts included here, CFS, FMS)

Possible risks and side effects of natural progesterone:

Because progesterone creams contain the hormone identical to that produced by the human ovary, side effects are usually minimal. If experienced these may include breast tenderness and swelling, fluid retention or slight vaginal bleeding. Dizziness, nausea, fatigue, headaches and light headedness have been reported occasionally and usually disappear with adjustment of dose. (I class these side effects as Estrogen Dominance Wake Up Crisis, EDWUC).

Progesterone is the hormone essential for promotion and maintenance of pregnancy. Ovarian output of progesterone in the non-pregnant state is 25-30mg daily during the luteal phase. The placenta output during the third trimester of pregnancy is 340-400mg per day. Where as progestogens are contraindicated in pregnancy. Whilst progesterone exhibits no adverse effects on the foetus.

Types of HRT regimes that might be offered by your doctor:

- ESTROGEN ONLY - usually only recommended for women who have had a Hysterectomy (can be natural or synthetic)
- ESTROGEN + PROGESTOGEN - usually recommended for women with intact uterus to protect the endometrium (lining of the uterus)
- SEQUENTIAL OR CYCLIC TREATMENTS - estrogen taken 7-14 days followed by progestogen 10-14 days, resulting in a period after the progestogen dose is taken. Usually recommended for perimenopausal women to control menopausal symptoms and to regulate bleeding whilst protecting the endometrium.
- CONTINUOUS COMBINED - estrogen and progestogen continually to prevent the thickening of the lining of the uterus without incurring a bleed. Usually for

women 2 years post-menopause who do not wish to have a period in their therapy.

- PROGESTOGEN - oral pill, injection or IUD (coil, vaginal ring) combination varies for specific purposes and treatment such as contraception, perhaps Endometriosis, PCOS.

Note: Women with a history of gall bladder disease, Liver Disease or dysfunction, blood clots, severe migraines, PMT, high blood pressure, excessive weight and smoke should consider natural hormones as a preferable choice to HRT.

How is conventional HRT usually taken?

- Tablets
- Skins patches - (can include natural or bio identical estrogen or natural testosterone), combination patches (have natural estrogen but synthetic progestogen)
- Creams and gels (natural estrogen)
- Implants (hormone or contraception)
- Injections (testosterone / progestins)
- Pessaries
- IUD, Estring (estrogen)

How is NHRT usually taken?

I recommend you take a closer look at chapter 9, 'Cream Usage and Guidelines' for more and 'What to be aware of with your Natural Progesterone and the different deliverance systems'. Transdermal creams, vaginal gel, pessaries, losenges/troches, patches (testosterone or estrogen), progesterone capsules (not in Australia) in chapter 11.

Alternative therapies and changing tactics and trends

Drug companies (via your doctor's surgery) scare women into believing that diseases such as Osteoporosis and Heart Disease are inevitable consequences of menopause. They advocate that while alternative therapies may relieve some symptoms of menopause for some women, they are not HRT and do not replace the vital hormones required by the body to function well and prevent diseases.

They claim that many of these over-the-counter medications and products derived from soya beans, wild yam, evening primrose, red clover, etc., are not researched or tested to the same standards as conventional drugs and the effects of these remedies, long term, have not been established. They warn us they will not protect us long term.

Not true, according to NPAN. I have seen many successes where women have adopted alternative therapies without the need for hormone replacement. These over-the-counter remedies (knowledge of which dates back centuries) have provided women with effective alternatives that enhance hormonal health and balance, rejuvenated their energy and stamina, supported their metabolism, aided weight loss, and counter-balanced depression, anxiety, and insomnia.

This has been as simple as incorporating a balanced phytoestrogenic formulation, increasing their essential fatty acids, supporting liver and adrenal functioning through vitamin, mineral and liver formulation, acknowledging their body type, and eating foods that are compatible to their hormonal and metabolic characteristics. I have also noted in many women a drop in cholesterol, blood pressure and fluid retention. So while drug companies may claim there's no proof, NPAN certainly has empirical evidence to the contrary and so do millions of women worldwide. It is evident that the alternative health industry is threatening the drug industry as they ruthlessly compete harder to win back their market place, placing more pressure on Doctors and raising the TGA standards in quality control alternative therapies (as seen with PAN. Laws and regulations are becoming more stringent and therapeutic claims censored unless substantiated with trials to back). The health shops battle to survive and more Doctors are introducing nutritional practitioner only lines (products) into their surgeries and practice. I hope the day will not arrive that we have to go to our Doctor to get a prescription for a satisfactory dose level of Vitamin C!

Let's state up front that not every woman approaching or in menopause needs hormone replacement therapy, be it via any of the natural hormones or conventional synthetic HRT. Their diet, exercise and lifestyle can carry them through, disease-free, to old age.

These fortunate people are free of disease, have good bones, and maintain hormonal harmony from the foods they eat which contain plant hormones known as phytosterols that have a balancing effect upon their cell receptors.

In a body functioning optimally, hormones are manufactured by the ovaries, adrenal glands, fat tissue, thyroid and pineal glands. Only when the sex hormones are out of balance in the body is there a need for hormone replacement therapy. And at this point you would thoroughly consider all your options.

I see so many women entering menopause or postmenopausal who were asymptomatic but were placed on HRT as a preventative measure, only to be faced with a host of new health issues ranging from weight gain, high cholesterol, headaches, fluid retention, irritability, etc., none of which were pre-existing prior to HRT.

This is where it is our responsibility to always ask if a drug treatment is prescribed to you, to question the reasons and look at the side effects. Drug information sheets can be obtained. If you cannot get information on medication don't touch it or accept it until you have satisfactory knowledge. I was one of these women.

I naively trusted my Doctor to give me an implant in his surgery on a visit before doing my homework. Feeling I did not wish to waste his time, let alone questions my then 38 year family General Practitioner. He had studied with my father and had looked after our family all those years since his death. I trusted this Doctor as a family friend holding my best interest at least - so I thought. When I arrived home and told Garth, he went off his brain. He was panic stricken. Stating 'I was not a candidate for that implant having fine bones only 6 1/2 stone in weight'. The dose was that of a person 3 times my size. Garth was concerned for my bones (which incidentally probably contributed to my Osteoporosis). The following day I was very ill which continued for 3 months. The implant shut down my pituitary gland.

Garth bought me home drug information which I read with horror. Had my Doctor provided me with this first I would never have contemplated such treatment which he claimed would enhance my fertility chances. I now know there is extra money when 'surgical procedures' are conducted in your General Practitioner's surgery. So be careful. Make a second appointment before you allow yourself to be coerced into a decision that you may regret.

Women who are considered low risk and possibly do not require any hormone replacement therapy are women that:

- Have good bones - medium to heavy bone structure
- Do not have Osteoporosis (or family history)
- Do not have Cardiovascular Disease (heart, stroke, embolisms) (or family history)
- Do not smoke
- Do not suffer depression
- Do not use drugs that might increase bone loss (steroids, thyroid medication, diuretics, antacids)
- Have an intact uterus and ovaries (no history of Tubal Ligation) or gynaecological problems*
- Correct weight to height ratio, do not have a fatty liver*
- Good cholesterol and blood pressure reading, normal functioning thyroid
- Exercise regularly, yoga, pilates, meditate*
- Have a healthy diet rich in fresh fruit and vegetables, low-saturated fat diet,
- Do not enter early menopause*
- Have no estrogen dominance symptoms or history of PMS*
- Have a happy disposition and good relationship, sexually active*
- Have no symptoms of Hot Flushes, dry vagina or Osteoporosis*.
- There are new studies negating reasons to place women on HRT regardless if you are high or low risk category

These lucky souls can cruise through menopause benefiting on these phytoestrogens and Vitamin supplementation alone however minimal natural progesterone can still offer wonderful benefits and many women in this category chose to use it as the icing on the cake! * My observational extras.

My girlfriend of 54 years is one that comes to mind. She looks like a 40 year old and has an exercised, amazing body having practiced yoga for 20 constant years. Has had 5 children and never suffered an illness or hormonal symptoms in her life and is still regularly menstruating. Interestingly when she divorced and obtained my book I thought it was odd and assumed it was for her friend! She proclaims and reveals now, that she has been on 20mg of progesterone day 12-26 for the past 18 months and is loving it. So much so she has found a man who is 35 and states 'she is in her prime'.

Regarding hormone replacement therapy, I am confused about which form of hormone replacement therapy I should use.

These days anyway, most women are confronted with the question of hormone replacement therapy whether it be a young girl prescribed the Contraceptive Pill to control period problems, pain, or contraception, or whether it's a woman being prescribed synthetic HRT to treat perimenopausal or postmenopausal symptoms. **The most important thing to remember here is that you have options.** That the decision is entirely up to you, based on accurate information, your health requirements and lifestyle.

You need to conduct a little research - don't accept everything you read or hear - and if hormone replacement therapy is a likely choice, think about natural-to-the-body forms of hormone replacement therapy NHRT) that include progesterone, estrogen, testosterone, pregnenalone and the corticosteroid (the 'super' anti-aging hormones). These bio-identical hormones are less imposing on the body and kinder on your liver. I personally do not have enough experience or observational data on the usage of prednisolone, corticosteroid, natural thyroid or DHEA, so I leave this area to the experts specialising in all bio identical hormones (Dr Sandra Cabot and others have a handle on this and these hormones are for more accessible in the USA than Australia). To find out more read her book 'Hormone Replacement The Real Truth' by Dr Sandra Cabot.

I've always advocated progesterone as the starting hormone before looking at the introduction of other hormones into the equation. I think I get a little nervous at the prospect of throwing the Endocrine system into chaos. I also do not suggest women start off with a hormonal mixture such as progesterone, testosterone or DHEA or Triest. The reason I urge women to begin quietly with progesterone separately to gauge the benefits and to assess how well this hormone/being a pre cursor to the other hormones (bar DHEA) goes along the building cascade pathway (see diagram) in building the other hormones. This enables control and true assessment and opportunity for adjusting dose requirements. If the cream is mixed with all the hormones it is difficult to adjust doses, as I've witnessed with so many, and it leads to expensive repetitive saliva assays and many visits to the Specialising Doctor and more compounding cream mixes, attempting to tailor dose to the individual.

Down the track this may be a more economical option. When your body is balanced but certainly I err with caution at the beginning when natural hormone replacement is commenced. You need to get a handle on maximising your progesterone performance first.

Ovestin vaginal cream can also be introduced if vaginal dryness and bladder problems persist. Again you can control application and administration according to need and response. The state and condition of your vagina ie. Not so dry will assist your dosage amount requirements. Vaginal estriol will not impede on your progesterone performance or cloud your interpretation of response.

I have seen and spoken to far too many women out of control on mixed hormones to be convinced of its initial predictability. Get you creams separated if compounded by a pharmacist. It may be more expensive (most cases rebatable) but far more user friendly when you are mastering balance and in the long term more cost effective.

One case comes to mind - Julie, under her Doctors supervision following her blood tests, was given a cream containing progesterone, testosterone, DHEA and Triest. She was not gaining balance and was placed on (with her Doctor's knowledge) Vitex 1000mg to assist modulation. Two months later, she rang, screaming down my phone, 'what is this Vitex doing to me?'. 'My testosterone and estrogen levels have gone through the roof!' Angry and frightened. I calmly told her 'to go back to my book and refer to the hormone cascade pathway and note that DHEA is a pre cursor to producing testosterone then estrogens. So perhaps this was the reason for such high levels not the Vitex'. It is also interesting to note here, Julie 47 years, has functioning ovaries but is under weight and a vegan who does not eat enough protein and has Fibromyalgia and CFS. She does not assimilate the little nutrition she eats, bleeds heavily (perhaps due to too much estrogen and interference in her prostaglandins and blood clotting factors coupled with suspected iron deficiency) and has been in poor nutritional status for years. I also suspect her eating patterns (I'd class starving) have interfered with her pituitary gland given the fact that Vitex had no benefits on her in its expected influence on this gland for modulation. Naturally she was told to stop Vitex, read my book, go back to her Doctor. I felt she was using far to much DHEA and testosterone in proportion and relationship to progesterone. The scales in my opinion were clearly lop sided towards the estrogen dominance side.

CHAPTER 17

Estrogen, Phytoestrogen & Xenoestrogens

- *What is estrogen?*
- *What are estrogen receptors?*
- *My doctor says I need estrogen and yet I've read there are different forms of estrogen. I am confused.*
- *Do I need estrogen if I'm still having regular periods?*
- *Do I need estrogen if I am not having a period?*
- *What is Amenorrhea?*
- *What are the causes?*
- *What is the safest form of estrogen to use if I have to use an estrogen?*
- *I want to use Natural Progesterone cream but my doctor wants me to take a tablet. I'm totally confused.*
- *My doctor wants me to stay on estrogen for my bones and heart but I get headaches and other problems. I don't know what to do.*
- *Suggested guidelines when coming off estrogen replacement therapy*
- *I have been on estrogen for Hot Flushes but would like to use progesterone. Will I need to stay on my estrogen?*
- *I qualify for some estrogen because I am still having Hot Flushes and vaginal dryness but I'm not sure when I am meant to be taking it.*
- *How can I reduce my estrogen dominance naturally?*
- *Guidelines of an estrogen reduction program*
- *What are phytoestrogens?*
- *Other benefits of phytoestrogens*

- *Why do estrogen dominant symptoms return 3-4 months later on Phytoestrogens ?*
- *Supplement with a PREMIUM phytoestrogen formulation*
- *What is the difference between phyto-hormones and xenohormones?*
- *How do I reduce my exposure to xenoestrogens and xenohormones in my environment?*
- *What are some of the foods containing natural estrogen?*
- *Who would benefit most from estrogenic foods?*

What is estrogen?

Estrogen is a group of sex hormone secreted primarily by the ovaries. It is responsible for female characteristics such as the development of breasts and female curves, as well as for menstruation. There are several types of estrogen and the main ones that we know are estradiol, estrone and estriol. These naturally occurring estrogens are found in the blood and in the body.

Too much estrogen in the body:

- Builds up uterine lining
- Stimulates breast tissue
- Increases body fat
- Create salt and fluid retention
- Causes depression, headaches/migraines
- Interferes with thyroid hormone
- Increases blood clotting
- Decreases libido
- Impairs blood sugar control
- Increases risk of endometrial cancer
- Increases risk of Breast Cancer
- Slightly restrains bone loss
- Reduces vascular tone
- Promotes estrogen driven diseases - cancer, Fibroids, Endometriosis

What are estrogen receptors?

Like progesterone, it is the physical structures on the cell membrane that attract estrogen and respond to its effect (i.e. delivers specific messages to the body). There are many estrogen receptors throughout the body.

There is only one progesterone receptor which means there is only one type of progesterone, but there are several types of estrogens.

My doctor says I need estrogen and yet I've read there are different forms of estrogen. I am confused.

Yes that is correct. There are three 'classes' of natural estrogen that are produced in our body: estradiol, estrone and estriol. They are all natural and found in the blood. They are made by the adrenal glands and in the ovaries. There is only one 'class' of progesterone produced by the body.

However, there are several man-made estrogens on the market, although doctors refer to estrogen as if it is one specific hormone - which it is not. Some estrogens are natural in configuration while others are synthetic. One particular synthetic estrogen product is harvested from pregnant mares urine (PREMARIN).

You might be prescribed a combination of all three types, or perhaps just the one in the treatment of hormone imbalance. Estradiol seems to be the most popular amongst doctors.

NPAN's approach is to primarily tackle the estrogen dominance symptoms with progesterone cream, and any residual problems after 4-7 months such as continual hot flushing, and dry vagina may warrant estrogen supplementation. Where women are petite, slim and small-boned and/or exhibiting signs of Osteoporosis, they may need to consider intelligent use of estrogen in conjunction with progesterone.

Furthermore, don't discount the huge benefits of phytoestrogens in the overall picture of estrogen therapy and natural choices. Also worth mentioning here is testosterone which is capable of producing the 3 estrogens – estradiol, estrone and estriol. The hormone cascade diagram demonstrates this. Please refer to and read section on phytoestrogens.

Some women are taking small amounts of natural testosterone for improvement of their libido, mood, depression and/or building and maintenance of bone growth (where Osteoporosis is evident). Interestingly many who are using natural testosterone seem to not require estrogen substitution. Perhaps this is because of the way it can convert to produce estrogen. And they may just resort to topical estriol creams e.g. ovestin (minute doses) for treatment and maintenance of vaginal dryness.

Lawley Pharmaceuticals in Australia manufacturers of Pro-Feme also make natural testosterone and natural estrogen cream.

Website http://www.lawleypharm.com.au

Do I need estrogen if I'm still having regular periods?

If you are menstruating, regularly or irregularly, it's indicative that the body has enough estrogen to build up the uterine lining, resulting in a period when hormone levels fluctuate. So therefore you cannot technically be estrogen deficient. When a woman's estrogen levels drop low enough, she will stop having her period, signaling, in most cases, the end the of her reproductive epoch (menopause). This is activated/initiated when the ovaries have no more eggs left to ripen.

Following this theory, many women question the need for extra estrogen therapy offered by their doctors while they continue to menstruate, completely overshadowing progesterone in this equation.

Women ask a similar version of the same question, "do I need estrogen after my periods stop?" Even at menopause after menstruation ceases, it is possible for a women be estrogen dominant. Even a woman with low estrogen levels can have estrogen dominance symptoms if she doesn't have any progesterone.

Remember a woman's ovaries continue to produce estrogen (lesser amounts) after menopause.

Hormones are also manufactured in our glands such as the pituitary, thyroid, and adrenals. HORMONES ARE MADE FROM CHOLESTEROL WHICH IS MANUFACTURED IN

THE LIVER. (Derived mainly from our food sources essential fatty acids, Omegas 3, 6)

THIS IS ONE VERY GOOD REASON WHY IT IS IMPORTANT TO HAVE A HEALTHY LIVER TO OPTIMISE HORMONE BALANCING.

A women is never totally estrogen deficient even after menopause or where the ovaries are removed but she is near zero in progesterone levels. Estrogen is also converted by another hormone stored in lower body fat and we also get estrogen from our food source particularly estrogen laced foods.

Do I need estrogen if I am not having a period?

The question often arises here for the need of estrogen in young women who have stopped menstruating that are not menopausal, or have not commenced menses. Often estrogen is prescribed to promote menstruation.

A cessation of periods can be due to a number of reasons but basically it still means the risk of endometrial cancer when estrogen is low enough to halt menstruation.

What is Amenorrhea?

The absence of menstruation in a women during the usual menstruating years for more than 6 months is called amenorrhea. It is categorised as primary or secondary for purposes of diagnosis and treatment. Taken from Ruth Trickey's book with permission 'Women Hormones and The Menstrual Cycle'. A recommend guide to read.

Causes can be primary or secondary.

PRIMARY:
* Where menstruation has not commenced by age 17
* When physical maturation such as breast development has not commenced by 14

Or
* When the period has not started within 2 years of physical maturation commencing.

SECONDARY:
* Cessation of the period for 6 months or more during any of the years between the onset of menstruation (menarche) and menopause

Or
* Cessation of the period for more than 3 menstrual cycles when the cycle is longer than usual, for example when a women has a period only every 2 months

What are the Causes?
PRIMARY:
* Uterine causes (obstruction preventing menstrual flow - conditions affecting uterus and cervix, destruction of endometrial tissue).

- Hypothalamic amenorrhea
- Pituitary causes
- Failure to ovulate (prolonged leading to Ovarian Dysfunction)
- PCOS
- Breast feeding
- Thyroid conditions
- Cushing's Syndrome
- Congenital Adrenal Hyperplasia
- Androgen-secreting adrenal and ovarian tumors
- Premature ovarian failure (cessation of ovarian function before age 40). Possible causes - autoimmune response or failure of ovarian tissue to respond to FSH and LH
- Destruction of ovarian tissue - impaired blood supply to ovaries, surgery eradication (Tubal Ligation, Hysterectomy, Ooporectomy)
- Possible drugs - Largactil, Stemetil, Stelazine and prolactin levels leading to menstrual irregularity or amenorrhea. Some antihypertensive drugs Aldoctone Aldomet. Some oral contraceptives. Chemotherapy - temporary or permanent damage.
- Possibly certain herbs - Vitex has been reported also.

What is the safest form of estrogen to use if I have to use an estrogen?

Because estrogen (estriol, estradiol and estrone) are natural to our bodies, in balance they are not hazardous. Unfortunately the problem arises when our body is out of balance and there are excessive amounts of estrogen, possibly not opposed by progesterone. *Estrogen is the proliferating hormone which encourages multiplication of cells. It is also the factor that is known to promote and cause certain types of cancer, particularly of the breast, ovaries and uterus.*

Estrone and estradiol are relatively potent estrogens that can relieve menopausal symptoms, but can also produce very nasty side effects, possibly leading to an increased risk of breast, ovarian and uterine cancer if given in high doses, and over a long period of time, say more than five years. Estradiol is believed to be the effective type of estrogen in slowing down bone resorption however a huge risk to take for Osteoporosis if there is a history of family cancer Fibroids. There is strong evidence that its performance and influence on bones is not of great significance in the overall picture. See Medical Reference page.

Because estriol is far less potent that the former two forms of estrogen, it's less likely to stimulate breast and uterine tissue. Estriol is much safer and produces less side effects. So it is advisable for women to use estriol in the forms of tablets or vaginal creams (including pessaries) if they are worried about the stronger estrogens and have a history of breast or uterine cancer in the family.

Overall, if a woman is menstruating, she has adequate levels of estrogen in her body. One would have to question why a woman would need to be on supplementations of estrogen when there are other ways of providing natural estrogenic effects in the body and treating conditions such as vaginal dryness. And women know that progesterone combined with phytoestrogens and diet often controls such symptoms as Hot Flushes and other menopausal problems (including vaginal dryness and discomfort in many cases).

I want to use Natural Progesterone cream but my doctor wants me to take a tablet. I'm totally confused.

There is no doubt your doctor is really confused, too, if he has implied a synthetic progestogen tablet contains natural progesterone. In fact, a good many doctors actually believe they are prescribing real progesterone, and we can thank drug companies for at least some of the confusion.

Far too many times from feedback a doctor is absolutely convinced he is prescribing an oral form of real progesterone when the medication it actually a patented synthetic progestogen (also referred to as progestin).

So how does this happen? How can a GP, of all people, be confused? Quite simple really. Doctors derive information and training on the drugs they prescribe from the pharmaceutical companies who manufacture them. If a drug is not produced by these multi-national companies, it's unlikely your GP will hear about it. Which begs the question why aren't these pharmaceutical giants mass-producing natural progesterone if there's a captive audience out there in the marketplace?

It all comes down to 'owning' a drug versus being on the same playing field as your competitors. Pharmaceutical companies are not permitted to 'patent' (or own exclusive right to) a naturally occurring medicine, molecule or that naturally occurring in nature. And progesterone falls into this category.

Natural progesterone is not produced anywhere in the plant kingdom. 'Natural' progesterone is actually manufactured in a laboratory with the aid of an enzyme. The substance diosgenin, found in the Mexican Wild Yam or Soy plants, has to undergo a series of chemical changes whereby it is synthesised or converted from its raw state into United States Pharmacopoeia (USP) grade progesterone. This progesterone is referred to as 'natural' because the end result represents the same molecule naturally occurring in the body. It can be introduced into the body with a relative margin of safety when there is a need to supplement progesterone levels.

Yet pharmaceutical companies aren't so much interested in what's natural to the body. They need to 'alter' the hormone from it's natural state in order to apply for and obtain a patent (i.e. can then own the rights to sell exclusively). And unfortunately for us women, in changing natural progesterone's original molecular configuration beyond its 'natural' state, these drug companies transform natural progesterone into a synthetic progestogen (or progestin), rendering it potentially toxic to a woman's body.

So to claim a progestogen / progestins is real progesterone is incorrect. And women along with their GP ought to be aware of this play on words designed to disguise the truth.

My doctor wants me to stay on estrogen for my bones and heart but I get headaches and other problems. I don't know what to do.

As hormones in Australia and New Zealand are scheduled an S4 drug by prescription only I cannot and do not advise women for or against estrogen in the form of HRT prescribed in combination form or on its own (usually prescribed if she has no intact uterus). This is by law, the Doctor's job. Nonetheless, by the time a woman contacts the Natural Progesterone Advisory Network she has, in many cases, already trialled HRT. She reports numerous nasty side effects and wants to know how she can get her hands on a safer alternative.

I suggest women research their options. You are entitled to be given access to all information relating to the drugs you are introducing into your body. Particularly an understanding of its contra-indications (indications you shouldn't be using this particular drug).

Get on the internet and do your research. Make an informed choice when it comes to your health. Don't leave it all up to your healthcare professional. Because it's often a fact your doctor doesn't know what he doesn't know. My network exists out of demand because woman out there are prepared to put in the time it takes to become informed and, in so doing, regain control of their health and well-being. My organisation has never been advertised. It has been driven by the power of women networking and word of mouth.

There is growing medical evidence that HRT is perhaps not all it's cracked up to be. Clearly, some medical claims are based on myth and not fact, and the jury is still out on whether HRT is as safe as the drug companies would have us believe. But I can tell you, if the hundred upon hundreds of women contacting my Advisory Network are anything to go on, women are no longer prepared to take a passive role in their health regime. I commend them!

Suggested guidelines when coming off estrogen replacement therapy

I like to **warn** women who have been on estrogen therapy for a long time, t*hat it's not wise to go "cold turkey" and stop their estrogen as their body is conditioned to a high estrogen threshold.* A sudden drop in estrogen can actually cause Hot Flushes and can contribute to rapid bone loss as the body tries to adjust. I suggest you begin by cutting your estrogen dose in half, and then again by half in a few months time, until you find the lowest possible dose that keeps you free of symptoms.

If you are using natural progesterone in conjunction with an estrogen reduction program, remember to take your break from estrogen at the same time as you break from progesterone.

Just be aware that progesterone will amplify estrogen receptors, that's why I suggest you initially halve your dose (or stop for 4-8 weeks) of estrogen when introducing progesterone back into your body. In effect, the body is still interpreting estrogen at high levels. As progesterone becomes more effective and your body adjusts so, in turn, will the body synchronise with the gradual reduction of estrogen. Please read Estrogen Dominance Wake Up Crisis in Book 2 'Natural Progesterone More Secrets Revealed' it is explained with more depth with a slightly different angle. Also refer to the use of phytoestrogens in this section as well as weaning off estrogen.

Some women do go "cold turkey" and feel great for 2-3 months, and then fall into a hole. The reason being, they are initially over-riding estrogen dominance symptoms with progesterone and also they have reserves of estrogen in their body fat. The sudden slump comes about because when they have used up all their body's reserves of estrogen. Symptoms such as Hot Flushes, weariness, anxiety, palpitations, insomnia, bladder infections, dry vagina and Cystitis, may surface. Don't abandon progesterone.

If this occurs it is perhaps advisable to re-introduce a small amount of estrogen in gel or cream not tablet or patches as dosage adjustments is more difficult to achieve to restore equilibrium to the body and to abate symptoms. Then, if inclined, a gentle reduction program using your symptoms as a guide.

Some women can come off estrogen altogether, whereas some cannot. They may require a small amount along with their progesterone. Many women prefer to try phytoestrogenic formulations and high intake of plant foods containing phytosterols and find this sufficient without the need to take estrogen replacement therapy also essential oils (flaxseed and evening primrose) are most beneficial here. It is important to incorporate the above suggestions even if you are using estrogens.

If progesterone alone does not abate symptoms of Hot Flushes and vaginal dryness after four to seven months (incorporating phytoestrogens), it's usually an indication that some form of estrogen is required. Best you get your hormone profile checked out.

Changing your estrogen may be helpful. The reason being a small number of women find the patch form of estrogen delivers too high a dose, dumping in body fat. These women prefer to take transdermal estrogen where they can control dosage at low levels. And, of course, there are those women who still successfully take low oral doses of estradiol (0.25 - 0.5mg per day three out of four weeks) or 2-4mg of oral estriol along with their progesterone cream as opposed to Premarin that is reported to be less kind in side-effects for a lot of women. A more popular form of natural estrogen therapy emerging is the **Triest combination** incorporating the three estrogens in proportion, compounded by a select few pharmacists (ALL FORMS OF ESTROGEN REQUIRE A SCRIPT IN AUSTRALIA). Sandrena gel manufactured and readily available familiar to your Doctor is also proving a convenient form of estrogen. Be aware that it is Estradiol but bypasses the liver unlike oral estrogen (synthetic).

I have been on estrogen for Hot Flushes but would like to use progesterone. Will I need to stay on my estrogen?

As a rule of thumb, estrogen levels should be halved upon beginning progesterone supplementation. This is to allow for heightened estrogen sensitivity in your body that generally follows once progesterone has been introduced. As you progress over a number of months, you may find that your body needs less and less estrogen. In fact, some women wean off estrogen replacement therapy altogether.

Women without ovaries continue to make estrogen from their body fat and, because natural progesterone makes the estrogen receptors more sensitive, they may find that they can stop estrogen replacement therapy completely after 5-6 months. Occasionally down the track 12-18 months they may need to revisit small administration irregularly.

With the reduction of estrogens and the introduction of phytoestrogens via diet or vitamin supplements, women usually find that estrogen supplementation is no longer required to control Hot Flushes beyond a very small amount of estrogen cream (not Vagifem this is an Estradiol estrogen) to maintain vaginal tissue health, and to protect the vagina lining from degeneration. Estriol helps the epithelial lining cells to be more healthy (it is the mild form of natural estrogen).

If a woman genuinely requires estrogen therapy, then she is advised to use the minimal amount to maintain hormonal balance and health. This applies particularly to thinner women who are at greater risk of Osteoporosis and Hot Flushes. I recommend patches or cream rather than tablet form so the body does not have to break it down via the liver.

Natural estrogens are estrone, estradiol and estriol. Premarin which most women are familiar with is not a natural estrogen. Actually the drug 'Premarin' comes from PREgnant MAREs urINe = PREMARIN. Think about that next time your doctor suggests synthetic estrogen therapy and consider those poor pregnant horses and the conditions in which they maybe kept. It is little wonder the drug companies hate me and other women and animal lovers who refuse to take this out of sheer principle.

I qualify for some estrogen because I am still having Hot Flushes and vaginal dryness but I'm not sure when I am meant to be taking it.

Use estrogen on the same days that you use progesterone cream, leaving 5-7 days without either hormone. It is advisable to find the lowest dose that controls symptoms. Estriol is the least harmful of estrogens available, and is usually prescribed to treat vaginal dryness and prevent bladder problems. If you take estrogen on your progesterone break you may become estrogen dominant.

Refer to areas covering Bladder Problems and Vaginal Dryness (Chapter. 14), and libido in my second book.

How can I reduce my estrogen dominance naturally?

If you do not wish to use progesterone but still have estrogen dominance symptoms, you can lower your estrogen by several methods. Weight loss and a liver cleansing diet are perhaps the greatest key issues here in reducing estrogen (as excess hormone accumulates and stores in fat tissue, thus the fatter you become the more estrogen you store).

Dr. Sandra Cabot a doctor and nutritionalist of 30 plus years specialises in this and the associated problems of a fatty dysfunctional liver. Visit her websites, (see reference page). Prime attack is by reducing and preventing excess calorie intake, avoiding refined carbohydrates and sugars, maintaining a high fibre diet and keeping good gut/bowel elimination, supplementing high fibre products such as rice and bran, and looking after your liver because estrogen excretion occurs in the liver and it's vital to have an optimally functioning liver to rid the body of hormone waste, particularly estrogen. To help enable the liver and balance the hormones, there are nutrients that support the liver to help this process.

When the detoxifying pathways of the liver are working, the liver will eliminate contaminants, pollutants, insecticides, pesticides, food additives and hormones. This will reduce the impact on the body and the effect of xenoestrogens within the body as well. Drink heaps of water to flush the toxins and assist the liver to rid of waste estrogens thereby reducing the cycle of estrogen dominance. If it is not eliminated correctly it is reabsorbed back into circulation as xenoestrogens which further compound the problems.

Since toxins, pollutants and drugs are fat soluble, they can be stored in body organs over many, many years. It is here in some of these fatty glands that our hormones are made if these glands are full of bio accumulative non degradable toxins endocrine disruption occurs. Little wonder that women feel hormonal, overloaded, overweight, and end up with all sorts of immunity problems that may include allergies, sinus/Asthma problems, and food sensitivities. Particularly if they've undergone synthetic HRT or other forms of treatment.

The liver is capable, when functioning correctly, to convert the fat soluble chemicals into water soluble chemicals so that they may be easily excreted from the body via the watery fluids, such as the bile and urine and bowel.

Many symptoms of liver dysfunction could be mistaken for estrogen dominance and, in a sense, they are estrogen dominance symptoms since both go hand in glove.

Women complain of abdominal bloating, high levels of Candida, headaches, Irritable Bowel Syndrome, high cholesterol, Gallbladder Disease, high blood pressure, sugar cravings, insulin resistance, low thyroid function, and an inability to lose weight, together with unpleasant moods and frequent fatigue. These symptoms also signal hormonal imbalance. So when the connection is explained, it makes sense to work on your liver, watch your diet and to use appropriate hormone and phytoestrogen supplementation to bring about a holistic healing process.

Worth noting, synthetic hormones may place extra stress on the liver perhaps already overloaded, and may contribute to further imbalance.

I caution women not to throw too many hormones into their system and overburden their liver (including the pill and even medications). Nine times out of ten, once the liver is functioning optimally, progesterone supplementation becomes the icing on the cake. Some responses have been such that no hormone replacement therapy is needed, or 'least is best' doses become a reality.

Guidelines of an estrogen reduction program

- Commence progesterone therapy - to oppose effects of estrogen in the body (initially first 6-8 weeks higher dose is required)
- Reduce excess weight
- Maximise estrogenic benefits through phytoestrogens and phyto-sterols in your diet supplements containing numerous plant estrogens.
- Learn your body shape type - and eat accordingly
- Stabilise blood sugar levels which reduces insulin resistance and sugar cravings
- Address fatty and dysfunctional liver. See Liver Principles.
- Use appropriate nutritional supplements
- Increase metabolism through liver and thyroid function
- Reduce exposure to xenobiotics and xenoestrogens (garden sprays, household cleaning agents, hair dyes, acrylic nails, smoking)
- Reduce stress
- Get plenty of rest and relaxation
- Exercise regularly
- Reduce over-the-counter medications where possible (analgesia for example)
- Avoid antibiotics where possible
- Review your current medications with your Doctor. (For example oral contraceptive pill, ERT, antidepressant, cholesterol, antihypertensive - all these exert overload on the liver and can retard or inhibit successful weight loss and hormonal balancing.
- Drink heaps of pure water
- Avoid foods that may be high in steroid estrogens i.e. non-organic chicken, grain fed animals, replace with foods high in plant estrogens.
- Eat organic where possible
- Improve lymphatic drainage (deep tissue massage, recipe for diuretic juicing) found in Dr Sandra Cabot's 'Raw Juicing Can Save Your Life' and refer to the section in book 2 on Lymphatic Herbal Teas.
- Improve bowel function, avoid constipation. Increase fibre and bowel transit time.

- Eliminate toxins - colonic treatment
- Give yourself permission to take time out - relax with yoga, Pilate's or meditation
- Eat more vegetables and adopt a juice regime
- Avoid stress triggers where possible and learn to say 'no'
- Reassess your job
- Address chronic infections (Candida, Thrush)

What are phytoestrogens?

Phytoestrogens, phytosterols are plant sterols (also referred to as natural isoflavone plant hormones) that come from the plant kingdom which have an estrogenic or female effect on our body. The traditional 'eastern' diet contains greater quantities of legumes (for example, beans, chick peas, soy) which are rich in natural plant estrogens called isoflavones, tubular plants are exceptionally high.

Isoflavones have been shown to play an important role in maintaining health before, during, and after menopause, and particularly in relieving menopausal symptoms such as Hot Flushes. It is well known that populations that consume abundant and regular amounts of dietary phytoestrogens have a lower incidence of Breast Cancer and other hormonally sensitive cancers, Heart Disease, menopause symptoms and Osteoporosis.

There is significant research into estrogenic substances found in plants and foods, and their effects upon hormonal disorder and balancing. Indeed, phytoestrogens have been widely used and recognised for their medicinal value and treatment in helping relieve many of the symptoms at menopause.

Foods high in beneficial plant hormones *can include alfalfa, apples, aniseed, brewers yeast, barley, beetroot, cabbage, carrots, chick peas, clover, corn, cow peas, cucumbers, fennel, linseed, garlic, green beans, green squash, hops, oats, olives, olive oil, papaya, parsley, plums, potatoes (sweet), red beans, pumpkin, legumes, peas, lentils, red clover, rhubarb, rice, rye, sesame seeds, soya bean, sprouts, split peas, sunflower seeds, nuts, wheat yams, cherries, wild yams.*

Some herbs *containing beneficial plant hormones are dong quai, hops, sage, red clover, fennel, liquorice root, wild yam, bladderwrack, horsetail herb, sarsaparilla.*

NPAN certainly does not profess to understand the complexity of phytoestrogens. I simply acknowledge the large majority of women who liaise with NPAN and appear to understand the value of phytoestrogens in their health regime, and their invaluable usage in hormone balancing.

In fact I would go so far as to say y*ou cannot use progesterone successfully without phytoestrogens.* A nagging point I hone in on with my women and one I do not wish you to overlook. *Herein lies one of the secrets of getting the best mileage out of your progesterone therapy along with Magnesium (which I believe assists chemical conversion of this hormone) allowing greater availability in its performance and its multifactorial tasks.* And it is important to continue your phytoestrogens (whether in diet intake or supplementation or both) during your break off progesterone.

Please acknowledge that phytoestrogens are the silent partner to the success of progesterone therapy. **Phytoestrogens have application in progesterone therapy** *because they actually help reduce the impact of estrogen dominance when progesterone is reintroduced into the body (when you start and when you return from your break). The reason is simple. Phytoestrogens help tone down the symptoms of estrogen wake up. Phytoestrogens will be taken up by estrogen receptors.* This will block the impact of more potent estrogens produced by the body or the environment, and subsequently reduce the impact of estrogen dominance.   Whenever progesterone is introduced and the receptors have been refreshed/revitalised/restored and upregulated. It will invariably restimulate and wake up the estrogen receptors. *Phytoestrogens tone this 'wake up' down.*

All women using progesterone cream or experiencing hormonal imbalance should give due consideration to the benefits of food and supplements rich in phytoestrogens. Their benefits are just incredible. It's why I vehemently encourage young teenagers / women to first try plant hormones to reinstate hormonal balance before they resort to the introduction of hormone therapy to balance their estrogen dominance. This is particularly relevant to women who have intact ovaries and are ovulating. Perhaps they've neglected their diet, maybe they aren't exercising, maybe they are unknowingly exposed to xenoestrogens, chemical agitators, or just plain stressed.

While I encourage women to combine phytoestrogens with progesterone therapy, I do caution them to not go over the top with the use of soya products. *Some soya products are not fermented, rendering them less effective. Just be wary. These products can interfere with digestive enzymes.* Asian countries have learned how to use soya products in balance, in correct proportion (properly prepared - formulated), and to always eat them in conjunction with other food combinations.

There are many packaged soy products - many not so healthy because of wrong fats and sugars. Just because it says soy does not necessarily imply healthy. Learn to read labels.

Other benefits of phytoestrogens

- Helps keep the skin and mucous membranes more youthful.
- Helps boost dwindling estrogen levels.
- Stimulates estrogenic benefits in the body by stimulating estrogen receptors on the walls in the skin, breast and vagina.
- Stimulates progesterone activity (estrogen and progesterone need the presence of each other to work effectively they are a pigeon pair).
- Has balancing or modulating effect thus can protect cells from over stimulation from sex hormones.
- Protects body from cancer promoting estrogens by excreting some blocking effects upon receptors (i.e. occupies the receptor preventing stronger estrogen getting onto that receptor)

- Reduces estrogen dominant symptoms
- Helps reduce imbalance of excessive male hormones (androgens) by exerting feminine influence in conjunction with the use of progesterone.
- Helps tone down estrogen dominance and calms the body giving it a message that 'I'm okay, I have plenty of estrogen' because all the receptors are full.

The question always arises **'if I am so estrogen dominant, isn't it unwise to use lots of phytoestrogens. Won't this make me more estrogen dominant and increase all my symptoms?'**

Absolutely not! I can understand why this is difficult to grasp and I will endeavour to explain it as if I was talking to you in person. As I write most of my style and repetitious writing. I acknowledge in my work that if a question is still being asked and has not been understood it needs revisiting. Much of this revised book has been padded and repeated in areas based on questions still asked and on feedback. I need to know that you can journey in confidence and full of understanding. So let me get back to phytoestrogens. If you have grasped this contradictory principle i.e. Reduce estrogen dominance by increasing phytoestrogens. Skip on.

It is my understanding that even Doctors don't get it as seen time and time again. Whilst Doctors are backing off from estrogen (quietly) they are more frequently suggesting phytoestrogen formulas such as Remifemin (drug company pushed and backed with studies on Red Clover) to abate Hot Flushes, uncomfortable menopausal symptoms. When the women return 3-4 months later out of control again, complaining of severe estrogen dominance, they panic and tell them to stop phytoestrogens. These women arrive at NPAN very confused. What their Doctor may have missed in this equation, is the need for progesterone. Phytoestrogens (wild yam included) will not make progesterone. Whilst phytoestrogens minus progesterone will temporarily tone down symptoms. It is usually short lasting as progesterone deficiency emerges.

Why do estrogen dominant symptoms return 3-4 months later on phytoestrogens?

Phytoestrogens 3-4 months later become ineffective and *many women cannot successfully treat menopausal symptoms and estrogen dominant symptoms with phytoestrogens alone if they are truly progesterone deficient.* Progesterone is a different hormone to estrogens. They both have different roles to perform in the body and need each others presence in (balance) to synchronise and stimulate each other efficiently and effectively. In the absence of progesterone or too much estrogen, estrogen dominance prevails and runs amok producing havoc and unpleasant symptoms.

The key is ratio balance. The higher the ratio indifference between these hormones the worse symptoms become due to that dominant hormone being the leader (Testosterone can be a dominant player as seen in some instances) causing andrenous symptoms (male characteristic symptoms such as male pattern baldness and hair growth (moustache, chin hair etc).

There is only one progesterone receptor (thousand scattered of which are found throughout our body) but there are several different estrogen receptors (again thousands scattered throughout the body).

The body cannot differentiate the difference between real estrogens (be it estradiol, estrone or estriol) toxic estrogens as in xenoestrogens or plant estrogens, however what gets on those receptors first will determine the message that is going to be delivered to the body. (Just like if synthetic progestins take up the progesterone receptor space first - the message is different to real progesterone).

Plant estrogens (phytoestrogens) are safe estrogens, I liken them also to tricking estrogens and where they are so powerful in benefit is *they stop more potent estrogens getting in as they have already occupied that receptor space (blocking action).*

This consequently tones down or calms down the impact of stronger estrogen dominance induced symptoms and can be likened to a protector or guard man at the door. *The more plant estrogens occupying the receptors and the more calming effects* and less likelihood of unwanted toxic estrogens entering. Of course you still need to eliminate these from circulating in the symptom through diet, weight loss and liver work etc, as no one is exempt from xenoestrogens and if overweight, manufacturing and storing excess estrogen reserves. I tell my women to imagine a supermarket carpark, lots of spaces to be had. Any empty spaces will be occupied by any form of estrogen. This does not mean if you are eating and supplementing with phytoestrogens that your body won't get the benefits of real estrogen. It does because cars leave once the shopping (the task) is completed and thus making receptors (car spaces) available for the next occupier (more estrogen). The aim is to make phytoestrogens the major occupier of the car park.

This will tone down estrogen dominance, sending the message that the park is full, giving the body estrogenic benefits and calming the body, telling it that all is okay and thereby eliminating the need to panic and inducing estrogen balance. The fully occupied receptors sends feedback messages to the brain to not make more estrogen. The body does not feel the need to do this as it has interpreted it as adequately full and is satisfied by these tricking plant estrogens being present. (I call these estrogens *benign estrogens).*

Weaning off real estrogen can present problems being the pre conditioned high threshold that it has been used to (with stronger estrogen). Because the administered dosage puts the body in a pre menopausal state, the body has not learnt to adjust naturally to its own production and resources and is dependent upon additional administration top ups. *The aim here is to use phytoestrogens in conjunction with a reduction estrogen program allowing the brain and body to adjust naturally and let the body then progress into real menopause (not a halted state).*

Supplement with a PREMIUM phytoestrogen formulation

A good formulation would contain some, if not all the following ingredients:

Ascorbic acid

Calcium ascorbate

Bioflavonoids

Cholecalciferol

dl-alpha-Tocopheryl acetate

Calcium amino acid chelate

Calcium citrate

Calcium gluconate

Calcium orotate

Magnesium amino acid chelate

Zinc amino acid chelate

Folic acid

Phytomenadione

Pyridoxine hydrochloride

Thiamine hydrochloride

Riboflavine

A variety of phytoestrogens such as Black Cohosh

Wild Yam

Bladderwrack (kelp)

Dong Quai root

Liquorice root

Peppermint herb

Sage leaf

Sarsaparilla root

Rose hips

Horsetail stem

Alfalfa herb powder

Barley leaf powder

Carrot powder

Linseed powder

Pawpaw powder

Spinach powder

Soy protein

Brown rice powder

(NPAN women have discovered such a synergistic formulation called Femme Phase deriving multifactorial benefits combined with their progesterone cream usage). I have used Sandra Cabot's Femme Phase for 8 years (after trialling other comparatives along the way) and cannot go past it. Nearly all my women agree. I have hundreds of other women who have used Femme Phase for 7 1/2 years. We use two formulations (Femme Phase and Livatone Plus) and I have used them extensively in my consultancy work in hormonal balancing and thus leading to my association with Dr Sandra Cabot of more recent years. Book 2 'Natural Progesterone More Secrets Revealed', covers the ingredient dose guidelines.

What is the difference between phytohormones, phytoestrogens and xenohormones (xenobiotics /xenotoxins)?

The term phytohormones refers to plant substances that, when eaten, can be converted by the body into hormones. **Phytoestrogens**, for example, found in wild yam, soya, tofu, legumes will go on to mimic estrogen in the body. *These hormone-like substances are metabolised in the intestines and absorbed into the blood stream. They hold huge nutritional therapeutic value.*

Soya beans are a good example. Soya beans are one of the richest food sources of phytoestrogens which have a similar biological structure to naturally produced human estrogens. They contain the estrogenically active compounds coumestrol, isoflavones and lignans. *Of all the plant estrogens,* **coumestrol** *is the strongest and is most plentiful in soya beans.*

The term xenoestrogen refers to a foreign estrogen occurring in chemicals, petrochemicals and foreign substances (xenotoxins) that can also mimic estrogen in the body. *While the body interrupts/identifies it is an estrogen, it is a toxic form of estrogen, that invades the estrogen receptor sites, blocking more natural forms.*

Humans have evolved genetically in the context of what we eat. And we've been eating plants for many years. *The human body has the ability to bind the less toxic phytohormones to proteins thus reducing their effects and making them easier to eliminate more safely.* **This is not the case with synthetic xenohormones.**

Xenohormones (also referred to as xenobiotics / xenotoxins / xenoestrogen) *are foreign to the body and plant kingdom can be cell changing (cancer), and tend to have a very potent hormone-like activity in our body.* Nearly all xenohormones are synthetic petrochemical by-products present in our food, medicines, plastics, clothing, soaps, etc. These toxins build up in our body with disastrous effects, disrupting the endocrine system (dangerous).

Xenobiotics is a generic reference to substances with a hormone-like effect on the body, and **"xenoestrogens" specifically describe those with a estrogenic effect.**

Phytohormones (phytoestrogens) *have a balancing or modulating effect,* which means they can *protect our cells against over-stimulation from sex hormones* that are produced in the body, consumed in our diet or via medication and environment (safe form).

How do I reduce my exposure to xenoestrogens / xenohormones / xenotoxins (dangerous mimicking estrogens) in my environment?

Most women living in Western Industrialised countries will experience hormone related problems in their lifetime as a result of their exposure to petrochemical by-products present in their food, medicines, plastics, clothing, soaps, etc. *Too much estrogen in a woman's body without the balancing, protective properties of progesterone may be mirrored in the growing incidences of various cancers, PMS, Endometriosis, Fibroids, Infertility and early menopause.*

Humans are not immune to xenohormones / xenoestrogens, and our environmental exposure to these agents is increasing. It would be almost impossible to avoid them in this century and, as our modern technology advances, there grows an ever increasing danger, perhaps in plague proportion. The knowledge of the effects of xenohormones comes primarily from observing wildlife population exposed to chemicals in our waterways and through agricultural spraying. No living creature appears immune.

There are suggested links between exposure to environmental pollutants that mimic estrogen and the developing baby's tissue. Laboratory experiments, wildlife studies, and the human DES experience link hormone disruption with a variety of male and female reproductive problems that appear to be on the rise in the general human population - problems ranging from Endometriosis, Testicular Cancer, Infertility, disruption of menstruation, and in there somewhere is PCOS. The list is endless.

Hormonally active synthetic chemicals can alter the nervous system and brain, and impair the immune system. Synthetic chemicals can derail the normal expression of sexual characteristics of animals, in some cases masculinising females and feminising males. Some animal studies indicate that exposure to hormonally active chemicals prenatal or in adulthood increases vulnerability to hormone-responsive cancers, such as malignancies in the breast, prostate, ovary, and uterus (The book 'Our Stolen Future' details this).

It is argued that if a female embryo's ovarian follicles are compromised through exposure to these chemicals, this damage will not be apparent until after puberty.

Pregnant women should do whatever they can to protect themselves and their unborn child from exposure to xenoestrogens during gestation. Children, too, appear highly susceptible as their immunity system is immature. NPAN suggests women avoid buying plastic toys for their children, especially if they are at that age where they are prone to put everything into their mouth. Where possible, don't heat baby's plastic bottles in the microwave (it sheds plastic). Go back to using glass feeding bottles, and sterilise with boiling water rather than toxic chemicals.

Avoid foods such as non-organic chicken, avoid packaged and/or refined foods, and eat primarily fresh and preferably organic foods, taking care to wash produce thoroughly. Avoid storing food in plastics containers or plastic wraps. Instead store food in glass containers and never microwave or heat food inside a plastic container. Try and avoid plastic kettles (plastic lining disintegrates).

It is imperative to drink clean, filtered water. If you invest in a water filter be sure to change the filter whenever outlined by the product manufacturer otherwise this could create further problems.

One can only assume that pesticides, herbicides, fungicides, basically any substance that is used to kill fungi, plants, or bugs is going to be toxic to our body. Be aware, garden fertilisers, dog flea repellent wash, insect sprays and skin repellents may be highly toxic to you and your family and animals. Even oven cleaners are dangerous as seen with a 16 year old who worked in a chicken shop and had to clean the ovens daily, she had Endocrine Disease until she changed jobs.

If you're particularly susceptible to toxic fumes and are building a new home, do whatever you can to avoid laminated wood or wood veneers, or other materials that outgas chemicals. Glues and adhesives in particular are very toxic as in carpet laying. I have actually had women report severe haemorrhaging and heavy periods following the laying of new carpets.

Perhaps you're supersensitive to vinyls in cars, and vinyls on work benches (my husband is).

Women in the photography industry have also run into problems, specifically those working in the processing rooms of film laboratories and handling chemicals which are absorbed through their skin. Numerous hairdressers have come to me with cases of fibro-cystic breasts, Ovarian Cysts and polycystic ovarian syndromes, and I believe there may be a link between the chemicals and the fumes that they are exposed to in this industry.

Rural women who work on the land have displayed thyroid problems such as multi-nodular goiter. Observation suggests there's a link between chemicals used in farm management which may be adversely impacting the endocrine system. Otherwise, these women have lived a very healthy, active and organic lifestyle. It has also posed to me the questions of mineral deficiency using rain water only all their lives?

Certain hair dyes and hair products can contribute to xenohormone exposure in the body. I suggest, therefore, women try to use all natural products. If you know you are sensitive then perhaps refrain from dying your hair or applying unnecessary chemicals to your skin, eliminating exposure to fumes and skin. Acrylic nails is another one, too many incidents of disruption which I can no longer dismiss.

A small number of women in the plant nursery industry come to me with hormonal disorders and cyst problems. Could this be the result of exposure to toxic sprays, fertilisers and other substances?

Opt for detergents, soaps and shampoos that are echo-friendly. Avoid solvents and if you must use them protect your skin as they enter the blood stream quickly through the pores (200 to absorption rate). It is also important not to breath in fumes, to use masks were possible, and avoid exposure to paint fumes, car fumes, nail polish fumes as they can actually cause symptoms like Hot Flushes, heavy bleeding, and imbalances, as reported by far too many women.

There are certainly solvents in nail polish and nail polish removers used widely among the young teenagers who are vulnerable to reproductive damage. I caution women with hormone imbalance to be wary of the chemicals used to apply & remove false nails.

Through group meetings and my ongoing consultancy I have observed women with high levels of estrogen dominance who have undergone breast implants using foreign substances. It's crossed my mind there may be a correlation between their high level of estrogen dominance and a likely reaction to these foreign particles. Of course, there could be other underlying aspects, but there certainly seems to be a very strong link or suggestion that foreign objects implanted in breast cell tissue may lead to xenoestrogen exposure. As women are reluctant to remove these. Understandably so I stress the huge importance of ongoing protection using Livatone Plus, Femme Phase, MSM, Selenium, Vitamin C, Vitamin E and progesterone.

I reiterate here that progesterone cannot possibly protect us against the onslaught of xenoestrogens in our environment. Whilst progesterone may help tone down estrogen dominance symptoms and perhaps confer some protection, unless you directly address your exposure to xenoestrogens you'll always be vulnerable to endocrine disruption and associated complications. This is where continual liver function work and support is vital. Revisit Liver Principles.

For extensive information and references on xenohormones, please visit Dr. Theo Colborn's website: http://www.ourstolenfuture.org/. And of course Dr. Colborn's book, Our Stolen Future is an authoritative on the subject.

What are some of the foods containing natural estrogen?

There are many foods and herbs that are natural sources of plant estrogen referred to as phytoestrogens, and these can be very beneficial in helping control menopausal symptoms. Not only are these foods of estrogenic benefit, but they are also high in vitamins, minerals, fibre, essential fatty acids and low in saturated fat. Not surprisingly, consuming generous amounts of these phytoestrogens on a regular basis enhances general hormonal health and well-being and sound nutrition.

Foods range from hops, fennel, linseed, garlic, olive oil, olives, parsley, peas, plums, potato, pumpkin, soya beans, split peas, sunflower seeds, yam, wheat, rhubarb, red beans, red clover, rye, sage, sesame seeds, alfalfa, apples, bakers yeast, barley, beets, carrots, chick peas, clovers, corn, cow peas, cucumbers, liquorice, the list is endless. Gravitate towards dark leafy vegetables to.

Those women who have wisely incorporated phytoestrogens in their daily routine have reported benefits in helping reduce Hot Flushes, joint pains, fatigue, headaches, skin irritations such as itchiness and dryness, promoting bone building, improved immunity and cardiovascular systems, and vaginal dryness.

Who would benefit most from estrogenic foods?

Everyone, men included! Because our Western diet is lacking adequate amounts of raw vegetables, fresh fruit, and salads.

There is a 'class' of woman in particular who are high in androids or male hormone, and run an andrenous pathway that, using the assistance of phytoestrogens, helps feminise and balance the over-abundance of male hormones.

Typically, women who have Polycystic Ovarian Syndrome, women who have an android body shape type, who have hair loss or male pattern baldness, acne, carry excessive body weight around the stomach and abdomen often involving a fatty liver and insulin resistance, need to balance their body with forms of estrogenic foods and progesterone.

The Weight Control Doctor (http://www.weightcontroldoctor.com) talks about specific metabolic and hormonal characteristics in relation to your body shape and the right food for your body type.

I encourage women to be aware that these are the foods of life that will help to maintain and balance your hormones, and reduce your symptoms of hormonal imbalance. Foods that can be tailored to your specific body shape. There are foods that will derail your hormones just as there are fats that heal and fats that kill.

Men are not exempt here! Particularly for prostate health maintenance and protection. They too are exposed to high levels of estrogens and xenoestrogen and are also experiencing hormonal/endocrine disruption. I see too many men accompany their wives on their consultancy appointment only to end up addressing all their problems too. It has been an eye opener and I am convinced they too go through menopause (andropause). As I write this I am laughing to myself and humoured as to why it was called menopause? Surely it should have been named womenopause - whatever, they are welcome to this one since a man probably named it menopause. Did it refer to end of an era for men? i.e. sex being a medieval attitude of end of menses and reproduction and mistresses being the accepted way of life for these women glad to be rid of child bearing duties and ignore husbands extra curriculum! Can anyone enlighten me here? Whatever, *menopause means end of menses* when reproduction ends. But I have news - life can truly begin at this phase as so many of us have discovered. I trust you will join us on this wonderful journey of enlightenment and empowerment and not necessarily a break from men!

CHAPTER 18

Men & Teenagers: Progesterone Usage

- Men and Progesterone Usage

- Why would men need to take progesterone?

- Will progesterone help men with Osteoporosis?

- Suggested application sites

- Teenagers and progesterone usage

- Strategies to help correct hormone imbalance in teenager

- What are the circumstances that would require hormone replacement therapy in teenagers?

Men and Progesterone Usage
Why would men need to take progesterone?

I have certainly received my share of calls from men interested to learn how progesterone can be incorporated in the treatment of male-related illnesses that are linked to hormone imbalances. Sadly I am of little value to them in providing much information on progesterone usage in men. One of the primary functions of progesterone in men is to make testosterone and I have no doubt would have all the multifactorial benefits that women experience. Men are also exposed to the dangers of xenoestrogens as much as females and they too are suffering endocrine disruption as a result of this.

Progesterone in men is vital to good health. It is the primary precursor of their adrenal cortical hormones and testosterone. Men synthesise progesterone in smaller amounts than women do but it is still important.

THE LATE DR. JOHN LEE WRITES IN HIS JANUARY 1999 MEDICAL NEWSLETTER that as men get older their testosterone levels fall and their estradiol core levels go up.

The hormone testosterone undergoes changes that stimulates prostate growth. More testosterone is changed (by 5-alpha-reductase enzyme) to dihydrotestosterone (DHT), stimulating prostate growth. Since progesterone is a potent inhibitor of 5-alpha-reductase, the decline of progesterone in aging males plays a role in increasing the conversation rate of testosterone to DHT.

Basically, The Late Dr. Lee suggested men undergo progesterone replacement therapy using a maintenance dose of 8-10mg a day and 1-2mg per day of testosterone to protect against prostate cancer.

Regular FAI (Free Androgen Index) blood assay readings to check testosterone levels is recommended. Your doctor would be very familiar in interpreting this test as opposed to saliva readings. Bio identical hormone replacement therapy in men is beginning to get huge attention (ha, ha). Transdermal testosterone has become very popular and emphasis is now on testosterone trials in men and women. Men are definitely suffering endocrine disruption and it thrills me, not because I wish them to suffer or get a taste of their own medicine but it means medical mind shift may melt quicker as more and more men demand help and natural hormone supplementation.

If it is any gauge of a growing awareness and frustration amongst men, I would like to share a story. I recently had a phone call from a very irate male who was finding it difficult to get a prescription for transdermal testosterone and DHEA. He was on fire telling me (yelling) how ridiculous the system was and how unjust. ('Boy', I said, 'we've been trying to tell you guys this'). Women have been putting up with these barriers and obstacles for years. Tell me about it! He had saliva results proving a need in all hormones but could only find one Doctor in his area 'specialising' at $275.00 a visit. He was a pensioner. He had arranged with a compound chemist (new at the game) who had already made up his concoction of DHEA and testosterone and said he needed a script to release it. He then went on to state the cream would only last 6 weeks in expiry time. My alarm bells went off and heckles rose (more exploitation and now men!). I first enlightened him to seek an experienced, reputable compounding pharmacist who new how to correctly formulate and one that had studied hormone compounding and knew the value of correct bases. No cream should 'go off' in 6 weeks if correctly formulated and packaged! The manufactured testosterone Andromen® has a life span of 2 years provided it is stored in the right conditions. And the preservatives in it are in accordance with most standard formulations meeting and manufacturing regulations with quality control.

I secondly told him, in Australia his pharmacist friend was very presumptuous in telling him 'just go to a Doctor and get a script to match his recipe'. Thirdly I apologetically told him 'I was not in a position to refer him to my Doctor' which was what his pharmacist said. Just ring Jenny. I have spent years earning my credibility and trust working along side Doctors and am not going to allow myself or my privileges in helping women, be jeopardised by people who assume they can short circuit 8 years of consultancy work and bypass women who are prepared to work with my systems. As fragile as they are at least we are getting more and more Doctors (and even bulk billing ones) on side with respect and trust in my work and the women allowing them the benefit of their doubt by trying and using this still so unknown bio identical hormone to main stream medicine. They are nervous and skeptical, waiting to be disproved in their opinion with founded trials and research data and backup trials.

My Doctor only sees and prescribes once he knows women have been consulted (2 hours) assessed, informed and have read my book. He does not wish to end up with egg on his face from uninformed women/men who run off on a tangent and think they know it all only to end up back in their Doctors surgery complaining and putting them off side, spoiling it for others. I explained to this gentleman that I do not consult men as I do not have the knowledge and expertise in there hormonal health. I do however consult men on weight control and only if they are accompanied by a spouse or partner. I did however refer him to Dr Sandra Cabot's clinic for other options in obtaining a script and correct interpretation of his saliva readings and specific dosage needs. With this episode I felt positive that it would be the men (due to their anger and their threatened libidos) who will bring about political changes, that I am sure. When women's lobbying has fallen on deaf ears, as I have discovered.

Information for Men and hormones.

The Late Dr John Lee wrote a book addressing this specific area and can be obtained from his website or by contacting Virginia Hopkins.

Will progesterone help men with Osteoporosis?

Possibly yes, the same principle applies because progesterone will help build new bone for men in much the same way it does for women.

Usage of plant ingested estrogens may play a great role here too and a good bone joint formulation, along with natural testosterone if low F.A.I. blood readings.

Remember testosterone and DHEA are also S4 drugs requiring a Doctor's script in Australia and New Zealand.

Suggested application sites for men

If there is a cyst or lump in the testes that has been tested and found to be benign then I would suggest you apply cream directly to the testes. A similar approach is adopted by women with Fibrocystic Breasts, and progesterone has certainly helped reduce if not eliminate lumpy breasts and benign hormone related Cysts.

I recommend that the sites of application mirror those adopted by women. Areas where the blood vessels are very close to the skin, avoiding fatty areas like the stomach and buttocks, and **avoid areas where there are more than a few hair follicles (ie hairy).**

Suggested areas for men where there is good blood supply is inside the groin, behind the knees, ankles, wrists, inside under your arms (not armpit), on the temples, forehead, neck, upper chest. It's not necessary to apply progesterone cream directly to the penis. (Libido and testosterone is covered in Book 2).

Too much cream may cause fluid retention, headaches and other associated symptoms so please use only small maintenance dose of 8-10mg a day. Men also suffer estrogen dominance wake up and benefit enormously from phytoestrogen foods. For example salads, nuts, legumes daily.

Please visit Lawley pharmaceutical website www.testosterone.com.au and even contact the manufacturer who does hold a TGA approved overseas export license.

Teenagers and Progesterone Usage

Problems already surfacing in the teenage years

Hormone dysfunction exhibited in our teenagers is indeed an alarming and growing concern. Painful periods, embarrassing acne, unexplained weight gain, aggression and moodiness, emotional instability, depression, girls with excessive body hair, reproductive disorders such as Endometriosis and Polycystic Ovarian Syndrome, cycles that fluctuate every month, 15 years old girls with severe PMS, girls coming into their menses age 10 years or earlier, cranky, irritable sons who can't seem to find any joy in the world. It is a universal problem affecting both sexes. Evidence is suggesting huge endocrine disruption is now erupting in ever increasing numbers of young teenagers and young adolescents. I have lost count of all the distraught mothers not knowing where to turn with their daughters and related hormonal problems. Many of which are falling on deaf ears. Doctors do not know any other way to assist other than referrals and when tests come back clear and negative, the oral contraceptive pill is offered. Mothers are adamant and do not want their average 12 year olds on the pill.

Hormone disruption is physically and emotionally crippling our teenage children. And we ought to be extremely concerned. Mums are bringing their daughters to me at NPAN on a weekly basis desperate for answers, and unable to find appropriate guidance for these problems that don't involve strong medication, synthetic HRT, the oral contraceptive Pill, anti-depressants, or antibiotics. There appear to be no satisfactory explanations forthcoming that would explain such bizarre hormonal disruption and abnormal behaviour patterns.

I've seen a range of sad cases from girls as young as 12 years of age having experienced a couple of years of menstrual problems. Girls as young as 12 with severe Polycystic Ovarian Syndrome undiagnosed till age 14 and yet so obvious when you look at the collation of symptoms they present (later confirmed with high testosterone levels and ultrasounds revealing Ovarian Cysts). Another extreme where an 18 year old girl has only experienced one period since her menstruation commenced at 12 years old. And no endocrinologist can offer an explanation other than low estrogen levels and to administer estrogen therapy.

In much the same way as I encourage women to assist themselves, mums and dads can help their teenager children establish healthy habits that will foster optimal hormonal balance, emotional and physical, during adolescence and beyond. I encourage mothers not to look for a quick fix medication. It is not that simple and often masquerades other problems needing addressing. The band-aid approach does not address real deep seated physical and emotional issues experienced in these vulnerable and impressionable years. It also encourages young adolescent children to seek drugs 'stimulants, mood alterers' to sort out their problems, with our consent and often with the message, 'If you're not okay take medical drugs to make you feel better'. In their minds there is often no difference between swallowing an antidepressant or smoking from a bong or smoking a joint or taking recreational drugs.' What's the difference in their head when they do not differentiate at this age, as young people do believing they are indestructible. I speak from first hand experience here and now having survived my own codeine addiction/dependency and my son's drug habits (now clean). I am very much wiser and more aware. I am also very resistant to the idea of children/young adults being placed on antidepressants and the Pill unless absolutely warranted. I beg parents to look at other options first. Dangerously young people are using antidepressants with alcohol and other recreational drugs not understanding the consequences of these actions and negating the benefits of being prescribed these medications for specific conditions.

Strategies to help correct hormone imbalance in teenagers

What are the circumstances that would require hormone replacement therapy in teenagers?

Basically, if you want to help your children correct hormone imbalance, you want to teach them about being healthy. Discuss what that means to them, and what strategies they ought to employ to get on top of their problems.

- Encourage your teenage children to eliminate carbonated, fizzy drinks from their diet. Teenagers don't appreciate that they are, in fact, laying down bone mass that will determine bone integrity when they're older. And these drinks literally leach calcium from their bones. Studies and surveys in nutrition at schools are proving children are actually malnourished due to high levels of carbohydrates and imbalanced nutritional dietary intake.

- Weight control is essential for good health and hormone balance. And there's growing evidence that a diet high in carbohydrates is not necessarily good for you. More attention should be given to our protein-carbohydrates-fats ratio to eliminate obesity and any likelihood of Diabetes Type II which is on the rise in Western cultures. You might also like to read Dr Sandra Cabot's book 'The Body Shaping Diet' and 'Syndrome X' for a better understanding of diabetes and diet.

- In a world where the 'remote control' rules, getting off our backside is a chore. Clearly, we're not getting the daily physical workout of yesteryear when physical exertion was a part of just about everything we did growing up (fun and play) when computers and televisions were limited. That's why it's imperative our kids exercise in some shape or form for good bone building, to naturally control weight, to improve mental alertness, to feel good about themselves, and get on top of dark moods and stressful situations.

- As parents, we can help significantly by providing nutritious, organic meals and snacks wherever possible. Think RAW foods, including vegetables, fruit and greens such as salads daily with cold pressed and olive oil dressings. Plenty of eggs - they are full on natural cholesterol, organic sulfur and protein. Get your family into juicing every day. Reform them slowly, and make it a way of life so they don't see it as being forced upon them and depriving them of their comfort foods.

Rule of Thumb

Avoid packaged and deep-fried food where you can. Essential oils (omega 3-6) are the building blocks of the body and as the term applies they are essential to the body for good health. They also nourish the brain. So serve your children the right oils (cold pressed) and avoid polyunsaturated fats and oils (including margarine). Avoid processed fatty meats, these include most deli foods, i.e., salami which also can be full of bacteria.

Adopt more liver foods.

Eating is a sociable occasion, so encourage your children to sit with you at the dinner table and share of themselves. This is a perfect opportunity for kids to develop a positive association with food and family. A healthy, appetising meal prepared with love and shared with the family should be something our kids look forward to on a regular basis. It's an opportunity also to assess signs of a possible eating disorder and the attitudes associated with the foods you might serve. Social pressure will influence young girls regarding fear of weight gain, and/or being a (selective) vegetarian to be seen as 'cool', but not getting a balanced vegetarian diet. For example, chicken in their mind is acceptable but, realistically, it's known to be laced with estrogen, antibiotics, and chemicals which may disrupt their hormone balance. Red lean meat provides iron so if they refuse red meat ensure they are getting plenty of iron. Green leafy vegetables, spirulina if necessary or iron supplement (liquid).

Explain the importance of clean (filtered) water in their diet each day - aim for at least 8 glasses. Invest in a water filter to encourage a higher intake of H2O. Tap water is often laced with chemicals and fluorides which puts more work on the liver to filter. And foul-tasting water discourages drinking.

Stress can be productive or destructive. And it can shift the balance of our hormones if it goes unaddressed. We need to teach our children how stress fits into their lives. How to harness & channel stress to reach for and achieve life-long pursuits. Parents need to look at their own stress levels and how it may be rebounding on their children. They also need to help their rechanneling of stress, anger and frustration appropriately (exercise helps so if necessary adopt a family interest that everyone enjoys in burning off pent up emotions and misdirected energy). Suppressed anger leads to depression. Often kids cannot locate their true problems (peer pressure, being bullied, image problems, poor self esteem, learning difficulties) and lash out where they feel safest, the parents and siblings. Exercise and fun activity release natural happy chemicals endorphins which are natural antidepressants. Sunlight is so important in the manufacturing of these chemicals (serotonin) everyone needs sun as an antidote so pick sunny holiday locations. It also promotes bone formation (Vitamin D).

Provide them with a safe place where open communication, honesty and freedom of expression can take place without fear of punishment, disapproval or rejection. Their self-esteem, self-worth and self-image are very fragile, and suppression through an inability to correctly express themselves reflects in their mental well-being and may come out in the form of ill health and imbalance. Parents often don't recognise stress and the pressure their teenage son or daughter is under (which may be of an external nature - peers, study and school problems) until it masquerades as physiological symptoms (such as depression or period problems).

Where possible, stay away from high sugar/refined foods, including white flour. Easier said that done in this day and age. Nonetheless, when it's pointed out how the body interrupts these foods and the burden it places on our metabolism, we think you'll find your teenage children surprisingly receptive to changes in their diet. Avoid that trap that we all fall into as parents of picking up those convenient, much loved fast-food meals ... and large bottle of soft drink. Protein stabilises blood sugar levels and prevents attacks of hypoglycemia (low sugar). Lack of good protein causes kids to reach for a quick fix energy hit. (Sugars, caffeine, chocolate, burger and chips). So it is important they obtain their energy correctly for brain food and growing energy. Give them more mixed (not salted) nuts and dried fruit snacks and fruit organic, homemade and whole grain biscuits and bread. White bread is full of refined flours, high in hidden fats and sugars and does not give long satiety. Pastas whilst are quick energy and yummy are carbohydrates so make sure there is less pasta and more meat or bolognase sauce along with a salad or vegetables. If you have to hide the vegetables in the sauce (puree). You can also purchase now corn pasta as a substitute.

Milk is not the only source of calcium. Look to other non-dairy sources such as soy products, green juice drinks like barley grass, wheat grass, seaweed, kelp, brown rice. Calcium is derived from many sources, although the general public believe it comes strictly from dairy intake. You'd be surprised just how many foods are calcium rich minus the saturated fats. Maybe you'd like to visit http://www.notmilk.com to learn more. If you are concerned for their growing bones use a good multi vitamin with high calcium levels or Calcium Complete or Super Calcium Extra (Vitamin Concepts) on their own. Both absorb brilliantly for most, and absorption is the key.

Don't be fooled by low-calorie diet drinks, they still have the same impact on the body as does refined sugars with the added lacing of aspartame which is a neuro-genic disrupter. More abuse on the developing body, liver and reproductive organs. We encourage you to visit http://www.doorway.com for more info on artificial sweeteners.

Teach your children to identify products that contain caffeine. Many people are unaware that certain fizzy drinks contain caffeine, particularly the older generation. The market pitches caffeine laced 'pick me up' soda drinks stimulants at our kids in the form of harmless fizzy drinks and stamina drinks. Little wonder Diabetes Type II is on the rise, aggravated by this high daily consumption of refined sugars. Adrenal exhaustion can result further down the track.

Nicotine, alcohol, and drugs generally are toxic to the body. And many of the drugs or medications that the kids are experimenting with (cocktails that include speed, amphetamines, ecstasy, marijuana, to name a few) are more harmful than they realise. Not only do they accumulate in the body, and often store in fatty organs such as the brain when the (overworked) liver is unable to break these toxins down, but it also breaks down their immunity system and compromises other bodily functions perhaps leading to psychotic, digestive or reproductive disorders.

NPAN highlights to parents how children too readily rely on headache tablets and household analgesics, and think nothing of the ramifications. When it comes to popping the headache tablet or period pain fix, teenagers do not think beyond the moment. A vicious cycle is established because they take the tablets to fix the headache which is often caused by toxicity and/or allergies, withdrawal from stimulants, and ebbs of sugar imbalances in the blood. Many of these painkiller tables are codeine-based which are addictive, and withdrawal may trigger more pain.

One mother was so concerned about the level at which her daughter was consuming painkillers for her headaches which, by the way, always followed a pattern, that she substituted the medication cupboard with bottles of magnesium. The outcome was quite remarkable. Her daughter, having experienced muscle relaxation, reduced stress and easing of her headaches, is now happy to resort to what she terms 'hippie' medicine. She's also aware of her need to maintain hydration with water rather than fizzy drinks. She also acknowledges smoking causes her headaches!

Introducing synthetic hormones into a teenager's body is going to create havoc, possibly leading to serious ramifications on breast and reproductive organs later on. So if your daughter is experiencing period problems, try natural alternatives before putting her on The Pill. The Pill might iron things out for a while, but problems can and do occur. For contraception and protection against STDs, using a condom is the safest option. Ensure your children are well educated in alternative methods of contraception never take this subject and topic for granted seek out educational books and services.

Exposure to xenoestrogens (foreign hormones that mimic estrogen in the body that are present in animal fats, particularly red meat and dairy fats, plastics, herbicides, pesticides, industrial by-products) can affect the reproductive organs of both teenage boys & girls. Xenoestrogens exaggerate the natural hormone surges at adolescence. For teenage girls suffering symptoms of estrogen dominance such as menstrual pain, early onset of menses, PMT, etc., the first line of defence is to eat foods rich in phytoestrogens to counteract these foreign hormones in the body.

Incorporate a daily liver tonic to help stimulate the liver into excreting some of the estrogen. Visit The Liver Doctor website for more info.

Encourage kids to become 'grazers' snacking on protein rich foods (which help balance their blood glucose and reduce their hunger pangs). For example, unsalted mixed nuts, seeds, hommus dips (chick peas) with celery or carrots. If your children are not getting enough protein intake per day, get them onto a high level spirulina - an excellent source of plant protein and iron. Offer the kids 'health' shakes that include raw eggs, soya, rice milk, bananas, without telling them what's in it! Add a protein powder to be base of this.

Teenage acne problems can be tackled with a whole food diet, exercise, minimal dairy and a good liver cleansing tonic that will assist elimination of toxins from the body and 2 litres of H2O and plenty of balanced omega oils as well as plenty of naturally rich antioxidant foods. Also educate your children about hygiene.

Nutritional and vitamin supplements are important if teenagers genuinely want to reach optimal health. And this can be encouraged through example. Get them to try one or two vitamins/minerals from your stock, see if they notice the difference. Vitamin C, a Multi B, and a Omega 3-6 are a great place to start in supporting the body. Once they're sold on the concept, help your teenage children to individualise a daily intake of core multivitamins and minerals that suits their specific needs. If need be, seek professional input (a dietician, natural approach).

Regular Health Checks. Get their health checked out, if they are not well make sure appropriate tests are run, e.g., blood profile (iron levels).

Herbs have incredibly powerful benefits in helping to balance and regulate hormone and menstrual cycles, addressing stress and sleeping disorders. And I certainly encourage parents to seek out a knowledgeable herbalist to guide and assist in this direction because often restoration can occur without the need for hormone replacement. For it is always best to let the body do what it can to resolve hormone imbalance naturally. Refer to side effects of oral contraception on pages 283, 306,346.

The question is often asked, what are the circumstances that would require natural hormone replacement therapy in teenagers?

My Network has witnessed favourable outcomes where natural progesterone has been incorporated in cases of:

- Polycystic Ovarian Syndrome
- Endometriosis
- Period irregularities
- Anovulatory problems
- Cyclic acne, Thrush

Severe PMS (which has failed to response to nutritional, herbal, and dietary methods). Mothers have adopted this approach, before undergoing stronger forms of hormone replacement therapy, because they are fearful of exposing their daughters at such a tender age until they feel satisfied they have given other options the full benefit of the doubt.

They are advised by their doctor that natural progesterone is not a standard form of treatment, that little is known about progesterone in the treatment of these diseases, suggesting these mothers are perhaps acting somewhat irresponsibly and/or irrationally. This places mothers in further conflict. I empathise with the emotional conflicts and issues faced by these mothers, nonetheless, I do make a point of clarifying that 'natural' progesterone is a form of hormone replacement therapy, and by supplementing their daughter's progesterone levels they ARE, in fact, tampering with their endocrine system. Unless this person is clearly not ovulating or is progesterone deficient with resultant estrogen dominant symptoms. A saliva hormone profile will reflect true progesterone levels and a blood test will indicate high testosterone levels as in suspected PCOS. Replacing a missing hormone in these cases is not tampering with their endocrine system. It is simply compensating an obvious deficit. For various reasons their ovaries function has become disrupted. So parents need appreciate this fact, and find a very supportive doctor who is willing to do regular tests, assessments and monitoring of their daughter's progress on progesterone supplementation. There may be biological/physical reasons beneath the surface needing further investigation but certainly putting back into the body hormone that is missing and should be there will not compound further damage. It will protect and support further disruption in my opinion.

PLEASE NOTE HERE: You must be absolutely sure your daughter is NOT on the Pill. Otherwise there is no point using progesterone.

Note, if your teenage son or daughter is overweight, no solution will be long-term until weight reduction is addressed, and the underlying problem identified. If you daughter's weight problems do not respond to dietary changes corresponding with hormone balancing, and you know she is not sneaking junk food, then we urge you to seek medical advice. Insist on a hormone profile testing all hormones, including progesterone because your daughter may not be ovulating. Ask to include blood profile, pelvic examination, ultrasound to assess the ovaries, further examinations should include bowels, breast, thyroid, liver function, blood sugar, likelihood of STDs. Don't overlook the possibility of glandular fever, Candida, or bowel parasites.

To counteract the androgenic symptoms (excessive body hair) experienced by teenage girls, incorporate a quality phytoestrogen supplement and feminising foods - refer to this chapter on phytoestrogens and nutrition in book 2. Natural progesterone supplementation may be required if hormone imbalance does not right itself. Eliminate all refined sugars and carbohydrates, and get on a weight reduction program. High levels of testosterone interferes with insulin and the manufacturing and metabolising of glucose, thereby causing further weight gain in the upper body, creating more testosterone which further interferes with ovarian function. Thus the vicious cycle.

Make sure your daughter is not on the Contraceptive Pill. I say this because I have had mothers bring their daughters to visit me, desperate for answers that might explain their daughter's hormone imbalance, mood swings, Depression, hair loss, weight gain, headaches, and so on. And upon further detective work, it has been discovered that these girls have been sexually active and placed themselves on the Pill without their parents' knowledge.

I also had a mother broach me for her daughter's genital herpes after commencing progesterone. She was adamant that the cream had caused this. Of course the Doctor confirmed her previous sexual activity was the cause not progesterone.

I see all sorts of scenarios and get into all sorts of situations. There are many times I just have to say it as it is, which can be very confrontational and threatening especially when it involves our child or children.

One sad and difficult case was a lady who came to see me for her own hormonal and weight issues. Nearing the end of our appointment I did not feel right. My gut was telling me something was not resonating and I felt I had not truly connected with this person and I felt the appointment was in vain. The phone interrupted me and conversation was around the callers usage of her "Ovestin".

My "Ovestin" package was sitting on my cabinet, as I'd accidentally left it there earlier that day. When I got off the phone apologising, this lady said 'oh, my daughter was on that'. Having done her profile, I realised her daughter was now 6 years old. My intuition was running. I asked her 'when and why?'. She said 'oh, when she was 4 for vaginal discharge'. I said 'that a child who has not reached puberty does not discharge for no reason'. She then went on to say that is what her second Doctor said and took her off it. Her next comment was 'I thought that cream was causing her to inappropriately and obsessively masturbate now constantly'. 'She is always red down there and I told her she's disgusting for masturbating on everything she could get in touch with' (wooden toy boxes etc). I gently explained perhaps she had been taught this, that the discharge had been introduced and the likelihood of sexual abuse could be a cause. Naturally the mother said 'No way, only her father has contact with her!' I handed her a card to follow up (if she wished) to the sexual abuse clinic and told her perhaps they could check out if there was or not anything sinister and if it so happened to be a severe case of natural masturbation and self contamination and self traumatic infection, then they could teach her (and the mother) skills to deal with it and redirect her daughters obsession into healthy physical outlets without growing up feeling guilt and shame ridden or embarrassed . Not to mention due to this promiscuous behaviour leaving her open to sexual predators. Because of the depth and complexities involved in this area with many men and women and the possible obstacles in hormone balancing and healing I have addressed this in the companion book and intend to delve further into this subject in a third book specifically on sexual abuse.

I mention just one of many tragic stories involving children and sexual abuse one in three women are victims and I feel it needs to be addressed. And no, Ovestin is not a standard treatment for children. I was shocked to hear this and shocked that the second Doctor did not take it further. Perhaps that "Ovestin" package and phone call was not coincidence but God incidence.

Always stay open to the possibility of your children being sexually abused (sudden behavioural changes, unknown gynecological problems. And if there is an element of doubt seek professional advice from experts in this area). I have had many intense and real situations involving adolescents and abuse. Horrible and confrontational as it is it's a mothers worst nightmare. I have taken off the blinkers in Book 2.

I also would like to mention cases of antidepressants, mood altering controlling drugs in adolescence. Far too many are placed on these which compound their surging hormonal problems and impact on their young liver.

One young adolescent boy was reluctant to use his regularly (yo-yo effect) as it interfered with his ability to sexually perform and interfered with his drinking weekends with his mates. He intelligently resourced for himself the drug indication and side effects leaflet and decided they were not for him, but did not have the maturity or know how to intelligently use them or wean off them. His mother kept dragging him back to the Psychologist who kept upping the dose as his moods were erratic.

This young man is closely known to me and I have discovered that he is suffering more from mother phobia and her attempt to control his life and moods. Now he has left home and he is happy and coping and is not as frustrated, angry and maybe was misdiagnosed by the Psychologist whom was a close friend of the mother.

How often we fall in the trap of wanting outside methods, institutions, experts or medications to fix or control our uncontrollable children. Not all cases and I am generalising. The point is sometimes we just may need to look in the mirror and take the cause effect of our own attitudes and behaviour.

For me when I confronted my son's drug habit (including everything but heroin, when they say they are not using drugs they often mean 'shooting up') and asked him why? He bluntly stated"Look at you and all those pain killers you're swallowing". This was my wake up call. I proceeded to get self help and sort my own habits out before I could adjust his. Thank the Lord, in time he responded change comes from within and the only power we have is that of changing ourselves. Women hold a golden key and can with faith and appropriate action can move mountains from a deep internal space and say absolutely nothing!

Incidence of Endocrine Disruption in younger women is becoming an epidemic.

Through figures and observation, this problem is growing alarmingly - in plague proportions. Statistics suggest obesity contributes up to 60% of polycyctic ovarian syndrome (PCOS) of all ages. Leading to 2:3 women experiencing Infertility as discovered in IVF programs (recently released by media). A loss of 10 kilos in many has made a difference between Infertility and successful conception. PCOS, weight gain and syndrome X (insulin resistance) are the culprits in hormonal dysfunction in so many women. Dr Sandra Cabot's revised update on her latest book "Hormones don't let them ruin your life", covers this in depth, also in her book "Syndrome X".

Principles for treating PCOS remain the same in all ages. Far too many mothers are reporting to me of this problem starting as young as 12 years. But they are not getting appropriate diagnosis, treatment or guideline management to deal with the problem.

CHAPTER 19

About NPAN and Jenny's work.

History and Activity of this Organisation NPAN.

The natural progesterone advisory network (NPAN) was conceived, founded and created by Jenny Birdsey from infancy in direct response to women's cries for help and the need for information!

Notwithstanding how we sourced our progesterone cream and in fact if it actually contained real progesterone or a synthetic substitute. There remained a million and one questions on how natural progesterone transdermal cream ought to be applied and used and how to interpret the signs and symptoms once progesterone therapy had commenced.

Outraged by what I discovered, it become all too apparent that these women along with myself needed an 'informed choice' and this could never be possible if doctors and pharmaceutical companies continued to deny women access to all the facts.

At the heart of NPAN's endeavours was a fervent understanding of each and every women's silent suffering.

For a time Wild Yam confusion reigned within the healthcare industry in Australia and New Zealand. The Therapeutics Goods Administration (TGA) initially allowed into Australia Progesterone Creams labelled under the banner of Wild Yam Creams but actually contained natural progesterone - an S4 drug - without sanctioning appropriate safety measures that would ensure women fully understand what they were buying and putting onto their bodies. Authentic natural progesterone creams were soon after subsequently banned. Women then faced the arduous task of locating a GP willing to write a prescription, sourcing a reliable cream after local supplies had dried up, sourcing a real progesterone cream then supplied by compounding pharmacists with no guarantee of efficacy. We were at the mercy of trusting that this was formulated correctly and then making sense of the effect this cream had on our bodies.

In my endeavour for further understanding and providing support for women in a similar situation I offered monthly support home meetings, a free phone service within Australia, to accommodate women's pleas for help and information. I also supplied free information packs in the earlier days to women and Doctors.

At times we were able to be in direct consultation with the Late Dr John Lee in the United States who assisted us in our quest for understanding on the usage of natural progesterone as we were obviously on our own and isolated from reliable information. As a group and through monthly meetings we acquired knowledge from each other and were to happy to put ourselves up for experimentation.

From here this is where my work and organisation started which provided the nucleus of my knowledge base to be expanded upon.

Jenny's activity in operating her NPAN organisation over the years.

Summary:

- NPAN began helping women in late 1996.
- NPAN became a registered business in 1998, solely owned, self funded and operated by Jenny Birdsey who is a non-practicing nurse and who's husband, Garth, is a clinical pharmacist & lecturer.

- Warning: NPAN has been officially registered and still is Jenny Birdsey's business it is now 2004 and in the last few years since 2001 NPAN has been fraudulently 'passed off' trading off by other unscrupulous operators. Which has created public confusion and the proliferation of misinformation that Jenny Birdsey in no way advises through her organisation. Do not be misconceived if you receive information via others.

- Jenny Birdsey and her organisation is the true and authentic NPAN and holds a worldwide trade logo.

- NPAN is the abbreviation of Natural Progesterone Advisory Network which people often get confused about.

- A network offering observational advice & support, consultancy and self published books.

- Has gathered information and analytical data to determine, where possible, the safety and reliability of various creams being used by women.

- Privately funded with additional help and assistance from some women through donations. Also continued support by her husband.

- No remunerations are derived from sale of progesterone creams, advertising or affiliated programs and MLM companies or sponsorship.

- Free phone consultations - labour and time with women callers has been in the past given freely. Phone consultancy is now by appointment and fees now apply.

- Active in lobbying the Western Australian Government to speed up legislation progress to make progesterone cream available in ALL states in Australia.

- NPAN work within the guidelines of the Therapeutic Goods Administration (TGA) in Australia.

- Promoted by word of mouth, driven by women throughout Australia and New Zealand, and has now expanded globally and guided by women's spiritual connectedness.

- Private, fee-for-service consultation made available by appointment. Email consultancy is currently being set up to accommodate international demand.

- Jenny Birdsey 's widely acclaimed book Natural Progesterone the Worlds Best Kept Secret has a sequel Book 2 Natural Progesterone More Secrets Revealed

- Jenny Birdsey's first book has been so sought after through word of mouth throughout the world through popular demand she has written a companion book to compliment this revised update of the 1st edition.

- A Resource Centre working in consultation with members of the Healthcare Industry (doctors, psychologist, herbalists, nutritionists, naturopaths, compounding pharmacists, community health centres, healthfood stores) and other holistic professionals.

- Working in association with Dr Sandra Cabot's 'Women's Health Organisation' incorporating Dr Cabot's weight control principles. NPAN is a separate organisation to Women's Health Advisory Health Organisation.(WHAS). NPAN or Jenny is not paid by Dr Sandra Cabot or WHAS.

- NPAN derives its funding from consultancy, seminar work, sale of nutritional supplements and books.

- Extensive circulation of 'Doctor's Packs' in the earlier days led to subtle infiltration of the medical fraternity to not only accept natural progesterone as an alternative therapy but establish alternative practices in women's hormonal health based on NPAN's intellectual property and observational data on cream usage and guidance.

- Jenny works in conjunction and/or cooperative association with many General Practitioners. Some of which originally sourced information from her organisation to begin their own involvement in practicing NHRT.

- Jenny continues advocacy through her seminar work and public speaking which is expanding by word of mouth.

- Consultancy is by appointment only. Due to limited hours her time to speak to women is very restricted and urges women to read the books rather than waste unnecessary time asking questions which are already addressed in her books. She also requests that if an emergency connection is required please use the business line only (between 9.00am - 10.00am), or visit her website.

- Jenny cannot guarantee that she will be able to respond to everyone

- Jenny's reputation in consultancy has extended to include clients in Germany, America, UK, South Africa and Sweden.

- Jenny's data and observation has been compiled from real case histories.

NPAN is collectively every Woman

Over several years, Jenny has personally met with hundreds of woman, spoken to hundreds of women over the phone, organised monthly meetings that led to the creation of NPAN enabling her to enrich information and data base collection.

Women often ask what are Jenny's qualifications. Here's Jenny's reply: "I am a registered trained nurse by profession but more importantly I am a woman on the same journey as themselves." I have had the ability to work through conflicting issues in conjunction with my hormonal imbalance, and understand why and how these emerged and where they all fit together.

I have also had the gift and opportunity to have been surrounded by some wonderful loving supportive women and men throughout the years operating NPAN, and for this I thank them. Without their contribution and continued encouragement, this Book and now my second book would not be possible.

NPAN now wishes to pass on this information because our journey has only just begun collectively as women. As more and more doctors embrace natural progesterone, it will give rise to further confusion and exploitation. Failure to educate women on the multi-factorial benefits and correct usage of progesterone according to symptoms may disempower women further.

If a doctor believes in the 'one size fits all' approach to progesterone therapy in the same way he or she prescribes HRT, it will not be as optimally effective as it could be. This is actually happening right now as I prepare this Book, and it gravely concerns me. I'm back to where I started from. Women are disempowered when denied full disclosure of the facts and ongoing support.

Women need to be made aware that the drug companies are going to be alarmed at the loss of their support in synthetic HRT and will do many things to recapture the market place. Already these trends are happening as more and more drug companies realise they are losing a very big part of the 'baby boomers' market. We will see, in the next few years, many trends in the guise of natural hormone replacement therapy.

The question is what form, what level, what dosage and what is right? Is the market pitch going to be at the expense of women once again. We have gone from Wild Yam confusion to topical natural progesterone (embraced by many women) to various forms of natural hormone replacement therapy (NHRT) in tailored doses, incorporating progesterone, estrogen, testosterone, pregnenalone, and DHEA.

Just take one look at the huge emphasis now placed on the management of menopause 'naturally' through the use of phytoestrogens in all areas of marketing from drug companies, to nutritional supplements, to everyday foods like breads, cereals, soy products, etc.

Giant multi-national drug companies will 'hone in' to recapture their market audience, and perhaps muddy the waters to further confuse women. NPAN has dedicated the many years to educating women and doctors in the differences between natural progesterone, wild yam extract cream and synthetic progestogen and they are still reluctant to listen.

Confusion will reign unless women become very aware, get educated, stand up for themselves and question their former treatment. Not allow themselves to be 'railroaded' by their doctors, or fooled by product packaging and cunning marketing ploys.

Will this trend give rise to all sorts of patented female hormone products supposedly derived from 'nature' but in fact far from it? Will women be more confused than ever? You bet. And exploitation right on its tail.

As we race head-on into this new era of anti-ageing hormone treatments, women are inevitably looking to NPAN for unbiased information that will help them make informed healthcare choices and confidence in reapproaching their Doctors, particularly since the HRT media scare and the surrounding controversy.

CHAPTER 20

Political Work instigated and conducted by NPAN, Jenny Birdsey.

Political activity - and Jenny's Lobby work

From 1998 over three years, some 7,000+ postcards and Reply Paid news article features have been signed and returned to the Health Minister of Western Australia - firstly Mr Prince and then Mr Day.

In November 1999 Jenny flew to WA to meet with the Health Minister, Mr Day, to discuss the desperate situation faced by women outside Western Australia. Dr Day cancelled his appointment with Jenny at the last minute. This appointment had been booked 3 months prior, and Jenny had flown across Australia specifically to represent women in need of access to a reliable manufactured progesterone cream (Jenny's attempts to meet with Mr Day in August 1998 were repeatedly overturned).

In Mr Day's absence and Jenny's refusal to leave without being heard, a meeting was granted with two health officials and a female solicitor. The meeting turned into a cross-examination of how women were sourcing progesterone cream on the black market, and questions insinuating misconduct on the part of Michael Buckley, the manufacturer of Pro-Feme. Not to be bullied, Jenny insisted that they get back on track and discuss what she came there for - women's hormonal health. The Western Australian government was made very aware on the day that they held the key to help fast-track a manufactured progesterone cream to all Australian women. At the conclusion of their meeting, officials made light of the Grandfathering Provision and their power to help women, going on to state that the matter belonged with TGA.

Just prior to the re-election of the State Government (end of 2000), material was being drafted in preparation to align WA drug laws with Australian Federal drug laws (all states within Australia would eventually have to comply). Tragically, around the same time, the existing Grandfathering Provision Act was overturned at Federal level. This move was initiated under the influence of the WA government, or at least this is what we have been led to believe.

If it wasn't such a big deal, then why did WA government officials enlighten Federal government of the loopholes of getting the product through faster using the Grandfathering Provision Act? Why, if they were in a position to help women, did they go out of their way to do the opposite?

Jenny sensed there was some form of personal vendetta or perhaps they were a mouthpiece for someone else. Upon reflection, one would have to question whether blocking the Grandfathering Provision Act, influenced by WA government officials, was sour grapes, political interests, palms crossed with silver, or outright sabotage of women's health. Whatever the reason - cynical, imagined or unfounded - the bottom line is, women are still suffering and women's health continues to be a low priority.

What is there to be gained by crushing a one-man pharmaceutical company who has invested every dollar he has in progesterone trials, when no other person or drug company or compounding pharmacist today in this country has been prepared to do likewise (because it's a non-patentable drug).

Without access to the Grandfathering Provision Act, the submission to TGA with trials will be far more stringent, time-consuming, more financially draining, and subsequent delays may take their toll.

Interestingly, the manufacturer of Pro-Feme has been granted an export license. This means theoretically you can legally import your Australian manufactured Pro-Feme cream from overseas, but you cannot buy it legally within Australia, except in Western Australia without employing certain loopholes and you must hold a script.

Coincidentally, around the time Jenny met with the Health Minister's off-siders, a reinforcing circulation from the WA Health Ministry was issued to all WA pharmacists (chemists) that they would incur a $40,000 fine if they were caught trading Pro-Feme interstate.

The manufacturer of Pro-Feme has realised how little regard government has for women's health and, for reasons of self-preservation, has focused trials on testosterone because clearly men hold the power.

In retrospect, had testosterone been the pilot, I believe that women would already have Pro-Feme, (already in the doctor's manual), on the pharmacists' shelves throughout Australia. A case in point, Viagra was one of the fastest tracked drug through legislation for market approval under pressure (from where?).

NPAN and the women collectively have supplied many doctors' packs and information packs on natural progesterone. Jenny and her organisation has handed out and lost hundreds of videos, books, and The Late Dr. John Lee tapes and have supplied information, doctors' lists, compounding pharmacists' lists all around the country, many of which have been sadly exploited and abused.

In providing women with a list of empathetic doctors willing to write scripts, these doctors were in turn harassed by some compounding pharmacists promoting their creams. This reflected badly on NPAN's professionalism and integrity and NPAN and Jenny were unjustifiably judged on many occasions for others' misconduct.

Update from Jenny

NPAN has seen a few publications use the organisation's resources and portray it as a free resource network. While I support most of these endeavours, I have been placed in a very embarrassing and costly position because women have simply assumed I am funded, that I provide free information packs, and that NPAN fills the gap that the publications have failed to address.

They fail to understand that NPAN is not a government-funded resource centre. Nor do I derive any kick-backs from the authors of these books, compounding pharmacists or prescribing doctors. Rather, I have given information and support out of love without thought of monetary gain, my time at the helm of NPAN as been completely voluntary in the past but due to shortage of funding I've been forced to charge for consultancy which ultimately means I can reach out and help more women.

Samples of lobby work efforts – the following articles highlight NPAN's activity for public awareness..

POLITICIANS MAKE WOMEN SICK

Advertisement published in Conscious Living Issue 50 and a local Western Australian Newspaper 98/99
Placed by Jenny Birdsey, NPAN for political lobbying.

Women fight for the right to choose healthcare

Australian women are suffering unnecessary pain, anguish, invasive medical operations and depression because politicians are too busy to change a simple law.

They agreed to pass new legislation ten years ago, but say they have more pressing matters. Obviously women's health is not important to them!

During this time women outside Western Australia have had no access to reliable quantities of natural progesterone therapies to treat debilitating hormone problems including premenstrual tension and menopause.

The lives of our sisters, daughters and mothers have been made a misery because our male politicians are 'too busy' to care.

Australian women are being treated as second class citizens by uncaring politicians. Please, help us to get them to do something NOW.

A natural progesterone cream called Pro-Feme is made in WA under pharmaceutical conditions and supplied on prescription by WA doctors.

Pro-Feme is the only pharmaceutically manufactured progesterone made in Australia. Applied as a cream, its progesterone replaces the missing progesterone in a woman's body. A deficiency in progesterone causes the debilitating symptoms of menopause, Premenstrual Syndrome (PMS), Osteoporosis (brittle bones), Endometriosis, Uterine Fibroids, Ovarian Cysts and depression.

The drug progesterone has liberated tens of thousands of women around the world from their pain and anguish and returned their wellbeing. It is a safe drug which is available over the counter in the US.

Desperate Australian women, fed up with being unable to treat hormonal symptoms properly, are resorting to buying progesterone on the black market from overseas and are administering it without medical supervision.

When doctors were worried that men would buy the sex drug Viagra on the black market, politicians worked in record time to pass the drug so that men could obtain it under medical supervision.

Are men's sex lives more important than a woman's quality of life?

Why should women be treated as second class citizens? Our pleas for change have fallen on politicians' deaf ears for two years. We need your help!

The WA Government is finally considering passing the long-delayed legislation that will allow progesterone cream to be available. Australia-wide.

Let WA's Minister for Health know that we want the legislative changes to happen NOW.

Please cut out this coupon, fill it in and post it in an envelope (no stamp required) addressed to:

Reply Paid 82510 (N/A)

Natural Progesterone Advisory Network

8 Normanby Street

East Geelong, Victoria, 3219.

It will be forwarded to the Western Australian Minister for Health.

Help women have more choice in determining their own health.

Dear Mr Day,

Your government holds the key to the health of tens of thousands of women. Western Australia is the only state in Australia where the hormone progesterone is available to women as a pharmaceutically manufactured cream.

A Western Australian company, Lawley Pharmaceuticals, makes a product called Pro-Feme which we cannot obtain.

Inaccessibility to this product is frustrating doctors and patients in the eastern states.

Please, please pass legislation to allow your Western Australian cream to be available to the rest of Australia. Most states passed legislation years ago to fall in line with Federal legislation. We need your state to do the same to allow us to obtain this vital product.

Let Western Australia know that you support progesterone being available Australia-wide by posting this coupon.

Signed:

Name:

Address:

Authorised by: Natural Progesterone Advisory Network

These political activities were examples of extensive lobbying and campaign work instigated and conducted by Jenny Birdsey involving thousands of women in 1998, 1999 and 2000. Some 7000 plus reply paid postcards were distributed and sent back to Mr Day by myself on behalf of NPAN. A handful were officially returned.

Grievance of inaccessability to WA's manufactured cream

This is an example of a letter written by an angry and concerned woman.
Placed in the paper along with others.

Supply: Why Can't I Get It Here?

Extract from a letter published in newsprint complaining about the drug law discrepancies between states within Australia.

Because of a state/federal discrepancy in the Therapeutic Goods Act, I no longer can buy natural progesterone (a hormone cream) from Western Australia.

Doctors put women on hormone replacement therapy – the fashion in medicine today – but it is wrong to overload us with estrogen and create more health problems when it is natural progesterone in which menopausal women are deficient.

Which politician (probably male) doesn't want me to practice preventative medicine so that I will not lose bone density and fracture my hip, get Breast Cancer or cervical cancer or have to take days off with migraines?

I was paying for my own continued health. Heroin addicts who have robbed, abused, violated society to support their illegal habits are given methadone and now heroin. Why? For their good health?

I can't get natural progesterone made from yams. Is it because it's secret women's business? Is it because pharmaceutical companies have vested interests?

Has WA seceded? Are WA women worth more than women in the eastern states? –
Ann, (Eastern States Aus.) August 9 '98.

CHAPTER 21

Resources

- *Sourcing and stockists of my books*
- *Recommending reading*

Resources

The Late Dr. John R. Lee, M.D.

The Late Dr. John Lee Medical Letter. The Late Dr. John R. Lee, M.D. was an international authority and pioneer in the use of natural progesterone cream and natural hormone balance. He was a sought-after speaker, as well as a best-selling author and the editor-in-chief of a widely read newsletter. His website offers a wide range of information about natural hormones and hormone balance for women and men, resources for finding out more, as well as a variety of books, audio and video tapes and other useful products. I understand Virginia Hopkins is overseeing.

Website: http://www.johnleemd.com

Progesterone Research Institute

The Progesterone Research Institute (PRI) is a non-profit organization dedicated to funding, supporting and promoting progesterone research. The Late Dr. John Lee was it's president.

Website: http://www.johnleemd.net/pri/pri_main.html

Saliva Hormone Testing

David Zava, Ph.D., ZRT Laboratory, (503) 469-0741, fax (503) 469-1305, e-mail dtzava@aol.com, ZRT Laboratory, 12505 NW Cornell Rd., Portland, OR 97229.

Website: http://www.salivatest.com/index.html

Great Smokies Diagnostic Laboratory, 63 Zillicoa St., Asheville, NC28801-1074, (800) 522-4762 (for doctors), (888) 891-3061 (for consumers).

Website: http://www.gsdl.com

Analytical Reference Laboratories (APA), 5 Leveson Street, North Melbourne, Victoria, Australia, 3051, (61-3) 9328-3586, fax (61-3) 9326-5004, 1300 554480 e-mail info@arlaus.com.au.

Website: http://www.arlaus.com.au

PATHLAB - 68 Burwood Highway, Burwood, Victoria, Australia, (61-3) 8831-3000 (Nutritional Laboratory Services)

Listing of Fertility Detector devices

Qvu-Tech

Website: http://www.ovu-tec.com

Lady Fertility Tester, NPT Ltd., Unit 15, The Metro Centre, Dwight Road, Watford WD1 8SS or Australia contact: 03 9439 5808 Med Direct (Pty)Ltd. P.O. Box 696, Eltham, 3095 Melbourne Victoria.

Website: http://www.med-direct.co.uk

Cleansing & Detoxification

The Liver Health Information Site: Comprehensive online resource for people interested in liver health, liver dysfunction and Liver Disease topics.

Website: http://www.liverdoctor.com

Dr Sandra Cabot's Weight Control Clinics

Weight Control Doctor: This is your "Weight Loss Lifeline" dedicated to all those people who seriously want to control their weight. Including overseas.

For all clinic updates visit: www.weightcontroldoctor.com

Dr Sandra Cabot Weight Control Clinics in Australia

• *Victoria - Jenny Birdsey*

A professional hormone consulting service as well as Dr Sandra Cabot Weight Control Clinic. Jenny has been personally trained by Dr. Sandra Cabot and conducts consultancy in weight loss programs.

Telephone: (03) 5222 7145 by appointment only. FEES APPLY.
(Phone between 9.00 -10.00 am Monday - Thursday)
Website: http://www.npan.com.au

• *Western Australia - Lyn Green*

Lyn Green, Naturopathy and Dr Sandra Cabot Natural Health and Weight Loss consultant

Telephone: (08) 9294 2433   Website: www.lyngreen.com
P O Box 1074 Midland WA 6936

• *New South Wales - Dr Sandra Cabot*

Dr Sandra Cabot, Natural Health and Weight Loss consultant
Telephone: (02) 4655 4666
Website: www.doctorcabot.com

Xenohormones

For extensive information and references on xenohormones, please visit Dr. Theo Colborn's website. And of course Dr. Colborn's book, "Our Stolen Future" is a classic on the subject.   Website: http://www.ourstolenfuture.org

Other invaluable websites:

http://www.co-cure.org   More on Fibromyalgia & Chronic Fatigue Syndrome.

http:/www.lawleypharm.com.au. Product information on testosterone usage

http://www.althysterectomy.org   Hysterectomy information and support

http://www.ccon.com/hers/index.htm   Hysterectomy Education & Resource Service

http://www.health-truth.com   Bladder Problems, Stress, Incontinence and Hysterectomy.

http://www.notmilk.com   To learn more about dairy products

http://www.nomorehysterectomies   Invaluable Hysterectomy information

Sourcing and Stockists of my books:

Direct

- Libraries
- Enquire at your book store to order
- Enquire at your compounding pharmacist to order
- To order online www.npan.com.au - Direct Merchant Bank facilities (secure ordering) or down load order form -
- Fill out and post order form at the back of this book.
- Fax Jenny Birdsey (03) 5222 7145

Stockists in Australia (July 2004)

- **Crossways Pharmacy**
  Cnr. Bagot & Rokeby Rds, Subiaco, WA 6008
  Telephone: (08) 9388 1777 Facsimile: (08) 9388 2481
  Email: crosswayspharmacy@bigpond.com.au
  Supply: Pro-feme®, Androfeme®, Andromen®, Natragen®
  Contact: Cliff Roberts and staff

- **Desana Pty Ltd**
  343 Cambridge Street, Wembley, WA 6014
  Telephone: (08) 9383 9997 Facsimile: (08) 9383 9164
  Email: info@desana.com.au
  Holistic Health Centre with specialising health care practitioners and a variety of treatments

- **Visionary Health**
  136 Beaumont Street, Hamilton, NSW 2303
  Telephone: (02) 4969 5081 Facsimile: (02) 4969 5091
  Email: info@visionarychemist.com.au
  Compounding pharmacist and associated practitioners on site

- **Shamley and Malouf's Pharmacy**
  128 Beaumont Street, Hamilton NSW 2303
  Telephone: (02) 4961 5987 Facsimile: (02) 4962 5060
  Contact: Roche Shamley or Allan Malouf

- **Naturopath and Dr Sandra Cabot Weight Consultant WA**
  Lyn Green
  Telephone: (08) 9294 2433 Web: www.lyngreen.com
  PO Box 1074 Midland WA 6936

- **Health Direction Pty Ltd WHAS**
  19 Little Street, Camden NSW 2570 P.O.Box 689
  Telephone: (02) 4655 8711 Facsimile: (02) 4655 8699
  Web: www.whas.com.au   Email: healthdirections@ozemail.com.au

- **Gooding Drive Compounding Chemist**
  Suite 6/166 Gooding Drive Carrara Qld 4211
  Telephone: (07) 5530 5888 Facsimile: (07) 5530 5896

- **Womens Hairloss Institute**
  (Medical and integrative scientific treatment of all female hair loss including topical Progesterone Prescription Pharmacy Compounded Scalp Lotions and Electrotrichogenisis)
  St Kilda Towers
  1 Queens Road (Suite 138) Melbourne 3004
  Telephone: (03) 9863 8814 Facsimile: (03) 9863 8822
  Web: www.whi.com.au   Mobile: 0408 559 403 Mike Kisylyczka

Updates and additions to this list can be found on www.npan.com.au

Recommended reading

I urge women not to blindly accept claims that one form of hormone replacement therapy, be it synthetic or natural, is your only choice. I suggest you do some research which is not at all difficult on the Internet. Books I have found to be very informative and openly recommend are:

- Dr. Margaret Smith on HRT, "Mid-Life Assessment - A Handbook for Women"
- Katharina Dalton, "Once a Month. Understanding and treating PMS" MD Hunter Publishers
- The Late The Late Dr. John Lee's book written by Jessie Hanley and Virginia Hopkins

    "What Your Doctor May Not Tell You About Premenopause" "What Your Doctor May Not Tell You About Breast Cancer"

    and his books "What Your Doctor May Not Tell You About Menopause", and "Men and Hormones".
- "Passage to Power" by Lesley Kenton
- Dr Sandra Cabot's books:

    "The Liver Cleansing Diet"

    "Hormone Replacement Therapy And Its Natural Alternatives"

    Revised update of "Hormones Don't Let Them Ruin Your Life"

    "Boost Your Energy" by Dr. Sandra Cabot MD.

    "Can't Lose Weight? You could have Syndrome X, the chemical imbalance that makes you store fat" by Dr. Sandra Cabot MD. (New Release)
- Sherrill Sellman "Hormone Heresy"
- Kimberly Patterson "Natural Progesterone"
- Dr Vicki Hufnagel "No More Hysterectomies"
- Christianne Northrup "Womens Body, Womens Wisdom", "The Wisdom of Menapause".
- Ruth Trickey "Women, Hormones and the Menstrual Cycle - Herbal and Medical Solutions from Adolescence to Menopause". www.allenandunwin.com

There are stacks more on the bookstore shelves, many of which have been written by doctors who do support alternative natural therapy or give a balanced view. Dr Margaret Smith recognises NHRT but more importantly has written a book to alert the medical fraternity how to use synthetic HRT wisely. An invaluable handbook to understand proper use of HRT. Dr Sandra Cabot, on the other hand, has come to adopt a more liberal approach to what she terms New Age Hormone Replacement Therapy.

Dr Cabot incorporates 4 principles of NHRT in conjunction with 'liver' health. These are:

Use bio-identical hormones

Get these hormones into the blood stream, bypassing the liver and gut

Preserve the delicate balance of hormones, fine tune

Individualise therapy to suit your weight, symptoms, bone density, blood profile, body type, age entering menopause

All the above share something in common - that hormones should be given in minimal doses. Their books imply, if not stating outright that synthetic HRT is perhaps overused and overdosed. NPAN always tries to be as balanced and open as possible. In so doing, I have come to realise that all forms of HRT, if used widely and conservatively, have their place in women's health. I am fully aware that this debate and information will always be evolving.

At NPAN, my fundamental focus is essentially natural progesterone. But I would not be telling women the full story if I failed to admit that there are other factors within a woman's personal hormonal profile and health regime that need to be considered for her ultimate health and success in healing. One needs to adopt a holistic approach rather than being biased towards any one treatment. I am constantly observing and broadening my knowledge such that what I publish in my 2nd revised edition may be adjusted or expanded upon tomorrow as new information finds its way to my Network. I will always remain open to new findings and women's experiences with natural progesterone and alternative treatments.

At NPAN, I believe natural progesterone is quite an incredible and remarkable hormone, discovered by millions of women worldwide. Nonetheless, if any of these women fail to understand the benefits and the interplay of other aspects that can increase the capacity and functioning of this incredible hormone, then they are not getting the best out of their cream ... or experienced optimal health.

CHAPTER 22

Sourcing Natural Progesterone cream

- *Health Care Providers and Australian Compounding Pharmacies that may assist you in sourcing Natural Progesterone and prescriptions*
- *Australian Compounding Pharmacies*
- *International Creams and Contacts*
- *Other USA and International Contacts*

HEALTH CARE PROVIDERS AND AUSTRALIAN COMPOUNDING PHARMACIES THAT MAY ASSIST YOU IN SOURCING NATURAL PROGESTERONE AND PRESCRIPTIONS

Australian Compounding Pharmacies

- **Australasian College of Nutritional & Environmental Medicine**
  http://www.acnem.org/

- **Analytical Reference Laboratories**
  5 Leveson Street North Melbourne Vic 3051
  PH: (03) 9328 3586   Fax: (03) 9326 5004
  Email: colmb@ariaus.com.au

- **Crossways Pharmacy**
  Cliff Roberts and his team supply Pro-Feme©, Andro-Feme©, Andromen©, Natragen©, within WA.
  Cnr Bagot and Rokeby Sts,
  Subiaco WA 6008
  PH: (08) 9388 1777 FAX: (08) 9388 2481
  Email:crosswayspharmacy@bigpond.com.au

- **Desana - Holistic Health Care Centre**
  This centre has practicing Doctor's as well as providing alternative therapies.
  (Dr Cathryn D'Cruz)   343 Cambridge Street, Wembley WA 6014
  PH: (08) 9383 9997 FAX: (08) 9373 9164
  cathryn.dcruz@desana.com.au or
  www.desana.com.au

- **Dr Sandra Cabot's Clinic Sydney**
  Level 1 Shop M103 and M104
  1-21 Bay Street Broadway 2007 NSW
  Provides a team of doctor trained naturopaths, trained in bio-identical hormones.
  For appointments and information
  (02) 4655 4666 or apply to WHAS Pty Ltd
  PO Box 689, Camden 2570
  PH: (02) 4655 8855 FAX: (02) 4655 8699
  www.doctorcabot.com

- **Menopause Institute Of Australia**
  PH: 1300 132 940
  www.menopauseinstitute.com.au

- **Professional Compounding Pharmacists**
  www.pccarx.com/contact.asp

- **Redwood Anti-Ageing**
  http://www.redwoodantiageing.com/

- **Visionary Health Compounding Chemist**
  - On site team of Natural Hormone Replacement Practitioners and prescribing doctors.
  - Compounding laboratory approved by NSW Pharmacy Board.
  136 Beaumont Street, Hamilton NSW 2303
  PH: (02) 4969 5081   FAX: (02) 4969 5091
  info@visionarychemist.com.au or
  www.visionarychemist.com.au

- **Renew You Medical Clinic**
  Dr Dzung Price, Dr Elen Apthomas
  Shop 13-14   221 Waterworks Road
  Ashgrove QLD 4060
  PH: (07) 3366 8955 FAX: (07) 3366 8933

  Suite 357   15 Albert Avenue
  Broadbeach QLD 4218
  PH: (07) 5539 0048 FAX: (07) 5539 0034
  www.renew-you.com.au

- **Gooding Drive Compounding Chemist**
  Suite 6/166 Gooding Drive Carrara Qld 4211
  PH: (07) 5530 5888 FAX: (07) 5530 5896

- **Roch Shamley, Kim Rumble, Alan Malouf Pharmacists**
  136 Beaumont Street Hamilton NSW 2303
  PH: (02) 4969 5081
  Servicing NSW and Australia

- **West Lindfield Pharmacy**
  Graeme Skinner
  30 Moore Ave Lindfield NSW 2070
  PH: (02) 9416 2642 FAX: 1800 66 33 63
  www.compoundingchemist.com

NATURAL PROGESTERONE CREAM AND PLACE OF PURCHASE
This list offers a guide as to where to obtain Natural Progesterone creams in Australia and overseas. If you reside in Australia or NZ you are required by law to hold a prescription to import Natural Progesterone cream for personal use.

Australian Compounding Pharmacies cont

- **Australian Compounding Pharmacy**
  16 Saint Mangos Lane, Melbourne VIC 3008
  PH: 03 9670 2882   FAX: 03 9670 9615
  http://www.compoundia.com/

- **Richard Stenlake Compounding Chemist**
  1st Floor, 76 Spring St., Bondi Junction NSW
  PH: 02 9387 3205   FAX: 02 9389 3821
  http://www.stenlake.com.au/

- **Shirley James Strathfieldsaye Pharmacy**
  32 Butcher St., Strathfieldsaye, Bendigo, VIC
  PH: 03 5439 3513   FAX: 03 5439 3514
  http://www.healthinbendigo.com.au/

- **Nation Wide Compounding Pharmacy**
  825 Glenhuntly Rd., Caulfield South, VIC
  PH: 03 9532 8555   FAX: 03 9532 8900
  nationwidepharmacy@bigppond.com

- **Thompsons Amcal Pharmacy**
  962-964 Main Road, Eltham, VIC
  PH: 03 9439 0799   FAX: 03 9439 2525
  eltham@amcal.net.au

- **Raju's Pharmacy**
  Gisborne Village Shopping Centre
  Brantome Street, Gisborne, VIC
  PH: 03 5428 2107   FAX: 03 5428 2793
  rajupharm@hotkey.net.au

- **Belvedere Park Pharmacy**
  284 Seaford Road, Seaford, VIC
  PH: 03 9786 2703   FAX: 03 9785 2420
  feldschuh@hcn.net.au

- **Dartnell's Pharmacy**
  376 Canterbury Road, Surrey Hills, VIC
  PH: 03 9888 5899   FAX: 03 9888 6911
  http://www.dartnellsphy.com.au/

- **Williamstown Pharmacy**
  81 Ferguson Street, Williamstown, VIC
  PH: 03 9397 6035   FAX: 03 9397 6093
  http://www.williamstownpharmacy.com.au/

- **Melbourne Compounding Centre**
  186 Victoria Street, Seddon, VIC
  PH: 03 9689 0833   FAX: 03 9689 0733
  http://www.compounding.com.au/

- **The Green Dispensary Compounding**
  Kensington Rd, Erindale, SOUTH AUSTRALIA 5034
  PH: 08 8431 6727   FAX: 08 8431 9540
  http://www.greendispensary.com/

- **Shamley and Malouf's Pharmacy**
  128 Beaumont Street, Hamilton NSW 2303
  Telephone: (02) 4961 5987
  Facsimile: (02) 4962 5060

- **Lawley Pharmaceuticals**
  (Holds an export licence for Australian manufactured cream. Cannot be purchased within Australia except in WA). Can export.

  672 Beaufort St, Mt Lawley, Perth, Western Australia 6050
  PH: 1800 627 506
  Email: lawleyph@arach.net.au,
  Website: lawleypharm.com.au
  Manufacturers of: *Pro-Feme*®-Progesterone supplement for women. *Andro-Feme*® - Testosterone supplement for the pre and postmenopausal woman. *Natragen*® - Oestradiol supplementation for women. *Andromen*® - Testosterone supplement for men.

- **Womens Hairloss Institute**
  (Medical and integrative scientific treatment of all female hair loss including topical Progesterone Prescription Pharmacy Compounded, Scalp Lotions and Electrotrichogenisis)
  St Kilda Towers
  1 Queens Road (Suite 138)
  Melbourne 3004
  PH: (03) 9863 8814   FAX: (03) 9863 8822
  Web: www.whi.com.au
  Mobile: 0408 559 403 Mike Kisylyczka

International Creams and Contacts

The following list is taken from The Late Dr John Lee's book 'What Your Doctor May Not Tell You About Menopause'

This is only a guideline of various creams that can be found on the market.

For continued updates and new cream additions on the market please visit my websites **www.npan.com.au** or **www.natural-progesterone-advisory-network.us**

PRODUCTS CONTAINING RECOMMENDED PROGESTERONE CONCENTRATIONS

Adam's Equalizer	HM Enterprises	Norcross, GA
Angel Care	Angel Care, USA	Atlanta, GA
Bio Balance	Elan Vitale	Scottsdale, AZ
Edenn Cream	SNM	Norcross, GA
E'Pro & Estrol Balance	Sarati International	Pasadena, TX
Equilibrium	Equillibrium Lab	Boca Raton, FL
Fair Lady	Village Market	Fond du Lac, WI
Femarone-17	Wise Essential	Minneapolis, MN
Fem-Gest	Bio-Nutritional Formulas	Meneola, NY
Feminique	Country Life	Hauppauge, NY
Gentle Changes	East Way, International	Indianapolis, IN
Happy PMS	HM Enterprises, Inc.	Norcross, GA
Heaven Sent	Answered Prayers, Inc.	Malibu, CA
Kokoro Balance	Kokoro, LLC	Laguna Niguel, CA
Marpe's Wild Yam	Green Pastures	Flat Rock, NC
NatraGest	Broadmore Labs, Inc.	Ventura, Ca
Natural Balance	South Market Service	Atlanta, GA
Natural Woman	Products of Nature	Ridgefield, CT
Natural Woman's Formula	Ultra Balance	Savannah, GA
New Woman	Pinnacle Nut, Inc.	Tulsa, OK
Nugerst 900	Nutraceutics Corp	Deerfield Beach, FL
OstaDerm	Bezwecken	Beaverton, OR
PharmWest	Pharm West	Marina Del Ray, CA
PhytoGest	Karuna Corp	Novato, CA
Pro-Alo	Health Watchers Sys.	Scottsdale, AZ
ProBalance	Springboard	Monterey, CA
Progessence	Young Living	Payson, UT
Pro-G	TriMedica	Scottsdale, AZ
Pro-Gest	Prof.® Tech serv., Inc.	Portland, OR
Progest-DP	Life Enhancement	Petaluma, CA
Progonol	Bezwecken	Beaverton, OR
Serenity	Health and Science	Crewfordvil, FL
Ultimate Total Woman	New Science Nutrition	N. Lauderdale, FL
Wild Yam Cream	Enrich International	Orem, UT

Products were tested by an independent laboratory assay prepared by Aeron Lifecycle, San Leandro, CA. March 1997.

Other USA & International contacts

- **American Academy of Environmental Medicine**
  PH: (316) 684 5500 FAX: (316) 684 5709
  Email: administrator@aaem.com
  http://www.healthreferral.com/
- **American Association of Naturopathic Physicians**
  http://www.aanp.com/
- **American College for Advancement of Medicine**
  http://www.acam.org/dr_search/
- **American Holistic Medical Assoc.**
  http://www.holisticmedicine.org/
- **Institute of Complementary Medicine**
  http://www.icmedicine.co.uk
  pracsearch.asp/
- **International Academy of Compounding Pharmacists**
  http://www.iacprx.org/
- **Menopause Clinician List for Canada**
  www.menopause.org/clinicianscan.pdf
- **Menopause Clinician List for USA**
  www.menopause.org/cliniciansus.pdf
- **Professional Compounding Pharmacists**
  PH: 800/331-2498 or 800/927-4227
  www.pccarx.com/contact.asp
- **Professional Referral Network**
  http://www.healthreferral.com/
- **Dr Sandra Cabot SCB/THD Inc**
  P.O Box 5070 Glendale AZ USA
  PH: 85312-5070
  www.doctorcabot.com
- **The Health & Research Inst.**
  661 Beville Road Ste. 101, Daytona Beach, FL 32119
- **Neways**
  150 E. 400 North, P.O. Box 651, Salen UT 84653. Endau Australia and New Zealand by law does not sell/distribute/ obtain or supply progesterone.

- **Vitality Lifechoice**
  Carson City, NV.
- **Alternative Medicine Network**
  16th St., #C-#105, Golden, CO 80401,
- **Arbonne International, Inc.**
  P.O. Box 2488, Laguna Hills, CA 92654, (800) ARBONNE
- **Life-flo Health Care Products**
  8146 N. 23rd Ave., Ste. E, Phoenix, AZ 85021, (888) 999-7440
- **Matol Botanical International**
  Quebec, Canada, (514) 639-3347
- **Pure Essence Labs, Inc.**
  1999 Whitney Mesa Drive, Suite A Henderson, NV 89014, (888) 254-8000
- **Restored Balance Inc.**
  42 Meadowbridge Dr. SW, Cartersville, GA 30120, (800) 865-7499
- **Lawley Pharmaceuticals**

The AIM Companies ™
Supply Renewed Balance to independent distributors. Does not apply in Australia and New Zealand.

- **Aim International, Inc.**
  3904 East Flamingo Ave., Nampa USA.
- **AIM Australia**
  Unit 6/ 137-145 Rooks Road Nunawading Vic 3110 aimaustralia@aimintl.com
- **AIM New Zealand, Inc.**
  Auckland, New Zealand info@aimnz.co.nz
- **AIM Canada** - Vancouver aimcanada@aimintl.com
- **AIM South Africa**
  Northcliff 2115 Republic of South Africa aimordersza@aimintl.com
- **AIM Hong Kong Ltd.**
  Phone 208-463-2622
  Fax: 800-901-479
- **AIM USA** - Nampa aimonline@aimintl.com

CHAPTER 23

Progesterone Drug Information Sheet

- *What drugs are not compatible with progesterone supplementation (or contra-indicated)?*
- *Medical References*

Progesterone Drug Information Sheet

Progesterone Product Information Leaflet provided by a recognised progesterone cream manufacturer in Australia, Lawley Pharmaceuticals.

It is standard procedure for drug manufacturers to provide your doctor with a Standard Product Information Leaflet on all prescription drugs he can legally prescribe or his patient might request. This is an example of the information your GP would reference when prescribing natural progesterone (an S4 Drug).

Description

Progesterone cream: Contains Progesterone BP (micronised) - a naturally occurring hormone - and dl- tocepherol acetate (vitamin E), in a white-vanishing cream base.

Pharmacology

Progesterone is secreted primarily from the corpus luteum of the ovary during the latter half of the menstrual cycle. Progesterone is formed from steroid precursors in the ovary, testes, adrenal cortex and placenta. Lutenizing hormone (LH) stimulates the synthesis and secretion of progesterone from the corpus luteum. Progesterone is multifactorial in its actions. Maintenance of secretory endometrium, precursor to steroid synthesis and a host of intrinsic biological properties make progesterone a hormone vital in providing a balance to oestradiol, the estrogenic hormone secreted by the ovary.

Progesterone has minimal estrogenic and androgenic activity. Orally administered progesterone is rapidly metabolised by the liver and the first pass effect is extremely high. The hormone is reduced to inactive metabolites pregnanedione, pregnanadone and pregnanediol in the liver, conjugated with glucuronic acid, then excreted in the bile and urine. Transdermal absorption of progesterone avoids this first pass metabolism.

Progesterone has a short plasma half-life of several minutes. Progesterone is extremely lipophilic and binds to plasma protein carriers, cortisol binding globulin (CBG) and sex hormone binding globulin (SHBG), red blood cellular membranes (1, 2) and fatty body tissue. 2-10% progesterone circulates unbound through plasma.

Progesterone administration achieves improvement in lipid and lipoprotein profiles and when combined with estrogen therapies indicates no increased risk of Endometrial Hyperplasia (3), (4) and may prevent breast epithelial hyperplasia (5).

The Mexican Wild Yam (Dioscorea Villosa) and the soya bean provide the lipid sterols, diosgenin and stigmasterol, from which natural progesterone is derived in-vitro.

Indications

Progesterone cream is indicated in progesterone deficient conditions, Postnatal Depression and Osteoporosis. Progesterone deficiency is associated with natural or surgical menopause, Premenstrual Syndrome (PMS), Breast Cancer, Ovarian Cysts, uterine Fibroids, Endometrial Hyperplasia and associated estrogen dependant malignancies, Fibrocystic Breasts and Endometriosis.

Progesterone is not a substitute for estrogen replacement therapy.

Contra-Indications

Progesterone should not be used by women with any of the following conditions:

Severe Liver Disease i.e. cholestatic jaundice, hepatitis, Rotor syndrome or Dubin-Johnson syndrome

Any unexplained or abnormal vaginal bleeding

History of herpes gestationis, jaundice of pregnancy

Known sensitivity to progesterone creams or any of their individual components

Adverse Reactions

Because progesterone creams contain the hormone identical to that produced by the human ovary, side effects are usually minimal. If experienced these may include breast tenderness and swelling, fluid retention or slight vaginal bleeding. Dizziness, nausea, fatigue, headaches and light headedness have been reported occasionally and usually disappear with adjustment of dose.

Use in Pregnancy

Progesterone is the hormone essential for promotion and maintenance of pregnancy. Ovarian output of progesterone in the non-pregnant state is 25-30mg daily during the luteal phase. The placental output during the third trimester of pregnancy is 340-400mg per day. Where as progestogens are contraindicated in pregnancy progesterone exhibits no adverse effects on the foetus.

Drug Interaction

Thyroid stimulating agents: Potential interaction exists in patients using thyroid supplementation. Progesterone may cause a potentiation of thyroxine's effects leading to hyperthyroidism. Normal T3 and T4 levels with elevated TSH suggests impaired thyroid hormone activity rather than insufficiency. Periodical TSH testing should be adopted on initiation or progesterone treatment in these patients.

Dosage and Administration

General Considerations

Distribution: Maximum absorption is achieved by application over a large skin area. Skin sites of choice are the inner arms, neck, upper chest, abdomen, and inner thighs on a rotating basis. Progesterone cream can also be applied to the breasts. Progesterone is first absorbed into the subcutaneous fat layer then passively diffuses throughout the body via the circulation. The rate which this is achieved is dependant on the amount of body fat. In general most significant physiological results are not experienced by patients until the fourth to sixth week of usage. In women using estrogen supplements the initial effect of progesterone is to sensitise estrogen receptors. A reduction in estrogen dosage may be required should breast swelling and tenderness, fluid retention or scant bleeding result.

WARNING: To date, progesterone creams have not been shown to be protective against estrogen-induced Endometrial Hyperplasia. Caution should be exercised and patients monitored if combination therapy is to be initiated.

In perimenopausal women with irregular menstrual flows the addition of progesterone cream may result in a return of menses. This may lead to the conclusion that progesterone caused the menses when in fact estrogen created the endometrial proliferation and the cessation of progesterone allowed for shedding of this proliferation. This effect is normal and there is no reason to cease using the cream.

Cycling: In a normal menstrual cycle progesterone is produced as the dominant hormone for approximately fourteen days per cycle. Receptor stimulation is not continuous. Aim of treatment is to mimic natural ovarian production as much as possible, thus monthly cycling is recommended. In post menopausal women progesterone should be used for 21-25 days per calendar month followed by a 5-7 progesterone free state. In perimenopausal women administration should be synchronised with normal corpus luteal progesterone production i.e. day 12 to day 26 of the menstrual cycle. If after initiating treatment menstruation occurs after 5-10 days it is recommended to cease application and re-commence 12 days later.

Eligibility: All women regardless of whether the uterus is intact or not, exhibiting signs of estrogen imbalance have a requirement for progesterone. Hysterectomised women are not exempt from using progesterone. Creams are available in two strengths: 1.6% and 3.2%. Dosage should be tailored to individual requirements and the patient reviewed on a regular basis. Dosage adjustments may be made by altering volume of cream applied or alteration of percentage strength prescribed. When applying progesterone, use the supplied measured applicator to achieve correct dosage. Squeeze the necessary amount of cream from tube onto applicator, then place the applicator with the cream side down onto the site of application. Massage cream over desired area until absorbed.

Overdosage

Toxicity of progesterone is extremely low. No specific antidote is available.

Presentation

- 1.6% cream containing 16mg/g progesterone BP 50Gm boxed tube.
- 3.2% cream containing 32mg/g progesterone BP 50Gm boxed tube.
- 10% cream containing 100mg/g progesterone BP 50Gm boxed tube.

Storage

Store below 25C. Do NOT freeze

Poisons Schedule

This item is listed under the S4 poisons schedule.

(Printed with permission - Lawley Pharmaceuticals, Western Australia)

Lawley Pharmaceuticals also manufacture:

- Testosterone Cream available for women (Andro-Feme® Cream)
- Testosterone Cream available for men (Andromen® Cream)
- Estrogen (Natrogen® Cream (Oestradiol).

I encourage you to visit their website for further product information. Website: http://www.lawleypharm.com.au.   Email: lawleyph@arach.net.au

ABOUT LAWLEY PHARMACEUTICALS MANUFACTURED PRODUCTS

I have personally used Lawley Pharmaceuticals manufactured transdermal creams for nearly 8 years, trialing others in-between and comparing along with other women in my NPAN organisation. Women often ring me for strength interpretation if they have sourced this product (Pro-Feme and or testosterone/ Andro-Feme) or purchased in WA.

A Doctor by law cannot write Pro-Feme or Andro-Feme unless she/he is registered in WA as this product is not federally legislated through TGA yet. It is only legislated in WA under their independent drug laws. But a Doctor can legally write progesterone 1.6%, 3.2% or 10% by 6 repeats. Or testosterone 1%, 2% and 5%.

Where you obtain your cream from is up to you and you are free to send it anywhere and to whatever compounding pharmacist you elect. You cannot buy bio identical hormones over the counter without a script. Nor will you buy any other manufactured progesterone cream in Australia apart from in WA (over the counter with a script- Lawley Pharmaceuticals is the only manufactured cream to date.) Because it is manufactured and quality batch controlled and packaged it is appealing and reassuring to women to use this product, however there are some very select few excellent compounding pharmacists throughout Australia. As the question has often arisen on dosage strength on Lawley Pharmaceutical products these are:

Pro-Feme   at 1.6% 1cm = 8mg

At 3.2% 1cm = 16mg

At 10% 1cm = 50mg

A plastic measuring ruler is supplied with the package and is measured out the same way as you do toothpaste.

A 10% strength is by far more economical as it is 4 times stronger as you require less on application, this is of particular concern to those of us who don't have private health insurance.

Andro-Feme at 1% 1cm = 5mg

This is the female version of testosterone and for men:

Andromen   at 2% 1cm = 10mg

Andromen Forte at 5% 1cm = 25mg

It is important where ever you source your cream from that you know your dosage per application. Check with your compounding pharmacist.

What drugs are not compatible with progesterone supplementation (or contra-indicated)?

Contraception:

Conventional hormone contraceptives that contain the progestins:
Levonorgestrel
Norethisterone
Cyproterone

Mini Pill
Levonorgestrel (Microlut/Microval)
Norethisterone (Micronor/Noriday)

Progestin Depots
Medroxyprogesterone (Depo-Provera/ Depo-Ralovera)
Etonogestrel (Implanon)
Levonorgestrel (Mirena) a hormone releasing IUD

Emergency Contraception
Levonorgestrel (Postinor)

Hormone Replacement Therapy
Medroxyprogesterone (Provera/ Ralovera)
Norethisterone (Primolut N)
Estrogen/ Progestin combinations
    Equine estrogens with progestins
    Estrogen patches with progestins
Dydrogesterone (Duphaston)
Tibolone (Livial)

Other Steroid compounds
Prednisolone
Prednisone
Cortisone Acetate
Cortisone based analgesics or injections

This is what I have discovered from my own work and the work of the late Dr John Lee.

Medical References
Compiled by Garth Birdsey *Bpharm Grad dip hos.pharm*
Assessed and researched for and on behalf of Jenny Birdsey

PROGESTERONE ABSORPTION
Topical

1: Cooper A; Spencer C; Whitehead MI etal. Systemic absorption of progesterone from Progest cream in postmenopausal women (letter) Lancet.1998 Apr 25;351(9111):1255-6

This is THE article that was given so much emphasis in the medical literature as proof that progesterone does not get absorbed topically. Several "leading lights" of the gynaecological world have repeatedly quoted this article as proof, even though there are some methodological problems with the assay used and the use of progesterone and topical oestrogens in the same patients. To get a better view of this article it is suggested that you also read the following discussions.

Lancet 1998 Sep 12;352(9131):905

Lancet 1998 Sep 12;352(9131):905-6

2: Leonetti HB; Longo S; Anasti JN. Transdermal progesterone cream for vasomotor symptoms and postmenopausal bone loss. Obstet-Gynecol.1999 Aug;94(2):225-8

3: Burry KA; Patton PE; Hermsmeyer K. Percutaneous absorption of progesterone in postmenopausal women treated with transdermal estrogen. Am-J-Obstet-gynecol.1999 Jun;180(6pt 1):1504-11

These two articles, coming a year later, give a different view. Interesting that they have been given scant attention by the "leading lights". Both give evidence of therapeutic effect from transdermal progesterone. One to give relief from the Hot Flushes and mood swings, the other to help protect the endometrium from estrogenic effects. Of importance the doses used were probably too low to affect bone loss, this is mentioned in the Leonetti article as is a mention of the 1 year follow up being too short.

Vaginal

4: Cincinalli E;de-Ziegler D. Transvaginal progesterone:evidence for a new functional 'portal system' flowing from the vagina to the uterus. Hum-Reprod-Update.1999 Jul-Aug;5(4):365-72

5: Levy T; Gurevitch S; Bar-Hava I etal. Pharmacokinetics of natural progesterone administered in the form of a vaginal tablet. Hum-Reprod.1999 Mar;14(3):606-10

6: Ross D; Cooper AJ; Pryse-Davies J etal. Randomized,double-blind,dose ranging study of the endometrial effects of a vaginal progesterone gel in estrogen-treated postmenopausal women. Am-J-Obstet-Gynecol.1997 Oct;177(4):937-41

7: Warren MP; Biller BMK; Shangold MM. A new clinical option for hormone replacement therapy in women with secondary amenorrhea: Effects of cyclic

415

administration of progesterone from the sustained-release vaginal gel Crinone (4% and 8%) on endometrial morphologic features and withdrawal bleeding. Am-J-Obste-Gynecol 1999;180:42-8

All these articles give evidence that vaginally administered progesterone is well absorbed, possibly better than trans-dermal. It also gives evidence that for those women who feel they must use an estrogen supplement, vaginal progesterone, in adequate doses will protect their endometrium from the estrogenic effects.

GENERAL ARTICLES ON PROGESTERONE USE

8: Wetzel W. Micronized progesterone: a new option for women's health care. Nurse-Pract. 1999 May:24(5):62-6,71,75-6

9: Langer RD. Micronized progesterone: a new therapeutic option. Int-J-Fertil-Womens-Med.1999 Mar-Apr;44(2):67-73

10: delignieres B. Oral micronized progesterone. Clin-Therapeutics 1999 Jan;21(1):41-60

11: Warren MP; Shantha S. Uses of progesterone in clinical practice. Int-J-Fertil. 1999;44(2):96-103

12: Wetzel W. Human identical hormones:real people,real problems,real solutions. Nurse-Pract-Forum1998 Dec;9(4):227-34

References 8-12 group together articles that discuss the rationale behind the use of progesterone as distinct from progestagens. The article from France (10) describes some considerable experience with progesterone, although it is oral progesterone that they use, so the doses are much higher. Still the responses are encouraging. Some 500,00 French women cannot all be experiencing placebo effects!

PHYTOESTROGEN THERAPY

13: Newall CA; Anderson LA; Phillipson JD. Herbal Medicines. A guide for health care professionals.

14: Mills S; Bone K. Principles and practice of Phytotherapy: Modern herbal medicine.

These two textbooks are both informative and very easy to read. They give balanced evidence both for and against the uses of various herbs in the treatment of menopausal symptoms. The Mills' book has a very informative section on wild yam, which will dispel all myths on its use and its ability to be transformed into progesterone by the body.

PROGESTERONE AND THE BREAST

15: Foidart JM;Colin C; Denoo X et al. Estradiol and progesterone regulate the proliferation of human breast epithelial cells. Fert.Steril. 1998 May;69(5):963-9

This article provides evidence that progesterone suppresses the estrogen induced proliferation of breast epithelial cells. Again progesterone protects against estrogen. In this study both estrogen and progesterone were applied to the breast as topical gels!

16: Cohen I; Beyth Y; Altaras MM et al. Estrogen and progesterone receptor expression in postmenopausal tamoxifen-exposed endometrial pathologies. Gynecol-Oncol.1997 Oct;67(1):8-15

Again further evidence that progesterone protects against estrogenic compounds. This time it is Tamoxifen. This article gives further proof that tamoxifen has estrogenic effects on the endometrium in menopausal women. This should ring alarm bells in women with Breast Cancers who are being treated with tamoxifen, especially if they still have their uterus!

17: Homberg L; Anderson H, for the HABITS steering and data monitoring committees. HABITS (hormonal replacement therapy after Breast Cancer- is it safe?), a randomised comparison: trial stopped. Lancet 2004;363:453-55

18: Chlebowski RT; Col N. Menopausal hormone therapy after Breast Cancer. Lancet 2004;363:410-11

The HABITS trial puts to rest the notion that after Breast Cancer treatment including that with tamoxifen you can use oestrogens to overcome the "menopausal " symptoms. All it did was increase the risk of recurrence! What is interesting in this study was that all HRT regimens used contained oestrogens and synthetic progestins. The risk was greatest in those women treated with tamoxifen or had HRT prior to the initial diagnosis of Breast Cancer. Of importance was that the trial did not include the use of placebo or alternative treatments for Hot Flushes!

HORMONE REPLACEMENT THERAPY AND THE HEART

19: The writing group for the PEPI trial. Effects of estrogen/progestin regimens on Heart Disease risk factors in postmenopausal women.JAMA.1995 Jan 18;273(3):199-208.

The famous PEPI trial, often quoted and often mis-quoted. It depends on which company you support or product you wish to sell. The conclusions of this trial are confusing as they say that unopposed estrogen is the best method, but do recognise the problem of Endometrial Hyperplasia. So the next best method is continuous estrogen with cyclicle medroxyprogesterone(provera). However they forget to mention the third arm of the study which used oral micronized progesterone which had the same results as the estrogen and provera arm! And they say the drug companies have no influence on publishing studies! If you can it is worth reading the comments that have followed this study.

JAMA 1995 Dec 6;274 (21):1676

JAMA 1995 Dec 6;274 (21):1675 and 1675-6

20: Heart and Estrogen/progestin Replacement Study (HERS) Research group. Randomized trial of estrogen plus estrogen for secondary prevention of coronary Heart Disease in postmenopausal women. JAMA 1998 Aug 19;280(7):605-13

This is an equally famous and land mark study. It really debunks the notion that conventional HRT protects menopausal women from Heart Disease. So it puts into doubt the use of HRT as a routine protection for Heart Disease in menopausal women, it may in fact be harmful in the first 12 months! As you would expect from such a study there are multitudes of letters and comments. 16 published comments and discussions followed in the 6 months after the study was published. So it really set minds working.

21: Kuller LH. Hormone replacement therapy and coronary Heart Disease. A new debate. Med-Clin-North-Am. 2000 Jan;84(1):181-98

22: Mercuro G; Pitzalis L; Podda A. et al. Effects of acute administration of natural progesterone on peripheral vascular responsiveness in healthy postmenopausal women. Am-J-Cardiol. 1999 Jul 15; 84(2):214-8

LONG TERM COMBINED OESTROGEN-PROGESTIN REPLACEMENT

23: Million Women Study Collaborators. Breast Cancer and hormone-replacement therapy in the Million Women Study. Lancet 2003;362:419-27

24: Hulley S; Furberg C; Barrett-Connor E; et al. Noncardiovascular Disease Outcomes During 6.8 years of Hormone Therapy. Heart and Estrogen/Progestin Replacement Study Follow-up (HERS II) JAMA 2002;288:58-66

25: Writing Group for the Women's Health Initiative Investigators. Risks and Benefits of Estrogen Plus Progestin in Healthy Postmenopausal Women, Principal results from the Women's health Initiative Randomized Controlled Trial. JAMA 2002;288:321-333

26: Lacey JV; Mink PJ; Lubin JH et al. Menopausal Hormone Replacement Therapy and Risk of Ovarian Cancer. JAMA 2002;288:334-341

27: Fletcher SW and Colditz GA Failure of Estrogen plus Progestin Therapy for Prevention. JAMA 2002;288:366-367

28: Wassertheil-Smoller S;Hendrix SL;Limacher M et al. Effect of Estrogen Plus Progestin on Stroke in Postmenopausal Women. The Women's Health Initiative: A randomised Trial. JAMA 2003;289:2673-2684

29: Rapp SR ;Edpeland MA; Shumaker SA et al. Effect of Estrogen plus Progestin on Global Cognitive Function in Postmenopausal Women. The Women's Health Initiative Memory Study: A randomised controlled trial. JAMA 2003;289:2663-2672

30: Shumaker SA;Legault C; Rapp SR et al. Estrogen plus Progestin and the incidence of Dementia and Mild Cognitive Impairment in Postmenopausal Women. The Women's Health Initiative Memory Study: a Randomized Controlled Trial. JAMA 2003; 289:2651-2662

All these references, 23-30, give compelling evidence against the combination of oestrogen and synthetic progestins. All used equine oestrogens (Premarin) and medroxyprogesterone (Provera). The combination proved to give no protection to women in regards memory, failing cognitive function and the progression of dementia. In fact it looks like the combination may accelerate the decline! I stress that this is long-term use, over 5 years. So compelling evidence for not being on such therapy for more than 5 years.

The editorial written by Fletcher and Colditz, put the whole argument into perspective. The combination of synthetic oestrogens and progestins provides little protection to menopausal women, rather they suggest, the therapy does actual harm.

SAMPLE IDEA OF A CHART

Month..........Date	1	2	3	4	5	6	7	8	9	10	11	12	13	14	15	16	17	18	19	20	21	22	23	24	25	26	27	28	29	30	31
YOUR SYMPTOMS																															
Menstruation																															
Heavy or Irregular Periods																															
Fatigue/Lack of Energy																															
Breast Swelling/Tenderness																															
Breast Cysts/Lumps																															
Weight Gain																															
Fluid Retention																															
Premenstrual Mood Swings (PMS)																															
Bloating/Water Retention																															
Diffused body Aches & Pains																															
Headaches/Migraines																															
Sleep Disturbances																															
Night Sweats																															
Hot Flushes																															
Cravings for Sweets (Chocolate)																															
Cold hands & Feet																															
Confusion/Disorientation																															
Irritability or Aggression																															
Alienation/Social Withdrawal																															
Guilt/Low Self esteem																															
Depression and/or Teary																															
Indigestion/Heartburn																															
Gastrointestinal Disorders																															
Anxious and/or Panic Attacks																															
Vertigo																															
Skin Problems (Creepy Crawley)																															
Loss of Libido																															
Endometriosis and/or Pelvic Pain																															
Fibroids																															
Bladder Problems																															
Thrush																															
Sinusitis																															
Acne																															
Other																															
Progesterone Dosage																															
Other (Vitamins, Minerals, etc)																															
Medications																															

A Woman's Guide to the use of Natural Progesterone

MONTHLY SCORE SHEET TO DETERMINE
PROGRESS / EFFECTIVENESS OF PROGESTERONE USAGE

Symptoms of Oestrogen dominance / Progesterone deficiency for a MENSTRUATING woman

Below is a list of the most common symptoms, please rate them as follows:

0 = Never;   1 = Rarely;   2 = Occasionally;   3 = Frequently or daily

Symptom	MONTH 1 Date:............ Rating		MONTH 2 Date:............ Rating		MONTH 3 Date:............ Rating		MONTH 4 Date:............ Rating	
	Pre Menses	Post	Pre Menses	Post	Pre Menses	Post	Pre Menses	Post
Heavy &/or irregular periods								
Fatigue or lack of energy								
Breast swelling / tenderness								
Loss of libido (sex drive)								
Weight gain-unexplained								
Bloating or fluid retention								
Generalised aches & pains								
Headaches/Migraines								
Sleep disturbance								
Hot flushes								
Night sweats								
Irritability or mood swings								
Confusion / disorientation								
Lack of self esteem								
Craving for sweets								
TOTAL SCORE								

Other symptoms, please tick any that you experience:

- ❏ Inability to lose weight
- ❏ Panic attacks / palpitations
- ❏ Crying for no reason
- ❏ Alienation or guilt
- ❏ Thrush
- ❏ Cold hands & feet
- ❏ Cold buttocks
- ❏ Foggy thinking / vagueness
- ❏ Irritated eyes – dry/gritty
- ❏ Acne Rosacea / skin problems
- ❏ Urinary tract infection/stress incontinence
- ❏ Breast Cysts / lumps, ropiness

- ❏ Allergy symptoms, ie asthma, hives/rashes, sinusitus
- ❏ Anxiety
- ❏ Memory loss
- ❏ Depression
- ❏ Mouth ulcers
- ❏ Hair loss / thinning
- ❏ Facial hair (upper lip, chin)
- ❏ Excess body hair
- ❏ Restless Leg syndrome
- ❏ Inability to orgasm
- ❏ Vaginal dryness / pimples

NATURAL PROGESTERONE ADVISORY NETWORK (NPAN)

MONTHLY SCORE SHEET TO DETERMINE
PROGRESS / EFFECTIVENESS OF PROGESTERONE USAGE

Symptoms of Oestrogen dominance / Progesterone deficiency for a NON MENSTRUATING woman

Below is a list of the most common symptoms, please rate them as follows:

0 = Never;   1 = Rarely;   2 = Occasionally;   3 = Frequently or daily

Symptom	MONTH 1 Date: .... Rating	MONTH 2 Date: .... Rating	MONTH 3 Date: .... Rating	MONTH 4 Date: .... Rating
Fatigue or lack of energy				
Breast swelling / tenderness				
Loss of libido (sex drive)				
Weight gain-unexplained				
Bloating or fluid retention				
Generalised aches & pains				
Headaches/Migraines				
Sleep disturbance				
Hot flushes				
Night sweats				
Irritability or mood swings				
Confusion / disorientation				
Lack of self esteem				
Craving for sweets				
TOTAL SCORE				

Other symptoms, please tick any that you experience:

- ☐ Inability to lose weight
- ☐ Panic attacks / palpitations
- ☐ Crying for no reason
- ☐ Alienation or guilt
- ☐ Thrush
- ☐ Cold hands & feet
- ☐ Cold buttocks
- ☐ Foggy thinking / vagueness
- ☐ Irritated eyes – dry/gritty
- ☐ Rosacea, pimples
- ☐ Urinary tract infection/stress incontinence
- ☐ Breast Cysts
- ☐ Allergy symptoms, ie asthma, hives/rashes, sinusitis
- ☐ Anxiety
- ☐ Memory loss
- ☐ Depression
- ☐ Mouth ulcers
- ☐ Hair loss / thinning
- ☐ Facial hair (upper lip, chin)
- ☐ Excess body hair
- ☐ Restless Leg syndrome
- ☐ Inability to orgasm
- ☐ Vaginal dryness, spotting

NATURAL PROGESTERONE ADVISORY NETWORK (NPAN)

Purchasing Nutritional Supplements

You are welcome to order nutritional products by requesting an order form.
You can do this by phone, fax or email
Business hours: 9.00am - 10.00am
Monday to Thursday only

Profits derived from this method of ordering NPAN nutritional programs or consultancy will assist jenny Birdsey's ongoing work and support the Natural Progesterone Advisory Network (NPAN) organisation.

Application for Order Forms
A current list will be forwarded to you

Name: _____

Address: _____

_____

_____ Postcode: _____

Phone: _____ Fax: _____

Email: _____

CONSULTANCY

Jenny Birdsey operates a professional hormone consulting service and Sandra Cabot's weight loss centre.

Preferential consultation is given to those who have previously read Jenny's books -
"Natural Progesterone - the world's best kept secret", and/or

"Natural Progesterone - more secrets revealed"

Jenny apologises that she is not in a position, nor does she have the time to answer non consultancy questions without a full disclosure of medical and hormonal history.

Appointments are required.

Jenny can assist women concerning:

- Hormonal balancing and associated hormone problems
- Weight management
- Nutritional concerns
- Body shape
- Syndrome X (personally trained by Dr Sandra Cabot)
- Individualised nutrition and hormone regimes

A consultation can be conducted by phone (usually evenings, 7.30pm), or in person at Jenny's consulting rooms, 8 Normanby Street, East Geelong, Vic, Australia.

By appointment only.

2 hour consultancy times available 10.00am-12.00noon, 2.00-4.00pm Monday to Thursday.

An extensive questionnaire will be sent for you to complete, with confirmation of appointment (soon to be available by email also).

To make an appointment phone between
9.00am-10.00am Monday-Thursday only
Phone/fax (03) 5222 7145
Int: 61 3 5222 7145

visit: www.npan.com.au

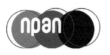 **NATURAL PROGESTERONE ADVISORY NETWORK (NPAN)**
8 Normanby Street, East Geelong, Vic 3219, Australia

Subject matter synopsis covered in Jenny Birdsey's companion book 2 "Natural Progesterone - more secrets revealed."

This is a book dedicated to womens courage. Acknowledgement and inspirational testimonials of special cases demonstrate this beyond doubt.

The philosophy of the NPAN organisation is basically about the empowerment of every woman on her journey to good health, seeking hormonal essence and restored balance. She is exhausted, fed up, bewildered, longing to find her way home to her true place of inner being and health.

Thousands of women empowered with knowledge on the use of Progesterone have discovered such a sanctuary can and does exist.

This companion book ensures that in times of despair and bewilderment, women are provided with further answers, strategies and solutions to overcome any possible obstacles that they may encounter on their unique journey.

Contents of "Natural Progesterone - More Secrets Revealed", covers in depth, hormones and their interplay, specifically in:

- Estrogen Dominance and Estrogen Dominance Wake Up Crisis
- Bleeding irregularities - all scenarios covered in detail
- Using Progesterone in conjunction with other hormones and adopting different deliverance techniques
- Using Progesterone in relation to modifying, influencing moods, depression, foggy thinking, Alzheimers disease
- Libido problems incorporating testosterone in men and women.
- Looking at sexual abuse with an open mind and its possible obstacles in attaining total healing and well being
- Incorporating strategies to complement hormonal balance including the usage of nutritional supplementation and diet, explaining how it fits into the bigger picture.
- Looking at body shapes, Syndrome X weight issues, the state of liver and other glands in correcting and achieving true metabolic and hormonal constitutional status.
- Clearing up confusion over the usage of different forms of contraception and other contraindicated medications. Grasping a greater understanding by addressing specific questions most commonly posed and different scenarios covering Infertility, Endometriosis, Breast Cancer concerns, Candida (thrush), Urinary Tract Infections, Stress Incontinence, vaginal problems, menopausal problems, perimenopausal problems, Irritable Bowel Syndrome, Polycyctic Ovarian Syndrome, Tubal Ligations and Hysterectomies.
- Clearing up more public misconceptions and looking at the usage of wild yam, Doctors patient relationship problems, resistance and attitudes
- Using Progesterone in animals

A condensed preview of topics covered in companion book 2 "Natural Progesterone - more secrets revealed".

Total contents to be found on website www.npan.com.au

Estrogen Dominance Crisis and Estrogen Dominance Wake Up Crisis (EDWUC): Causes and management
- How to use progesterone and what to be aware of with Estrogen Dominance Wake Up Crisis:
- The initial Wake Up • Wake Up is not permanent
- Signs of Estrogen Dominance Crisis 'Wake Up' or break through of progesterone benefits and
- Reasons for Crisis Recurrence
- Estrogen Dominance Crises in relationship to dosages
    Not enough progesterone and reasons for depletion:
    Managing deficiency due to "low dosage"; Too many breaks or too long a break and the pitfalls of taking too many or not enough breaks; Incorrect dosage due to irregular periods
    Too much progesterone: Causes and recognition of unnecessarily high doses; other causes
- EDWUC due to introduction of different hormones testosterone, DHEA and estrogen or reintroducing, changing various routes of administration
- Intravaginal application of progesterone, its benefits and side effects
- Other reasons for Estrogen Dominance Crisis: Recap

Other strategies in reducing and managing estrogen dominance wake up crisis
- How the liver filter protects you from toxic overload and reduces estrogen
- 8 Simple things you can do to detoxify your body
- Reducing estrogen dominance with nutritional support and diet, shopping lists

Determining The Right Dose for you and guidelines to follow with bleeding irregularities
- Tailoring the right dose and usage for Irregular Bleeding Patterns
- About cycling and mother nature's rhythm, synchronisation, the pattern of progesterone. Nature's phenomena
- Understanding progesterone and estrogen's role in menstruation
- What happens when progesterone is missing
- Bringing progesterone back to the body to restore menstrual regularity for those NOT in the premenopause phase
- How progesterone assists rhythm and restores balance in menstrual cycle and how to achieve regularity

Coping with changing period patterns and how to use progesterone
- Cycles that are now regular but have changed in length
- Experiencing estrogen dominance during the break
- Missing a period or not having periods. Amenorrhea

The premenopausal dance. What is it? Coping and what you can do
- Summary of important points in the usage of progesterone and irregular menstruation
- How would I know if I am in true menopause and what would my blood results read?
- What is the reason why the FSH reading is high in menopause
- Specifically tailoring dose and usage for irregular menstrual patterns, Amenorrhea, Menstrual Irregularities and reasons
- Can I use estrogen or the oral the oral contraceptive pill if I have amenorrhea and will it help bring my periods on?

Looking deeper into amenorrhea and possible solutions
- Progesterone usage for period regulation
- Non menstruation does not necessarily mean not enough estrogen - caution with estrogen use

Will progesterone assist in bringing back my periods?
- Yes, if not in true menopause
- Yes and no if you are in the pre menopausal phase

The premenopausal dance and using progesterone in this phase/transition
What happens in cases where a new cycle and pattern is re-emerging, what do I do?
The reasons and seriousness of obeying cyclic breaks

Public misconceptions

- Resistance to natural progesterone from doctors and other health professionals
- General problems and confusion around progesterone usage
- My attitude and observation of doctor's attitudes and reasons for their stance
- Explaining dilemmas in prescribing and obtaining a script
- Overcoming obstacles
- Food for thought - time to work together in the health industry

Not all doctors are fossilised and do not deserve to be put into the same category

- Good old fashioned doctor/patient relationship needs rekindling
- Restoring confidence and alleviating fears is one of the keys to doctors
- Pitfalls in not being honest with your doctor and/or naturopath
- Why do so many gaps exist between women and their doctors?
- Is technology intruding on our relationship with our doctors?
- What happens if I do not want to take any hormone replacement therapy but my doctor advises me that I should? Will tests help and what can I expect?

Balancing medication use and natural alternatives - pros and cons

- About my Wild Yam opinions
- Product misrepresentation on Wild Yam sales does still happen from time to time
- Wild Yam products are beneficial but not for progesterone deficiency

Sourcing progesterone cream in Australia from a compounding pharmacist

- Confusion on choosing the right progesterone cream and which compounding pharmacist to use
- Interpreting and understanding progesterone products with other ingredients
- An example of a progesterone cream and possible added ingredients
- Questions to ask, Deciphering answers you may get, Transport, Deliverance
- What proof would be indicative of a reliable compounded progesterone cream?
- Don't be frightened off by preservatives in cream
- Can a machine guide you in your choice of progesterone cream? Problems/questions that crossed my desk.
- Can I overdose on progesterone?
- What can I do if I suspect I have overdosed?
- Rule of thumb and guidelines

Other hormones and saliva readings and questions related to the need of progesterone

- What to expect on a saliva assay reading
- When is saliva assay for hormone profiling not suitable for accurate reading?
- Why do I have a low DHEA reading since progesterone, when all my other hormones are okay?
- What is the purpose of giving DHEA along with progesterone and what are the benefits?

Specific Questions

- If I have no symptoms and I am well and truly past menopause, could I benefit from progesterone? Pros and cons
- Are there some women who just cannot take progesterone
- Is it possible that progesterone is over related and a marketing scam?
- Will progesterone help my vaginal warts?
- Is progesterone addictive?
- How can I reduce my chances of breast cancer and will progesterone help?
- Is it important to take other measures in cancer protection and what are some?
- Is there any point taking good oils, essential fatty acids if I am on cholesterol drugs? Is it necessary to take Co-enzyme Q10
- Statin mechanism can impede Co-enzyme production. Solving the problem
- What may happen when Co Q10 production is reduced by statins?
- Medical opinions of incorporating Co-enzyme with statin anti cholesterol medication

Estrogen and Progesterone Questions and Answers relating to where they can be specifically useful or detrimental
- Most asked questions about estrogen's specific use with progesterone assisting problems such as stress incontinence, U.T.I. and vaginal dryness, cystitis
- Estrogen usage and other strategies in dealing with stress incontinence and bladder problems
- Is there any alternative option to improving vaginal dryness, discomfort and other problems, other than using estrogen
- Why is estriol safer to use than estradiol and estrone?
- Bladder problems, will estrogen supplementation help?
- Stress Incontinence: What exactly is it and the reasons?
- What is Biest and Triest Estrogen? Why is estrogen spelt differently and are they the same?
- Since I've started progesterone, my thrush has got worse. Why is this?
- Why is Estriol promoted for a helpful part of treatment in stress incontinence, urinary tract infections and thrush if I am already estrogen dominant?
- How does progesterone help control estrogen and why do they complement each other?
- How does the non real estrogen (plant estrogen) benefit progesterone's performance?
- So why do doctors insist on giving us more estrogen when we already have estrogen being manufactured and converted into fat cells in our body and stored, and also can derive estrogenic benefits in the shortfall by using less dangerous forms, such as through the use of diet phytoestrogens? When can supplementation of estrogen help?
- What you can do if you suspect you are overdosing on estrogen

Specific Questions and brief Answers to overcoming Specific Problems and Most commonly asked questions posed to me. Case Histories
- Estrogen dominance while menstruating
- PMS on progesterone
- Finding a sympathetic doctor and specific tests for body hair
- Severe weight gain and loss and stress ramifications
- Scared to go on HRT due to mother's experience
- Too young for hormonal problems?
- Dry eyes. Bloating. Cysts on ovaries
- Endometriosis and the use of estrogen post Hysterectomy
- Regarding men and progesterone and heart problems
- Antihypertensive medication and hot flushes on progesterone
- Testosterone dominance due to production of other hormones (Androstenedione) and weight storage
- Breast cancer concerns and lack of libido following Hysterectomy
- My hair has started falling out again while I have been on progesterone. Why?

Progesterone Usage in Depression and possible obstacles
- Question: My depression has returned on progesterone. Why?
- Other vitamins and mineral that may assist in supporting your depression and a word about Hypericum (St John's Wort) and other minerals
- Why is depression often difficult to diagnose?
- How would I know if my depression is due to hormonal balance?
- Can depression tilt or cause my hormones to become unbalanced
- Why you need to assist your body so progesterone can assist your depression
- What else enhances the serotonin levels and assist in overcoming depression?
- I am finding it difficult to come off my antidepressants. Why? (Casey's case)
- Testosterone usage for depression
- Libido problems on antidepressants

Progesterone in relation to modifying mood and influences and other associated issues such as:
- Moods, memory, foggy thinking, Alzheimers
- How do our hormones influence our moods?

- What else enhances the serotonin levels and assist in overcoming depression
- Depression, moods- foggy thinking - Alzheimers, specific problems
- How do our hormones influence and affect our moods?
- Progesterone's influence on pregnancy
- Progesterone's influence on PMS
- Other progesterone influences exerted in mood balancing and mental faculties
- Testosterone's influence on moods
- Estrogen's influence on moods and other important factors to consider
- Other important factors to consider
- I have memory loss and I'm scared I have the start of Alzheimer's disease
- Will progesterone help Alzheimer's or prevent me from getting it?
- A demonstration of hormonal imbalance, the resistant chemical imbalance: Penny's case of severe mood alteration

Libido
- Libido and issues around lowered sex drive
- Antidepressant use and other drug interference on libido
- Other influences: Ovarian failure or ovary dysfunction, OCP Hormonal imbalance, physical discomfort problems, physiological causes - self perception emotional issues
- Other possible reasons for lowered libido and deterants
- Using progesterone and testosterone to restore libido in men and women
- Low libido in men and some predominant reasons
- When women's libido exceeds a man's and its affects on the relationship intimacy and her self esteem

Testosterone
- Testosterone in relation to progesterone
- What is testosterone, who may qualify, general effects in women
- General observation of women who need to be cautious using testosterone substitution from women's experiences. Body types that resonate
- Commonly asked questions and problems
- General effects of testosterone in men and women, precautions
- Legality on testosterone

Oral Contraception Pill, side effects of OCP and progesterone usage regarding different forms of contraception
- Can I use progesterone with the pill?
- About Implanon and the usage of progesterone
- Answering the questions: Will progesterone surge ovulation during break time off progesterone while on Implanon?
- Can I get pregnant on progesterone and contraception?
- Forms of contraception being used. Contraceptive patch now available in UK
- US doctors to offer contraceptive patch
- About T-Frame, Mirena, implants, Oral Contraceptive Pill

Progesterone and Cortisol usage
Why can't I use progesterone if I'm on cortisol

General problems resurfacing while on progesterone
- Hair problems and other causes
- A dysfunctional thyroid gland or adrenals can contribute to hair growth changes
- Progesterone dose alteration during stress in relation to hair loss
- My nails have started to split again. Why?

General: Can I use progesterone on my animals?
Sexual abuse possible obstacle handicapping healing and hormonal balance

Fertility, Progesterone and Nutrition
- The need to correct nutrition and underlying problems in promoting fertility
- I am under a fertility program using progesterone receiving implantation of fertilised eggs but I keep rejecting them. Why?

Answering a common question posed and situation often seen.
- Analysing what her doctor was doing?
- What went wrong causing rejection ?
- Reasons why we are seeing more infertility and reduction in progesterone manufacturing
- Infertility can be multifactorial and not your fault
- Taking one step back and addressing underlying issues
- Suggested regime that some women have found to have helped them with infertility
- Dietary strategies, nutrition and lifestyle changes

Hormone correction, looking at it from other perspectives. Liver connection /principles, Weight, Syndrome X, Gastrointestinal problems and diet in relationship to hormonal imbalance
- Will progesterone help with Irritable Bowel Syndrome?
- Yes and No. We need to look at what is Irritable Bowel Syndrome.
- Symptoms, What causes IBS symptoms?, Testing for IBS
- Managing IBS involves treating the symptoms and self care. Guidelines/Management
- General Bowel Problems and their impact on Hormone imbalance

Syndrome X and weight
- The importance of addressing syndrome X: Weight Loss Principles and Hormone balancing
- What is Syndrome X and how is it related to hormonal imbalance and progesterone therapy?
- Progesterone and Syndrome X. Can progesterone help Syndrome X?
- Principles to acknowledge in restoring hormone balance

The Importance of incorporating nutrition for hormone balancing and where does it all fit
- How do I know if I am purchasing a reliable, safe, nutritional product and are there dangers?
- Nutrition in place of Hormone Replacement Therapy or Natural bio identical hormones
- Will Wild Yam creams help me if I do not wish to use natural hormone replacement therapy?
- Nutritional supplementation is not anecdotal
- What if I cannot afford much nutritional supplementation, what is the most essential to use with my progesterone? Tackling other concerns and apprehensions
- Liver Principles and healing naturally through foods/juicing with or without nutritional supplements

Nutrition and principles
- Principles of nutritional supplementation in hormone balancing
- Specific products I use in hormone balancing and why. My programs

Liver Tonics/Supplements
- The liver in relation to hormone balance and summary of multifactorial benefits
- What are all these ingredients required to assist the liver to function correctly and why isn't St Mary's Thistle enough? Guidelines of required liver detoxification ingredients

Essential Minerals: Magnesium, Selenium, MSM
- Magnesium - its other tasks and why it is so important in relation to hormones and other functions
- Possible causes of magnesium deficiency
- Selenium and hormone balancing and its important functions on other glands eg thyroid
- MSM: What is MSM and why it is so important?
- Summary of the beneficial actions of MSM
- How MSM may benefit people with osteoarthritis, arthritis and osteoporosis it's action may: and I believe from observational data
- MSM natural organic sulphur is not a sulphonamide
- Old fashioned grandma was right you know

Nutrition in adjunct with progesterone for osteoporosis and musculoskeletal problems of all ages
- Beneficial ingredients assisting in building up bone density may help reduce or slow the onset of arthritis
- Guideline formulations and purposes
- How important is calcium supplementation if I am taking progesterone
- What about caltrate and other calcium supplements

Metabolism and thyroid function
- Other beneficial ingredients and their role in metabolism:
- More about Tyrosine, Kelp, Brindle berry, Chromium and effects on weight
- Body type weight control supplements and ingredients for specific hormonal and metabolic constitutions of Lymphatic body type, Gynaeoid body type, Android body type, Thyroid body type

Sugar imbalances
- How specific ingredients may exert influence on blood sugar levels
- Associated problems concerning unstable blood sugar levels, sluggish metabolism and stubborn weight loss, cellulite, excessive appetite/hunger
- Why is refined sugar in large amounts so bad?
- What can I use instead of sugar to overcome sugar cravings?
- An alternative to sugar - Stevia

Immunity problems, adrenal exhaustion and hormonal disruption
- Why I have adopted the use of Olive Leaf Extracts to assist hormone balancing
- What I have discovered about this powerful product
- What to be aware of when starting and using Olive Leaf Extract: Blood detoxification
- All about it's wonderful beneficial properties that have been discovered by many women in our organisation and who may benefit including children
- A comment about Olive Life behaviour in addressing ailments such as colds, glandular fever

Strengthening the immune system and strategies that women have found to be beneficial

Co-enzyme Q10
- What exactly is co-enzyme Q10 and its roles? Why I believe in using it in my programs
- The manufacturing of a good co-enzyme Q10 (not synthetic)

Other important information includes:
- Multivitamins, Natural antidepressants, Liquid B, Liquid Iron, Vitamin C antioxidants and many more often overlooked assistors in healing and many missing factors

Herbal hormone modulators and regulators
- *Vitex* What is it?, Indications of use
- *Maca* Where does maca come from and what exactly is it? What's in it?
- Bowel function, Nutrients for gastrointestinal correction
- Probiotics
- Essential Fatty Acids (EFA's)
- Fitness fats (good fats that heal), Sources of essential fats, Functions of essential fats

Charts:
- The omega 3 and omega 6 pathways
- Chart guideline on toxic levels of vitamins
- Chart guideline on toxic levels of minerals

Other products found valuable by women
- Herbal teas, aromatherapy lotions, Bach flower remedies etc

General points on nutritional supplements and specific guidelines

JENNY BIRDSEY'S BOOKS ON
NATURAL PROGESTERONE

ORDER FORM

SEND TO: _____

ADDRESS: _____

_____

COUNTRY: _____ POSTCODE: _____

NO. OF BOOKS @ $39.95 PER BOOK:	BOOK 1 NO.	BOOK 2 NO.	$
ADD POSTAGE & HANDLING COSTS (Subject to change): • Within Australia $10.00 for one book - or even better value two books at same price • Outside Australia @ $17.00 per book • If paying by USA cheque, please add $10.00 US (Bank conversion rates).			$
AMOUNT PAYABLE:			$

MAKE CHEQUE PAYABLE TO: J Birdsey, NPAN

☐ Visa   ☐ Mastercard   ☐ Bankcard   ☐ Cheque   ☐ Cash Sale

CREDIT CARD NO: ☐☐☐☐ ☐☐☐☐ ☐☐☐☐ ☐☐☐☐

EXPIRY DATE: _____

CARDHOLDER'S NAME: _____

PHONE NO: _____ EMAIL: _____
(INCLUDE AREA CODE)

NATURAL PROGESTERONE ADVISORY NETWORK (NPAN)
8 Normanby Street, East Geelong, Vic 3219, Australia